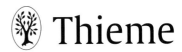

Breast Cancer

The Art and Science of Early Detection with Mammography

Perception, Interpretation, Histopathologic Correlation

László Tabár, M.D.
Professor and Director
Department of Mammography
Central Hospital
Falun, Sweden
University of Uppsala School of Medicine
Uppsala, Sweden

Tibor Tot, M.D., Ph.D.
Associate Professor of Pathology and Chairman
Department of Pathology and Clinical Cytology
Central Hospital
Falun, Sweden
University of Uppsala
Uppsala, Sweden

Peter B. Dean, M.D.
Professor
Department of Diagnostic Radiology
University of Turku
Turku, Finland
Visiting Professor
Brigham and Women's Hospital
Harvard Medical School
Boston, MA, USA

1590 illustrations

Thieme
Stuttgart · New York

Library of Congress Cataloging-in-Publication Data
Tabár, László.
  Breast cancer : the art and science of early detection with mammography / László Tabár, Tibor Tot, Peter B. Dean.
    p. ; cm
ISBN 3-13-135371-6 (GTV : alk, paper) -- ISBN 1-58890-259-5 (TNY : alk. paper)
1. Breast--Radiography--Atlases. 2. Breast--Cancer-Imaging--Atlases.
  [DNLM: 1. Breast Neoplasms--radiography. 2. Early Diagnosis. 3. Mammography--methods. 4. Radiographic Image Interpretation, Computer-Assisted. WP 870 T112b 2005] I. Tot, Tibor. II. Dean, Peter B. III. Title.
    RG493.5.R33T318 2005
    618.1'907572--dc22   2004025269

Important note: Medicine is an ever-changing science undergoing continual development. Research and clinical experience are continually expanding our knowledge, in particular our knowledge of proper treatment and drug therapy. Insofar as this book mentions any dosage or application, readers may rest assured that the authors, editors, and publishers have made every effort to ensure that such references are in accordance with **the state of knowledge at the time of production of the book.**
Nevertheless, this does not involve, imply, or express any guarantee or responsibility on the part of the publishers in respect to any dosage instructions and forms of applications stated in the book. **Every user is requested to examine carefully** the manufacturers' leaflets accompanying each drug and to check, if necessary in consultation with a physician or specialist, whether the dosage schedules mentioned therein or the contraindications stated by the manufacturers differ from the statements made in the present book. Such examination is particularly important with drugs that are either rarely used or have been newly released on the market. Every dosage schedule or every form of application used is entirely at the user's own risk and responsibility. The authors and publishers request every user to report to the publishers any discrepancies or inaccuracies noticed. If errors in this work are found after publication, errata will be posted at www.thieme.com on the product description page.

Some of the product names, patents, and registered designs referred to in this book are in fact registered trademarks or proprietary names even though specific reference to this fact is not always made in the text. Therefore, the appearance of a name without designation as proprietary is not to be construed as a representation by the publisher that it is in the public domain.

© 2005 Georg Thieme Verlag,
Rüdigerstrasse 14, 70469 Stuttgart, Germany
http://www.thieme.de
Thieme New York, 333 Seventh Avenue,
New York, NY 10001 USA
http://www.thieme.com

Cover design: Cyclus, Stuttgart
Typesetting by primustype Hurler GmbH, Notzingen
Printed in Germany by Grammlich, Pliezhausen

ISBN 3-13-135371-6 (GTV)
ISBN 1-58890-259-5 (TNY)   2 3 4 5

This book is dedicated to the task of finding breast cancer when it is still curable, and to the more difficult task of ruling out the presence of breast cancer in those women who do not have the disease.

Preface

For decades, early detection has been our most effective means of reducing the number of unnecessary deaths caused by breast cancer. Although the methods of early detection have improved and continue to do so, their application to the women who need them has always lagged behind. Not only has high-quality mammography been available to too few women, but there have always been too few radiologists skilled in detecting early stage breast cancer.

Radiologists who have taken the trouble to learn the many facets of normal breast radiological anatomy can interpret mammograms more effectively and with greater confidence. Also, knowledge of the pathophysiological processes leading to the pathological changes in the breast is necessary for the radiologist to master the intricacies of breast imaging. However, a wide gulf separates the pathologist's high-resolution images of a small, thin section of tissue from the radiologist's images of the entire breast at a lower resolution. We have endeavored to narrow this gulf by correlating mammography with subgross, three-dimensional pathology images and large, thin-section pathology images.

This book has been more than two decades in the writing, having gone through innumerable versions as we have sought to bring László Tabár's teaching courses to the printed page. It is our sincerest hope that this book will enable ever more radiologists to obtain the skills necessary to detect breast cancer at its earliest possible stages, while at the same time being able to assure the vast majority of the screened women that there are truly no signs of breast cancer on their images.

November 2004

László Tabár
Tibor Tot
Peter B. Dean

Contents

Introduction—The Normal Breast: Comparative Subgross Anatomy and Mammography   1

Introduction—The Normal Breast: Comparative
Subgross Anatomy and Mammography 3
Interrelationship between Histology and
Mammography 4
    Nodular Densities 16
Correlative Mammographic–Histological
Demonstration of the Four Building Blocks 16
    Ducts 17
    Fibrous Strands 22
    Vessels 23

Homogeneous, Structureless Densities 24
Radiolucent Areas 30
Overview of the Five Mammographic Parenchymal
Patterns 32
Mammographic Parenchymal Pattern I 33
Mammographic Parenchymal Pattern II 35
Mammographic Parenchymal Pattern III 36
Mammographic Parenchymal Pattern IV 37
Mammographic Parenchymal Pattern V 38

Chapter 1: Pattern I   39

Characteristics of Pattern I 40
Radiopaque Densities 46
    Nodular Densities 46
    Fibrous Tissue 54
    The Parenchymal
    Contour 56
Radiolucent Areas 62
Involution 66

Pathological Lesions in Pattern I Type Breasts 70
    How Do the Pathological Lesions Change the
    Mammographic Image of Pattern I Type Breasts
    and How Can We Perceive Them? 70
    Lesions with Convex Radiopaque Contours 71
    Lesions with Architectural Distortion 80
    The Evolution of a Tiny Spiculated Tumor 82
    Calcifications in a Pattern I Type Breast 84
    Mammographically Occult Lesions in Pattern I ... 86

Chapter 2: Pattern II   93

Characteristics of Pattern II 94
Linear Densities in Pattern II 95
    Ducts 95
      Atrophic Ducts and Their Branches 95
      Persistent Lobules in Pattern II 97
      Normal Ducts 98
      Ductectasia 99
Fibrous Strands 109

Blood Vessels 112
Pathological Lesions in Pattern II Breasts 114
    Spiculated Invasive Ductal Carcinoma in a
    Pattern II Breast 114
Microcalcifications in Pattern II Breasts 115
Screening Findings in Asymptomatic Women
with Pattern II Breasts 116

Chapter 3: Pattern III   119

Characteristics of Pattern III 120

Chapter 4: Pattern IV   123

Characteristics of Pattern IV 124
Adenosis 125
Sclerosing Adenosis 128

Fibroadenomatoid Change of the Lobule 132
Patchy Fibrosis 133
Pathological Lesions in Pattern IV Breasts 134

Chapter 5: Pattern V   141

Characteristics of Pattern V 142
Involuting Lobule with Fibrous Replacement 144
Calcifications in Pattern V Breasts 145
Perception of Noncalcified Lesions in Pattern V
Type Breasts 151
Relative Frequencies of the Mammographic
Patterns in the General Population 160

Distribution of Mammographic Parenchymal
Patterns by Age in a Screening Population versus
Clinically Referred Women 162
The Prevalence of Breast Cancer According
to Mammographic Parenchymal Pattern and Age ... 163
Summary 163

Chapter 6: Finding Breast Cancer When It Is Still Small: Rationale and Scientific Evidence   165

A New Era in the Diagnosis and Treatment
of Breast Cancer 166
    Detection of Breast Cancer in the Preclinical
    Phase 166

A New Paradigm: Prevent Breast Cancer from
Growing to Advanced Stages 168
The Most Important Task Is to Prevent Breast
Cancer from Developing to Large, Advanced Tumors 170

Contents

Nonpalpable, Screen-Detected Breast Cancer 172
Mechanism for the Impact of Screening 174
   Tumor Size 174
   Node Status 175
   Histological Malignancy Grade 176
The Relative Benefits of Downward Stage
Shifting 178
Mechanism for the Effect of Early Detection of
Breast Cancer: Comments and Conclusions 180
Summary 185
The Impact of Early Detection on Breast Cancer
Death 186
   Mammography Screening and Treatment in Early
   Stage Can Dramatically Reduce Mortality from
   Breast Cancer in a Population 186

Conclusion 187
Factors Influencing Early Detection 188
   Multiple Factors That Determine How Early in the
   Preclinical Detectable Phase Individual Malignant
   Tumors Can Be Detected 188
      The Nature of the Surrounding Breast Tissue ... 188
      Morphological Heterogeneity of Breast Cancer
      at Histology 190
      Morphological Heterogeneity of Breast Cancer
      at Mammography 194
      The Progressive Nature of Breast Cancer and
      the Variability in the Rate of Disease Progression
      According to Histological Type and Patient Age . 216
   Conclusions 235

Chapter 7: Finding Breast Cancer When It Is Still Small: Use of Systematic Viewing Methods   237

A Systematic Method for Viewing Mammograms ... 238
   Basic Philosophy 238
   Prerequisites 238
      Superb Mammographic Technique Is Essential . 238
      Viewing Conditions during Image Reading Will
      Have a Decisive Impact upon the Diagnostic
      Outcome 238
      Perception of Subtle Radiographic Abnormali-
      ties Can Be Enhanced by the Use of a Hand-
      held Mammography Viewer 238
   A Systematic Approach Is Essential for Viewing
   Any Diagnostic Image 239
Systematic Approach to the Analysis of the
Findings 240
   Asymmetric Densities on the Mammogram 240
      Systematic Work-up of Asymmetric Densities
      on the Mammogram 242
      Normal Fibroglandular Tissue 243
      Nonspecific Asymmetric Density with Architec-
      tural Distortion on the Mammogram 250

      Definite Pathological Lesion Causing an
      Asymmetric Density on the Mammogram 256
   Distribution of Histological Diagnoses at Open
   Biopsy 257
   Algorithm for the Work-up and Management of
   an Asymmetric Density on the Mammogram 258
Practice in Perception and Work-up of Findings 259
   Breast Regions with a Higher Frequency of Breast
   Cancer 259
      Lesions Localized in the Upper Outer Quadrant . 259
      Lesions Localized in the Medial Half of the
      Breast 318
      Lesions Localized in the Retroglandular Clear
      Space on the CC Projection 328
      Lesions Localized in the Retroareolar Area 346
   Characteristics of Lesions Regardless of Location . 358
      Lesions Causing Architectural Distortion 358
      Lesions Causing Parenchymal Contour
      Changes 394

Chapter 8: Large-Section Histology of the Breast   405

Introduction 406
Rationale for Large-Section Technique 406
   Prerequisites 406
Handling of the Specimen 407
Cutting with the Macrotome 412
Handling and Staining the Sections 413
The Final Product: The Large-Section Slide 414

Subgross, Thick-Section Histology Technique 420
   Steps of the Technique 420
Examples of Subgross, Thick-Section Histopathology
Images of Breast Tissue 423
Case Demonstrations 425
Conclusions 438

Chapter 9: Mammography Positioning Technique   439

References   467

Subject Index   471

Introduction

The Normal Breast: Comparative Subgross Anatomy and Mammography

Introduction—The Normal Breast: Comparative Subgross Anatomy and Mammography

Diagnosis and treatment of breast cancer in its earliest detectable phases results in dramatic improvement in the outcome of the breast cancer patient. Detection of the disease in its preclinical phase requires regular screening of asymptomatic women. The vast majority of mammograms are images of normal breast tissue. An understanding of how the underlying anatomical structure, in all its complexity and variability, is imaged on the mammogram is necessary for competence in excluding malignancy. This book was written to help the reader accomplish the following goals:

- **To increase specificity** through greater confidence in recognizing normal anatomy. This will enable the radiologist to avoid unnecessary call-backs, additional imaging, and interventional procedures.
- **To increase sensitivity** through improved skill in discerning subtle pathological changes.
- **To improve diagnostic performance** with the ultimate aim of decreasing anxiety among those who do not have breast cancer, and improving the outcome of breast cancer patients through detection and treatment in the preclinical phase.

As in other branches of radiology, we need to understand the detailed anatomy of the organ we are imaging as well as the capabilities and limitations of the imaging methods we use. It is our firm belief that competence in breast image interpretation can be best achieved by correlating the histology of the normal and abnormal breast with mammograms, ultrasound and other breast imaging methods. The importance of such correlation is reflected throughout this book. As was eloquently expressed by Ingleby and Gershon-Cohen in 1960: "**Very thorough knowledge of breast anatomy and pathology is a** *sine qua non* **for interpretation of breast films**."[2]

The continuously improving resolution in mammographic technique enables us to demonstrate breast abnormalities at earlier phases of their natural history. The different subtypes of in situ carcinoma, hyperplastic breast changes, and borderline lesions are detected at a far greater frequency than they were only two decades ago.

The **mammogram** also helps estimate the extent of the disease, information crucial for the therapist. Diagnostic imaging advances have placed new demands on the pathologist as well. The many **large-section histology** images presented in this book serve to emphasize the necessity for modifying current histopathological technique to improve communication among pathologists, radiologists, surgeons, and oncologists.

The gap between the resolution of the mammogram and the resolution of the microscopic image can be bridged. The **subgross, thick-section (three-dimensional) histological technique** is an extremely useful tool for helping radiologists, surgeons, and pathologists to understand the nature and extent of the underlying pathological processes. We have used this technique in many cases and these images have been included wherever appropriate.

Figures **I.1** to **I.5** demonstrate the interrelationship between large-section histology, subgross, thick-section histology, and the mammographic image.

Comparison of mammograms and 3-D histologic images with photographs of plants and other objects are included where appropriate. There are surprising functional and structural similarities among various biological entities. Demonstration of these similarities facilitates the learning process.

Interrelationship Between Histology and Mammography

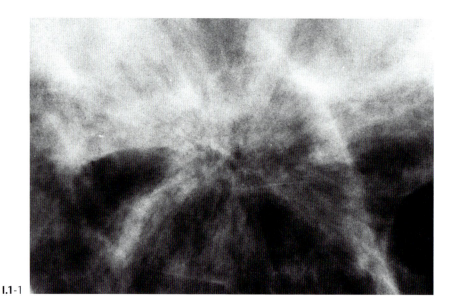

I.1-1

Fig. **I.1-1 Microfocus magnification mammogram.** Architectural distortion has altered the harmonious structure of normal breast tissue. The radiating structure does not contain straight, individually recognizable spicules and lacks a central tumor mass. Instead, there are several small, central lucencies. This mammographic image is characteristic of a radial scar.

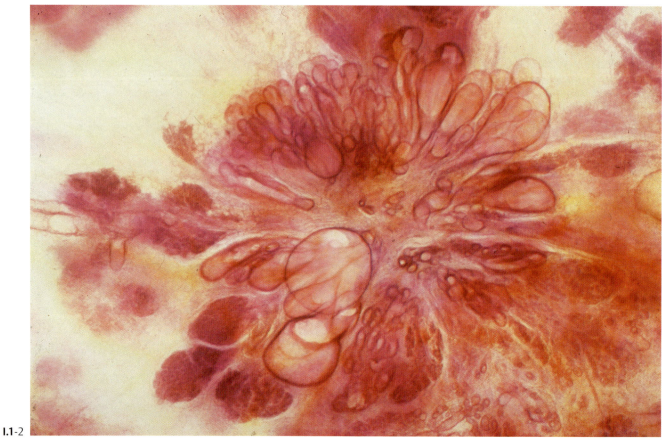

I.1-2

Fig. **I.1-2** This **subgross, thick-section histological image** shows the proliferating ducts arranged in a radiating fashion, accounting for the architectural distortion on the mammogram. **Histological diagnosis:** radial scar.

Fig. **I.1**-3 **Large-section histological image** of the radial scar, orcein elastic stain. The collagen stains red, while the elastic fibers stain black.

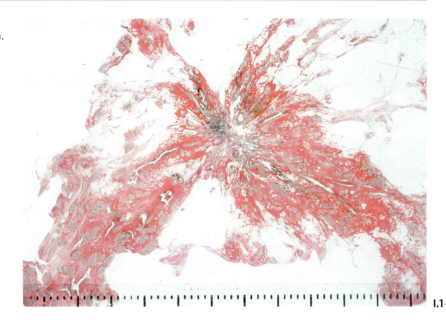

I.1-3

Fig. **I.1**-4 **Large-section histological image** of the radial scar; H&E stain.

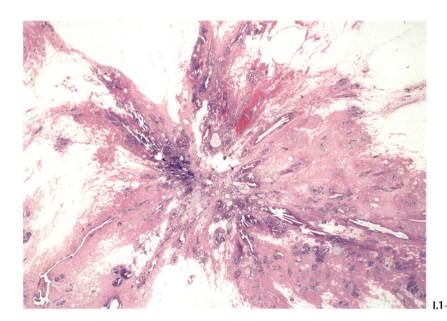

I.1-4

Fig. **I.1**-5 **Large-section histological image** of the radial scar; sirius red stain.

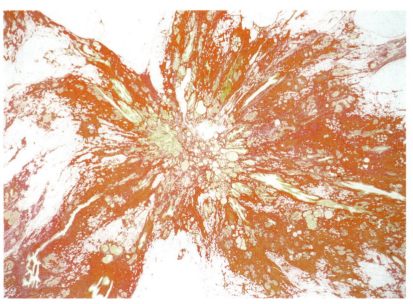

I.1-5

■ Mammographic–Subgross Histological Images of the Skin and Areola

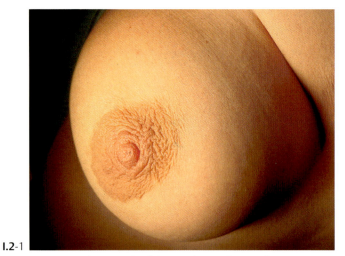

I.2-1

Fig. **I.2**-1   Photograph of the nipple–areola complex.

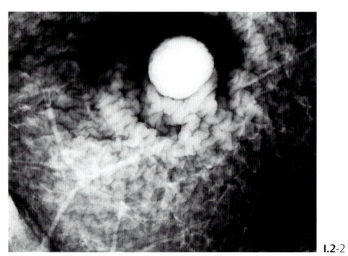

I.2-2

Fig. **I.2**-2   Radiograph of a mastectomy specimen slice demonstrating the skin, nipple, and part of the areolar region.

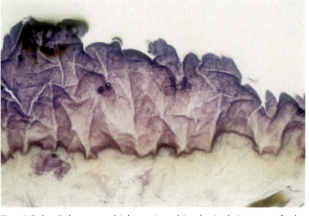

I.2-3

Fig. **I.2**-3   Subgross, thick-section histological image of the nipple surface.

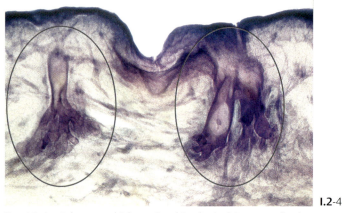

I.2-4

Fig. **I.2**-4   Subgross, thick-section histological images of sebaceous glands in the areola.

Fig. **I.3**-1 to 3   Subcutaneous tissue with a sweat gland and its duct originating in the skin of the areola. The areas outlined by the rectangles are enlarged on Fig. **1.3**-2 and **1.3**-3.

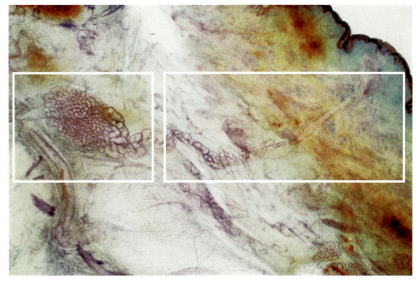

I.3-1

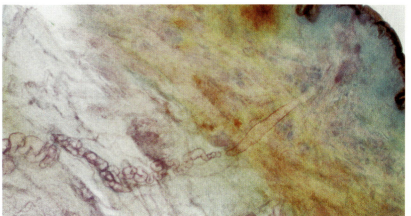

I.3-2

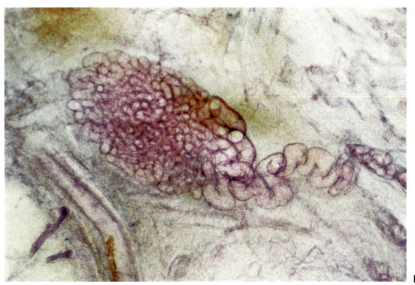

I.3-3

■ The Lobar Anatomy of the Breast

The female breast has about 12–15 **lobes**, each terminating in a major duct that empties into the nipple.

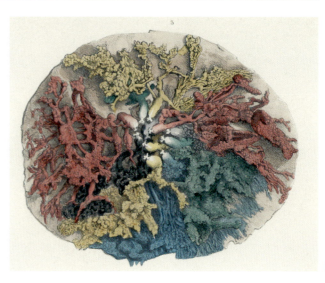

Fig. **I.4**   Colored wax was injected into the ducts by Cooper to outline the individual lobes. This image demonstrates that the lobes have different sizes and that they do not anastomose with each other, although they interdigitate. Galactography confirms this observation. There is no distinct anatomical or surgical boundary between the lobes. (Source: Cooper AP. On the Anatomy of the Breast. London, Longmans, 1840. Plate VI, Fig. 3).

I.4

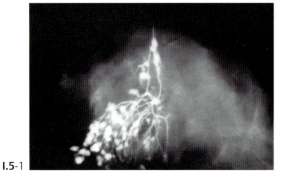

I.5-1

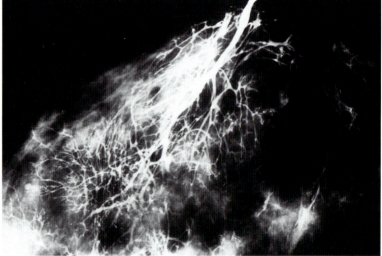

Fig. **I.5**-1 & 2   An excellent overview of the ductal system of a single lobe can be seen on the galactogram with the help of positive contrast media.

I.5-2

Fig. **I.6**-1   Subgross, thick-section histological image of a subsegmental duct with normal terminal ductal lobular units (TDLUs). Note the striking similarity to the California cedar.

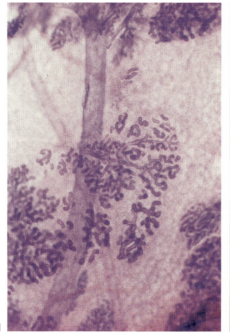

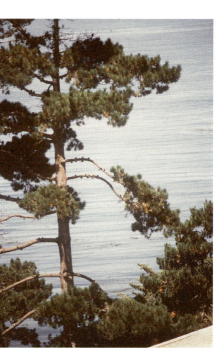

I.6-1

I.6-2

Fig. **I.7** Subgross, thick-section histology showing atrophic ducts and lobules in the retroareolar area.

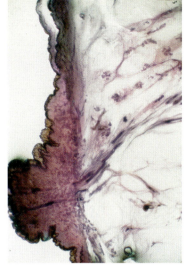
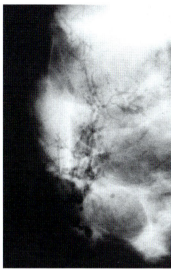

Fig. **I.8**-1 & 2 Occasionally the ducts and some of the lobules within a lobe will be seen on the mammogram outlined by air (negative contrast medium). The surrounding fibrosis enhances the visibility of the air-filled ducts.

I.7

I.8-1

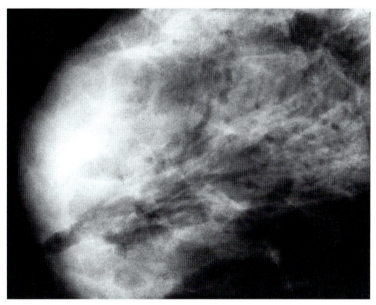

I.8-2

Fig. **I.9** The positive contrast medium on the galactogram outlines the atrophic ducts and their branches.

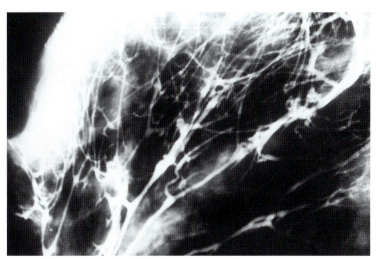

I.9

The size and extent of individual lobes vary widely, often extending well beyond the boundaries of a single quadrant. Galactograms in Figures **I.10** to **I.18** demonstrate some of these variations.

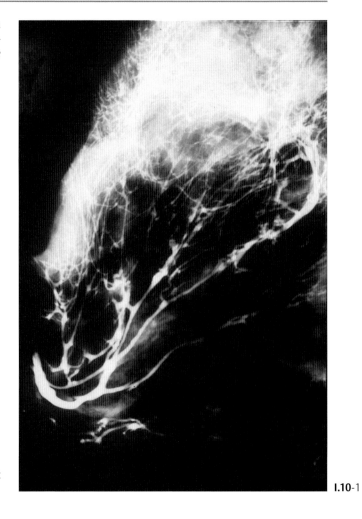

Fig. **I.10**-1 to 4 Bilateral galactograms of the same patient demonstrate variations in the size and extent of the lobes.

I.10-1

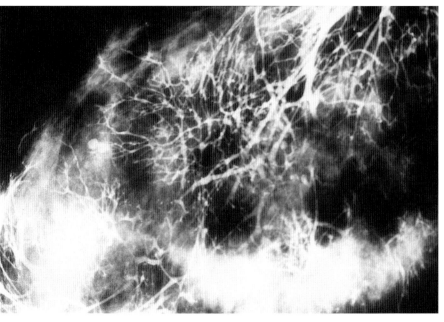

I.10-2

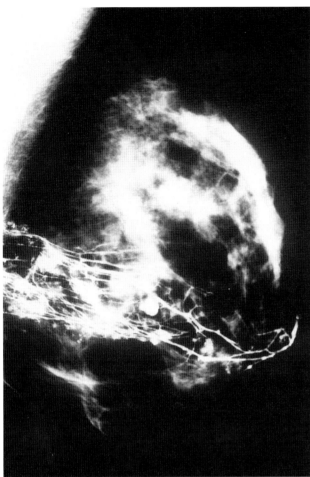

I.10-3

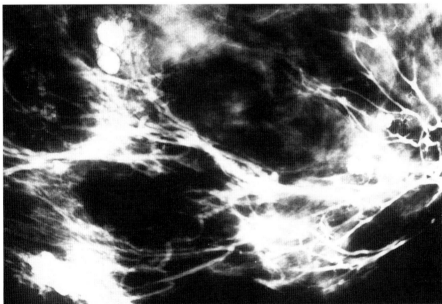

I.10-4

Figures **I.11** to **I.14** illustrate further galactographic demonstrations of normal breast lobes.

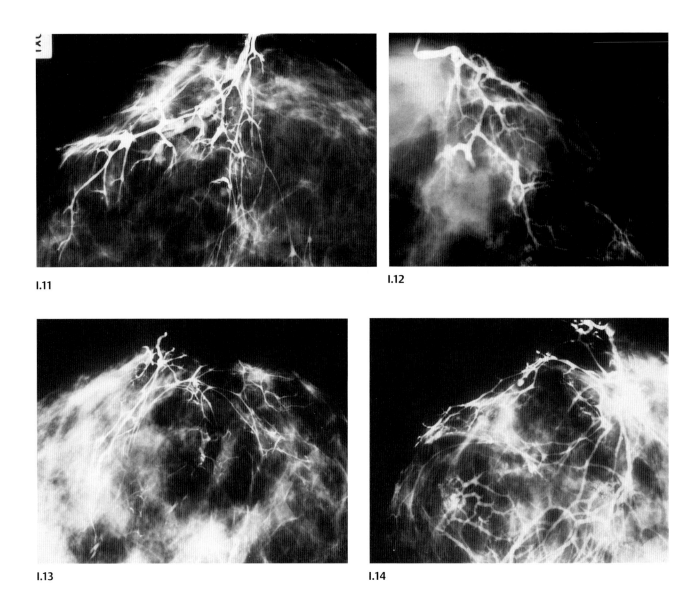

I.11

I.12

I.13

I.14

Figures **I.15** to **I.18** show smaller lobes with distended, fluid-filled ducts caused by multiple papillomas and duct-ectasia.

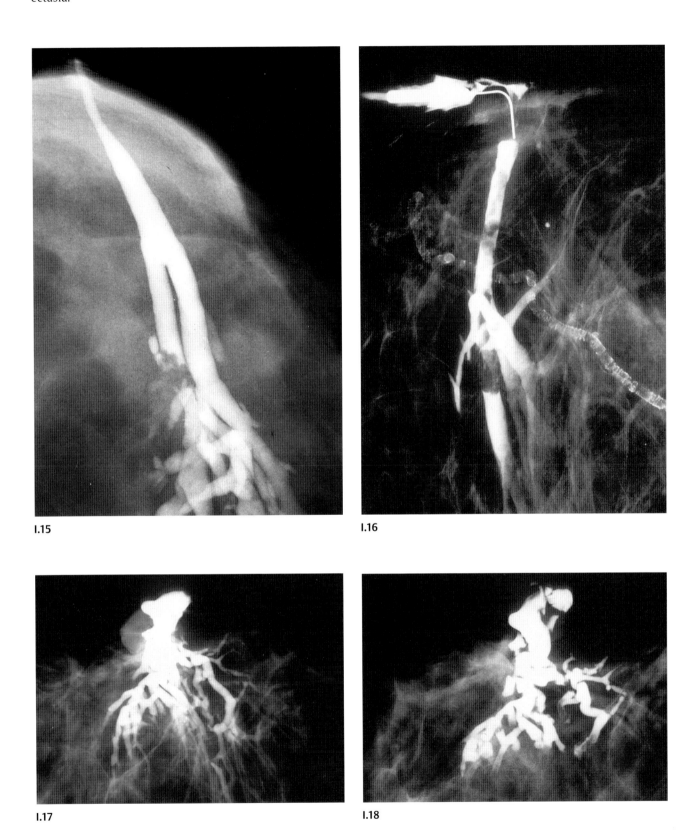

I.15

I.16

I.17

I.18

Although the ducts and lobules of one lobe tend to be localized within a volume of approximately one quadrant, the ducts of a single lobe may occupy portions of two or even three quadrants.

This **galactogram** in the craniocaudal projection shows the ductal structure of one lobe spreading over both the medial and lateral portions of the breast (Fig. **I.19**-1). This illustration suggests that the appearance of two or more seemingly independent tumor foci could still be located within a single lobe, bringing the term multicentricity into question (see Fig. **I.21**-1 to 9). Also, ipsilateral recurrences in such a lobe could be found far from the site of resection.

If the genetic transformation to breast cancer is localized to the epithelial cells of the diseased lobe, it follows that recurrence of the disease will appear in the remainder of the lobe after partial resection. Malignant tumors most often recur near the site of resection, but they can also recur at more distant sites within the same lobe.

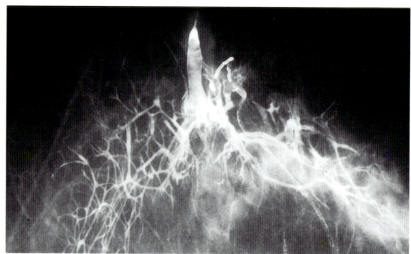

I.19-1

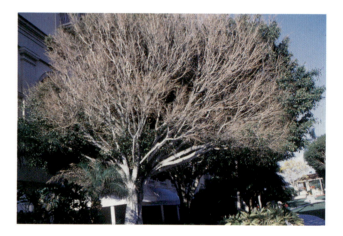

I.19-2

Fig. **I.20** Mammographic demonstration of a large lobe occupying more than one quadrant of the breast. First screening examination of a 40-year-old asymptomatic woman. Detail of the right CC projection shows innumerable casting-type calcifications characteristic for Grade 3 DCIS. The calcifications outline the duct system of a single lobe, spreading over a large part of the breast.

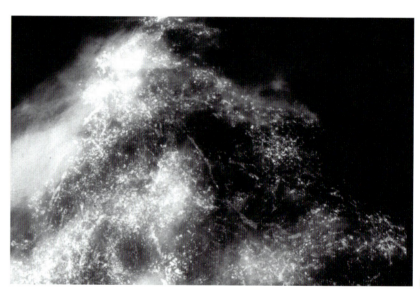

I.20

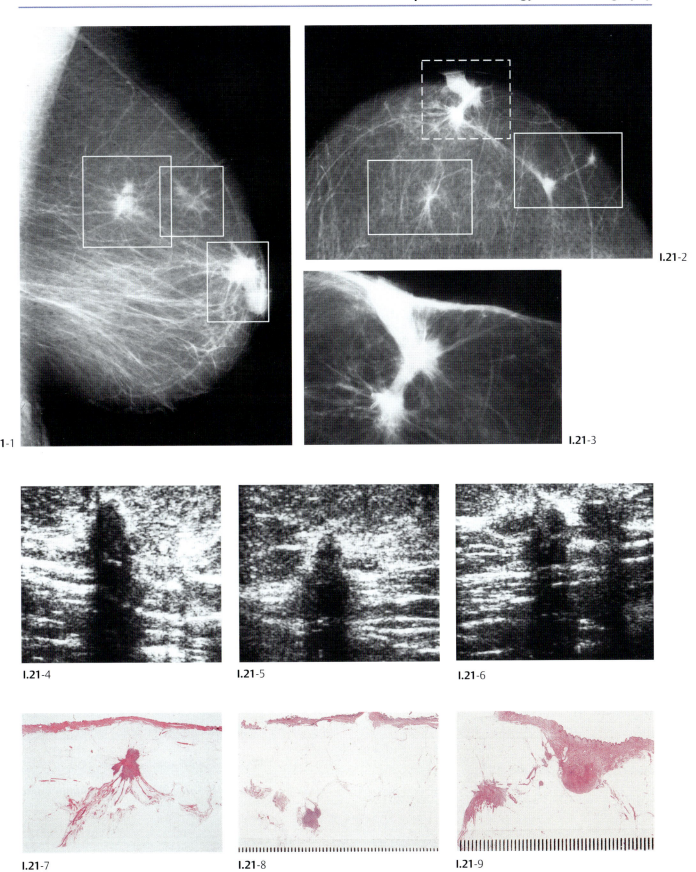

I.21-1

I.21-2

I.21-3

I.21-4

I.21-5

I.21-6

I.21-7

I.21-8

I.21-9

Fig. **I.21**-1 to 9   Mammographic, ultrasound, and large-section histology images of multifocal invasive ductal carcinoma, demonstrated on the same patient.

I.21-1   Left breast, MLO projection.
I.21-2   Left breast, CC projection.
I.21-3   Microfocus magnification view of dashed square in **I.21**-2.
I.21-4 to 6   Ultrasound images of the tumor foci in **I.21**-1 to 3.
I.21-7 to 9   Large-section histological images of same foci.

Correlative Mammographic–Histological Demonstration of the Four Building Blocks

The mammographic image is a reflection of breast anatomy and its occasional alteration by pathological processes. The vast majority of mammograms are images of normal breast tissue. The seemingly endless variety of mammographic images poses a challenge for the film reader because, unlike most organs in the body, there is great diversity in the histological structure of the normal breast. The relative proportions of the building blocks can vary considerably from one region to another in the same breast, in the same individual over time, and among different individuals. These variations are reflected on the mammogram.

The mammographic image is a characteristic mixture of the following four structural components or building blocks:

1 **Nodular densities**
2 **Linear densities**
3 **Homogeneous, structureless densities**
4 **Radiolucent areas**

The corresponding anatomy of these four building blocks consists of:

1 Terminal ductal lobular units
2 Ducts/vessels/fibrous strands
3 Supporting fibrous connective tissue
4 Adipose tissue

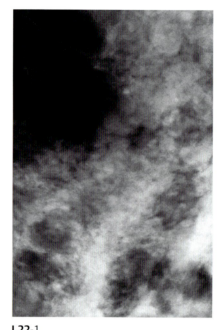

I.22-1

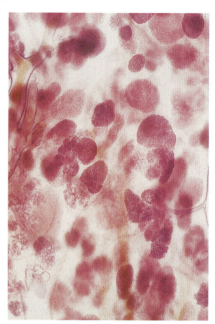

I.22-2

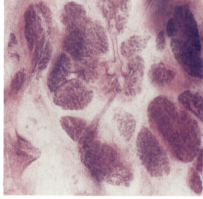

I.22-3

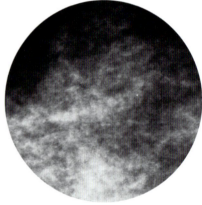

I.22-4

■ Nodular Densities

Nodular densities on the normal mammogram correspond to lobules, called more specifically the **t**erminal **d**uctal **l**obular **u**nits, or TDLUs (see Chapter 1, pages 46–53 for a detailed description).

Fig. **I.22**-1 to 5   Mammograms and thick-section histological images, both showing numerous lobules/TDLUs outlined by adipose tissue.

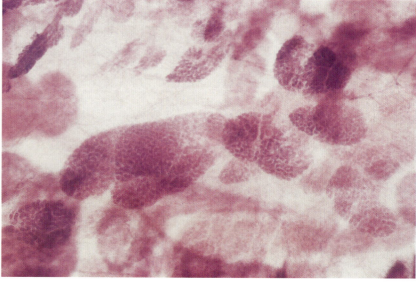

I.22-5

■ Linear Densities

Linear densities may be images of:
- Lactiferous ducts (Figs. **I.23** to **I.32**)
- Fibrous strands (Figs. **I.33** and **I.34**)
- Vessels (Figs. **I.35** to **I.38**)

Ducts

Figs. **I.23** and **I.24**   Thick-section histological images of *lactiferous ducts* with prominent pleating.

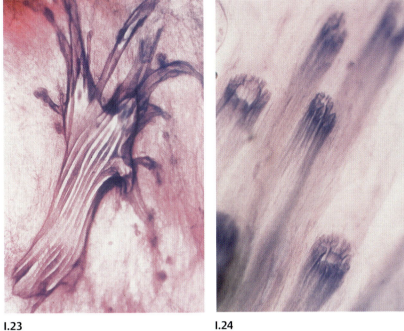

I.23

I.24

Figs. **I.25** and **I.26**   Retroareolar pleated ducts, longitudinal and cross sections (conventional histology).

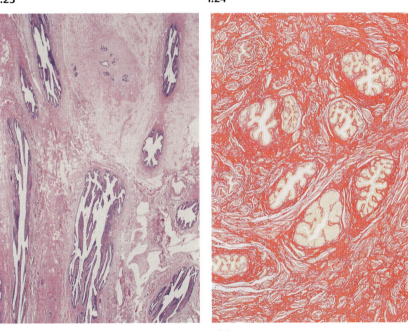

I.25

I.26

Figs. **I.27**-1 & 2   Galactography and thick-section histology showing the main duct and its branches in one lobe.

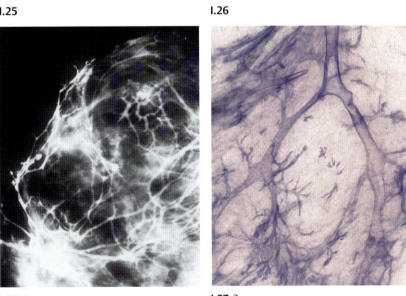

I.27-1

I.27-2

Linear Densities—Ducts

The 12–15 main ducts converge toward the nipple. The following subgross, thick-section histological images demonstrate the main ducts in the nipple and retroareolar region (Figs. **I.28** to **I.32**). Some TDLUs can also be seen just behind the nipple. Thus, malignant change can occur in the retroareolar region, as demonstrated in Figure **I.30**.

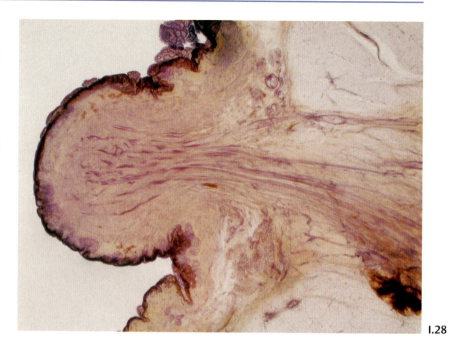

I.28

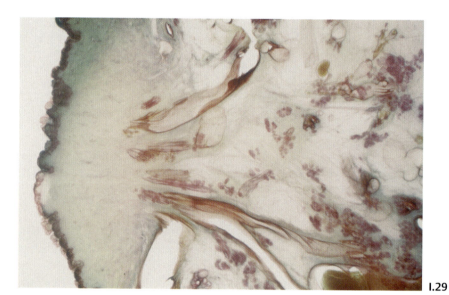

I.29

Fig. **I.30** Four foci of invasive lobular carcinoma are seen in the retroareolar region.

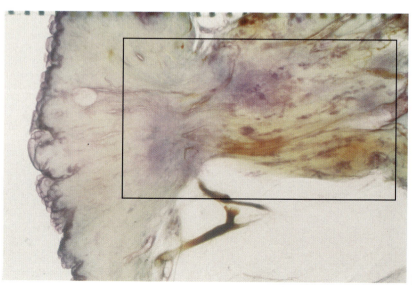

I.30

Fig. **I.31** Subgross, thick-section histological image of pleated ducts within the nipple in a sagittal plane.

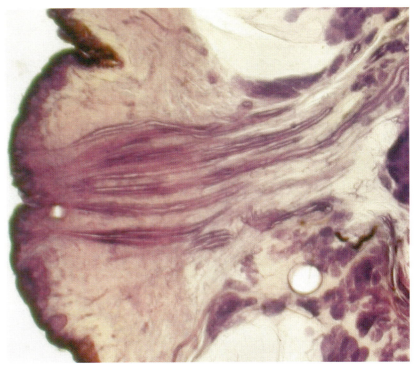

I.31

Fig. **I.32**-1 Subgross histological image of dilated retroareolar ducts.

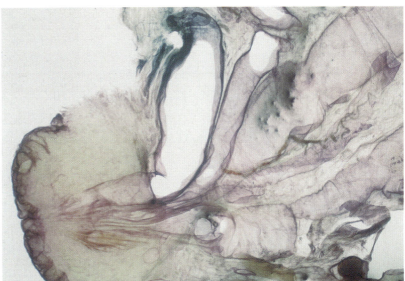

I.32-1

Fig. **I.32**-2 Specimen radiograph showing retroareolar ducts.

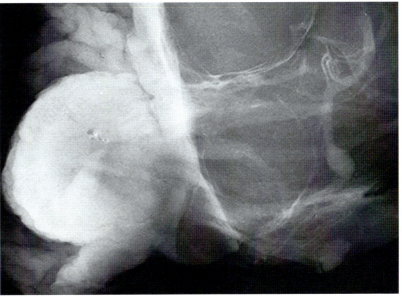

I.32-2

Mammographic and Subgross Histological Demonstration of Ducts and TDLUs

Fig. **I.33** Left breast, MLO projection, normal mammogram. Mammographic Pattern I with a large number of TDLUs (seen as small, round densities) and ducts (linear densities, seen mainly in the lower rectangle).

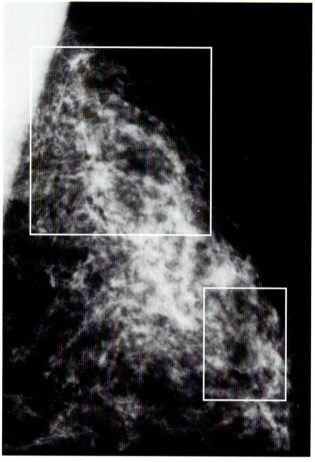

Fig. **I.34** Subgross, thick-section histological image showing numerous TDLUs of varying sizes along with dilated ducts.

I.33

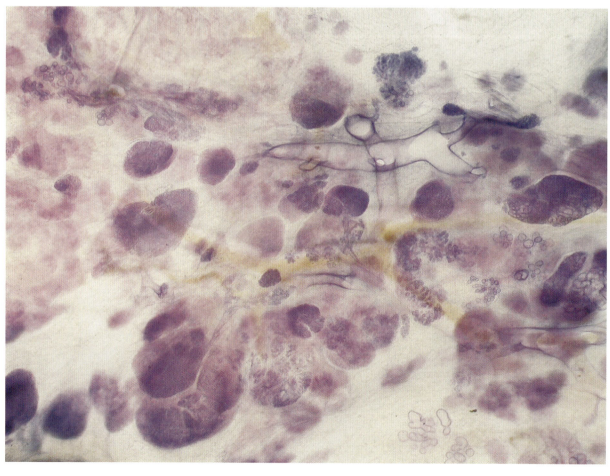

I.34

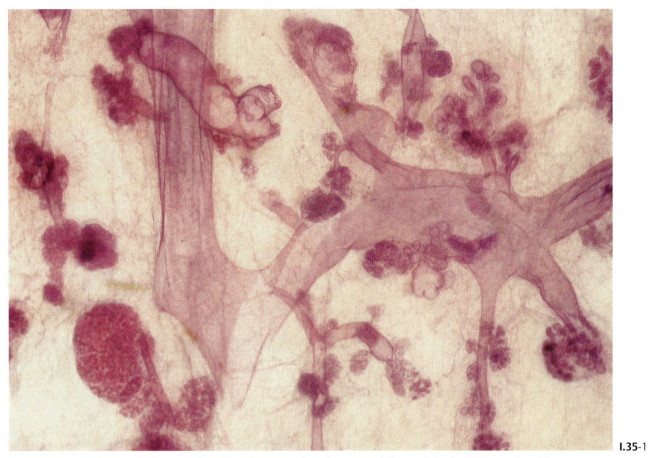

Fig. **I.35**-1 & 2   Subgross, thick-section histological images of a subsegmental duct with both atrophic and proliferative TDLUs.

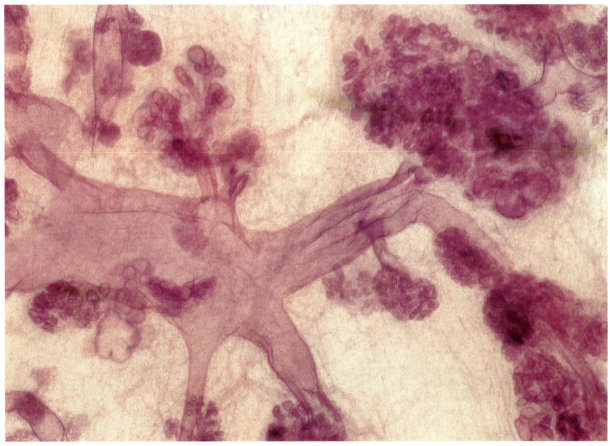

Fibrous Strands

Fibrous strands account for most of the linear densities on the mammogram and will be best visualized when surrounded by adipose tissue.

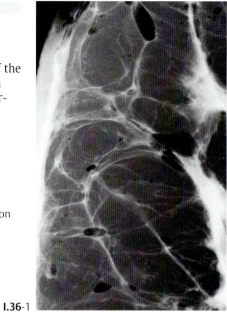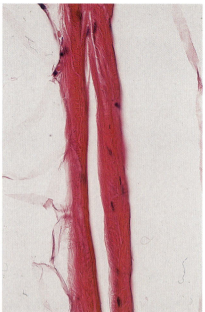

Fig. **I.36**-1 & 2   Fibrous strands as seen on specimen radiography and histology.

I.36-1

I.36-2

Fig. **I.37**-1 & 2   Radiograph of a mastectomy specimen slice and corresponding large-section histological image. Normal fibrous strands give a harmonious picture (rectangle), while the malignant tumor is obscured (arrow).

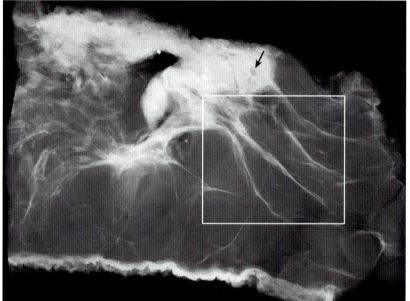

I.37-1

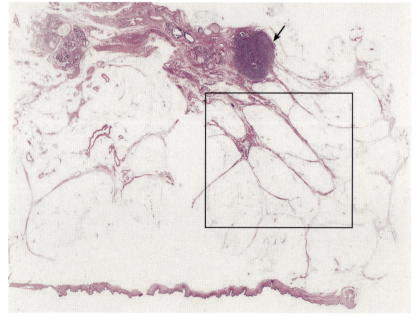

I.37-2

Vessels

Blood vessels account for some of the linear densities on the mammogram. Breast compression tends to accentuate the veins. Calcified arteries are particularly easy to recognize.

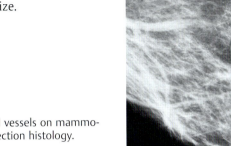
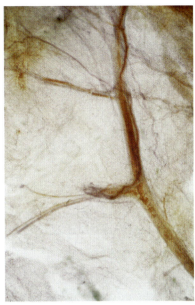
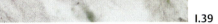

Figs. **I.38–I.41**   Blood vessels on mammograms and on thick-section histology.

I.38

I.39

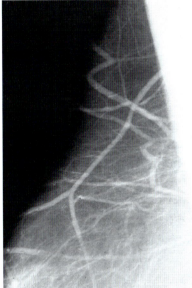
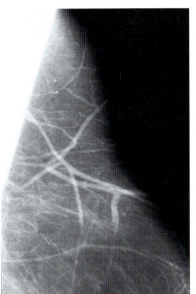

I.40-1

I.40-2

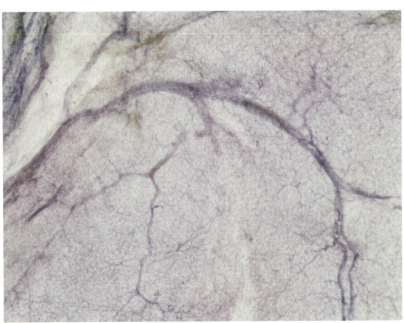

I.41

■ Homogeneous, Structureless Densities

Homogeneous, structureless densities correspond to fibrous tissue. This building block, together with adipose tissue, provides the supporting structure for the first two building blocks.

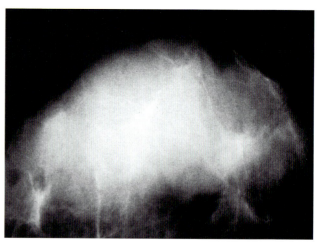

Fig. I.42-1 Mammogram, CC projection. The dense, structureless fibrosis obscures the underlying structure.

I.42-1

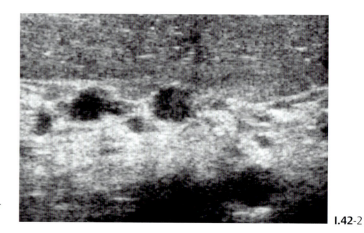

Fig. I.42-2 Breast ultrasound shows numerous cysts occult for mammography.

I.42-2

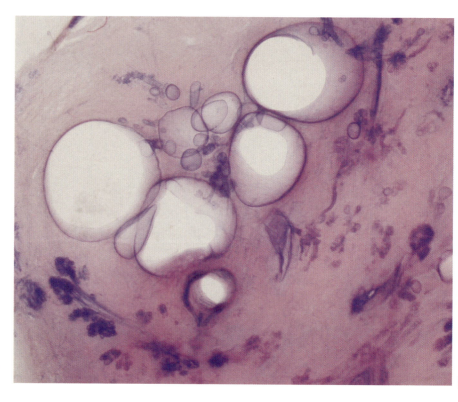

Fig. I.42-3 Most normal structures and noncalcified pathological changes, such as these cysts, can be completely obscured within dense fibrous tissue. Subgross, thick-section histology.

I.42-3

Fig. **I.42**-4 A distended TDLU containing "milk of calcium" is surrounded by fibrosis. Subgross, thick-section histology.

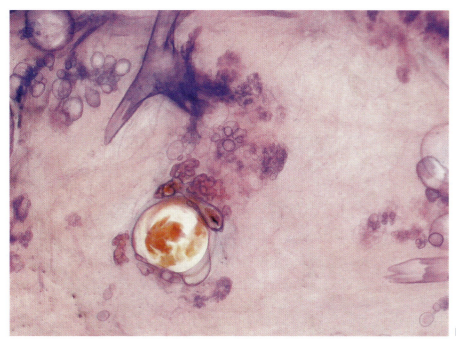

I.42-4

Fig. **I.42**-5 Normal TDLUs and adjacent, cystically dilated TDLUs within the dense fibrosis. Subgross, thick-section histology.

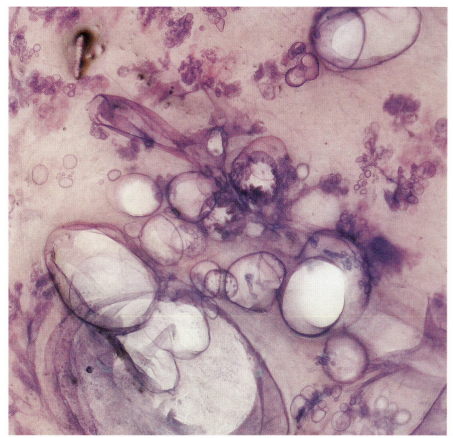

I.42-5

Homogeneous, Structureless Densities

Figures **I.43**-1 to 3 demonstrate the considerable heterogeneity in distribution and alteration of the structural elements, so characteristic for breast tissue. The normal TDLUs and ducts as well as their alterations due to hyperplastic breast changes can be hidden within the fibrous tissue surrounding them. This explains the occasional difficulties incurred when imaging dense breasts with mammography. Additional diagnostic methods, such as breast ultrasound, can provide better visualization of pathological structures in these cases.

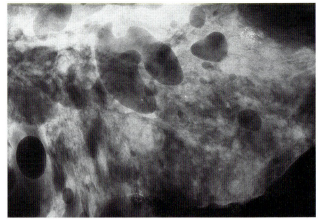

I.43-1

Fig. **I.43**-1   Specimen radiograph with numerous air-filled cysts (the corresponding thick-section histology is seen on Fig. **I.43**-2).

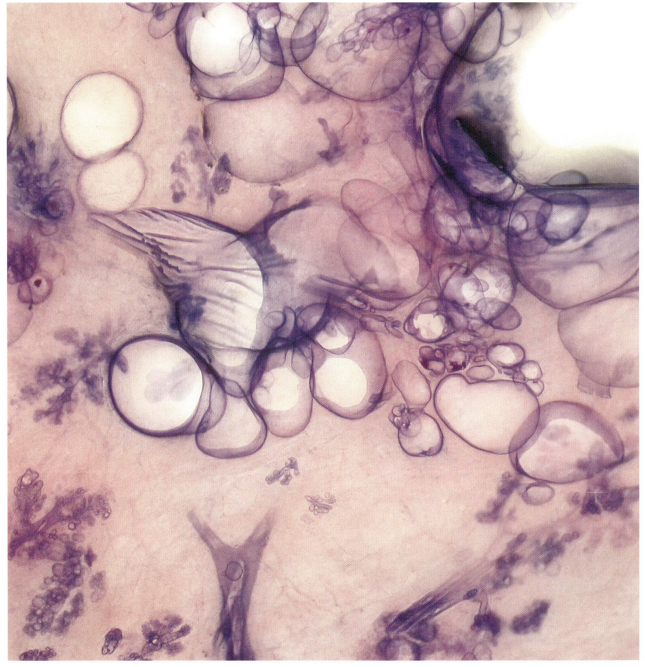

I.43-2

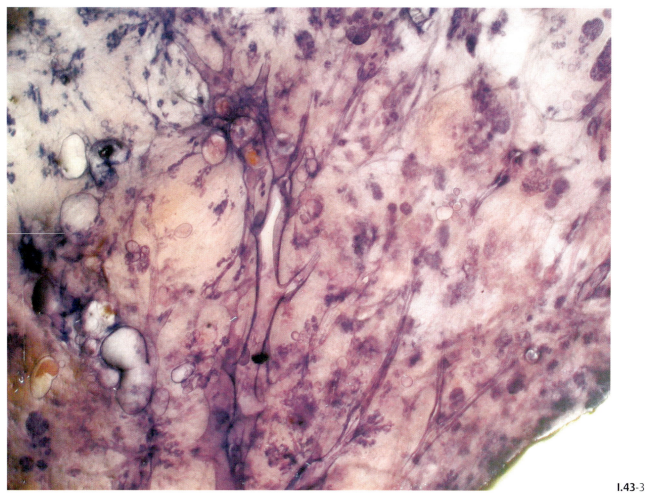

Fig. **I.43**-3   Subgross, thick-section histology image of breast tissue, containing all four building blocks in uneven distribution.

Homogeneous, Structureless Densities

Fig. **I.44** Detail of left MLO projection with focal fibrosis. The density on the mammogram is structureless, homogeneous, ground glass–like with concave contours.

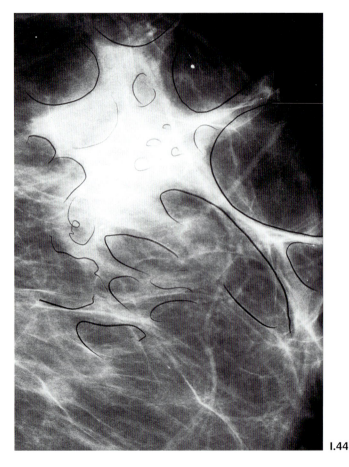

I.44

Fig. **I.45**-1 Specimen radiograph of a breast tissue slice containing a region of dense, structureless fibrosis with concave contours.

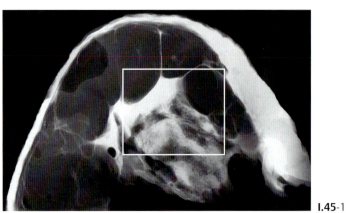

I.45-1

Fig. **I.45**-2 to 5 Large-section (H&E stain) and subgross, thick-section histological images corresponding to the specimen radiograph. The histological images demonstrate numerous atrophic TDLUs and ducts as well as a dilated duct, all of which are hidden in the surrounding dense fibrosis.

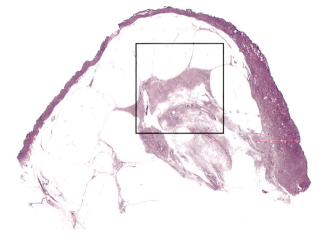

I.45-2

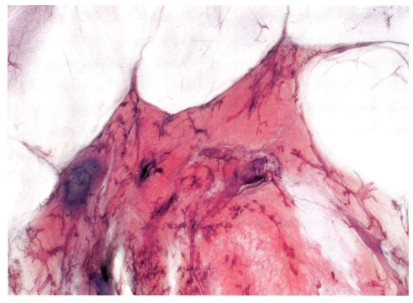

I.45-3

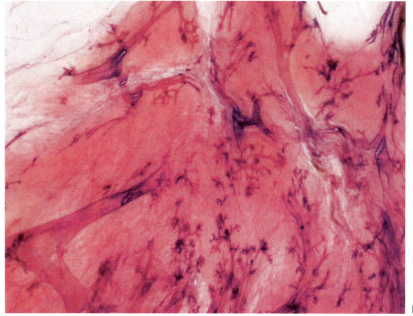

I.45-4

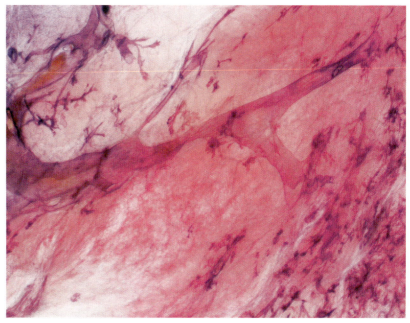

I.45-5

■ Radiolucent Areas

Radiolucent areas representing adipose tissue constitute the fourth building block of normal breast tissue.

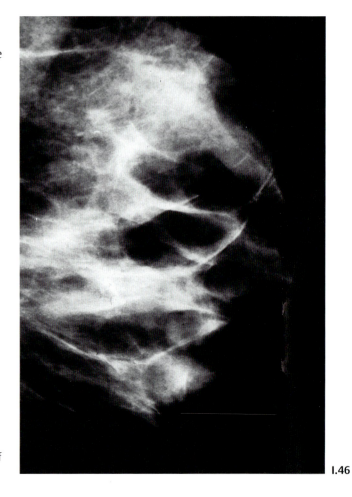

I.46

Fig. **I.46** Mammography showing oval-shaped regions of adipose tissue.

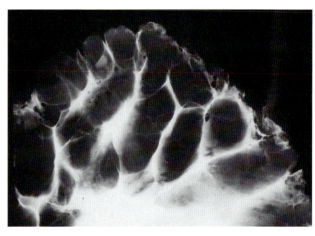

I.47-1

Fig. **I.47**-1 Sliced specimen radiograph demonstrating oval-shaped regions of adipose tissue interspersed with the remaining fibroglandular tissue.

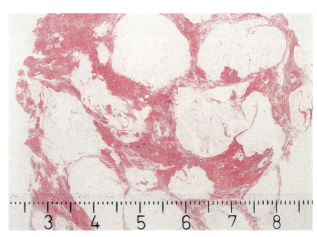

I.47-2

Fig. **I.47**-2 Large-section histology image showing the adipose tissue surrounded by fibroglandular tissue.

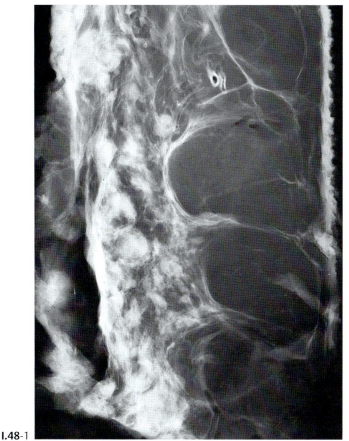

I.48-1

Fig. **I.48**-1   Radiograph of an operative breast specimen slice. Large areas of adipose tissue outline the Cooper's ligaments and the subdermis.

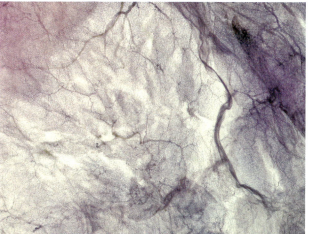

I.48-2

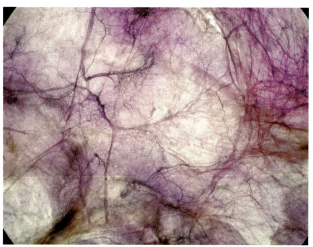

I.48-3

Fig. **I.48**-2 to 4   Subgross, thick-section histology images of adipose tissue and blood vessels.

I.48-4

Overview of the Five Mammographic Parenchymal Patterns

The challenge faced by the radiologist can be met by classifying mammograms into structural subtypes. In 1976 Wolfe described four mammographic parenchymal patterns and made predictions concerning the likelihood of developing breast cancer. His classification was based on radiological pattern reading.[5]

Further development and refinement required comprehensive mammographic–histological correlation. The application of comparative subgross anatomy and mammography has led to the development of a reproducible classification system with five mammographic parenchymal patterns.[1, 4]

In each of these patterns the mammographic image is a characteristic mixture of the four structural components or building blocks:

1 **Nodular densities**
2 **Linear densities**
3 **Homogeneous, structureless densities**
4 **Radiolucent areas**

Classifying the mammographic image of the normal breast serves a number of useful purposes, justifying our emphasis upon the utility of these patterns, as follows:

- Understanding the basic structural elements and knowing the capabilities and limitations of each imaging method will help us to recognize the normal mammogram and detect abnormalities with a high degree of certainty. This has become increasingly important as an ever-growing number of asymptomatic women undergo regular mammographic examination.
- The mammographic parenchymal patterns serve as an important means of communication among the specialists dealing with the diagnosis of breast diseases. In breasts with fatty replacement, such as mammographic Patterns II and III, perception and interpretation of the abnormalities will be relatively straightforward for all diagnostic modalities, including palpation, mammography and histology, requiring little help from the ancillary diagnostic methods, such as breast ultrasound.
- On the other hand, in so-called "dense breasts" (mammographic Patterns IV and V and often Pattern I), the efficacy of palpation and mammography may be considerably reduced, increasing the need for ancillary methods.
- Pattern I has a dynamic association with Patterns II and III, as it gradually undergoes involution. Conversely, hormone replacement therapy can reverse the direction of this process. Patterns IV and V remain largely unchanged during the woman's adult lifetime.
- One important practical implication is that the impact of hormone replacement therapy will be considerably influenced by the underlying breast structure. The differing response of women to a given regimen of hormone replacement therapy can be largely explained by the underlying structural differences and can be documented on the mammogram. For example, giving the same combination of estrogen and progesterone to women who have fatty involved breasts and to women who have dense, fibroglandular tissue may result in entirely different symptomatology and may lead to the development of different abnormalities.
- The mammographic parenchymal patterns are an indicator of risk for developing breast cancer. The risk of developing breast cancer is lower in women with Patterns I–III and higher with Patterns IV–V. There is an approximately 15-year delay in the development of breast cancer in the former group compared with the latter.[2]

Comparative subgross anatomy and mammography form the basis for this reproducible classification system with five mammographic parenchymal patterns. In each of these patterns the mammographic image is a characteristic mixture of the four structural components or building blocks.

Mammographic Parenchymal Pattern I

Mammographic parenchymal Pattern I is the most common mammographic pattern in premenopausal women. All four building blocks are fairly equally represented in this pattern (Chart **I.1**). With involution, it will change to either Pattern II or Pattern III. Hormone-replacement therapy tends to arrest and often reverse the process of involution.

Figures **I.49**, **I.50** and **I.51** show the variations of Pattern I on the mammogram.

See Chapter 1 for a detailed description of Pattern I.

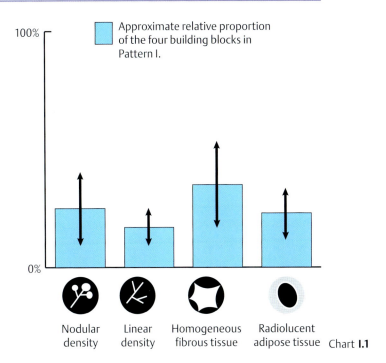

Approximate relative proportion of the four building blocks in Pattern I.

| Nodular density | Linear density | Homogeneous fibrous tissue | Radiolucent adipose tissue |

Chart **I.1**

Fig. **I.49**-1 to 4   Mammographic Pattern I with a predominance of adipose tissue. Mediolateral oblique (1 and 2) and craniocaudal projections (3 and 4).

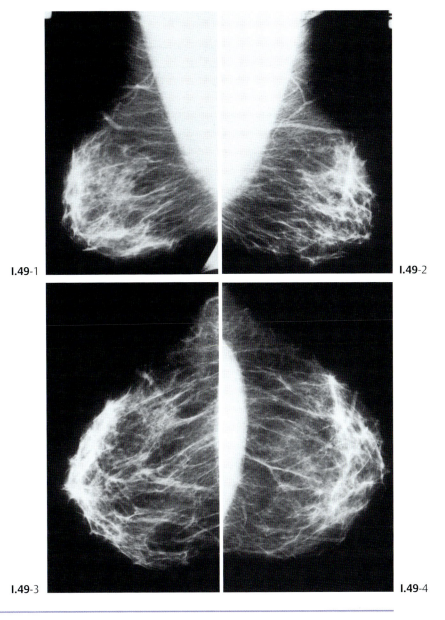

I.49-1

I.49-2

I.49-3

I.49-4

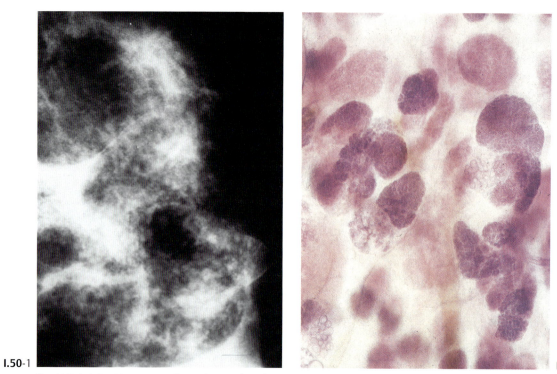

Fig. **I.50**-1 & 2   Mammographic–subgross histological correlation of Pattern I. The four building blocks occur in approximately equal proportions.

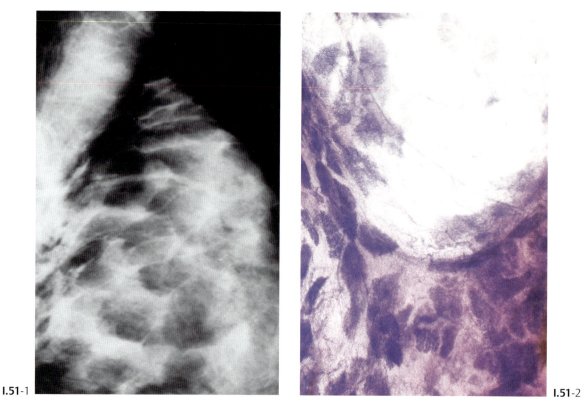

Fig. **I.51**-1 & 2   Pattern I with prominent fibrosis. Detail from a mammogram in the mediolateral oblique projection and thick-section histology, both showing spherical regions of fat surrounded by fibroglandular tissue.

■ Mammographic Parenchymal Pattern II

Mammographic parenchymal Patterns II (Fig. **I.52**) and III (Fig. **I.53**) represent the end results of the process of involution. The mammographic images are dominated by radiolucent adipose tissue and linear densities, making the detection of abnormalities relatively easy.
See Chapter 2 for a detailed description of Pattern II.

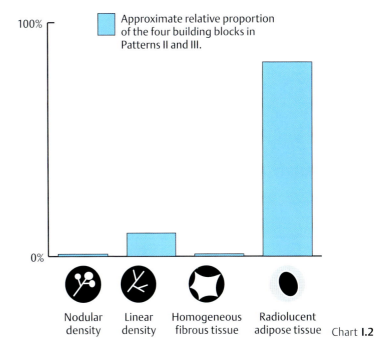

Nodular density · Linear density · Homogeneous fibrous tissue · Radiolucent adipose tissue

Approximate relative proportion of the four building blocks in Patterns II and III.

Chart **I.2**

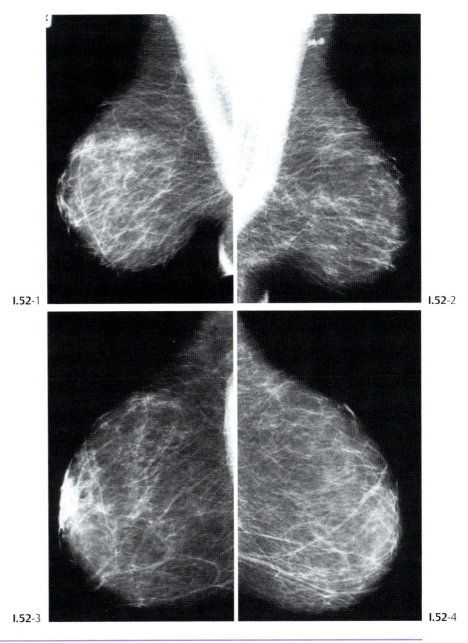

I.52-1

I.52-2

I.52-3

I.52-4

■ Mammographic Parenchymal Pattern III

Mammographic parenchymal Pattern III is very similar to Pattern II with the exception of retroareolar prominent ducts, often associated with periductal fibrosis.
Figure **I.53**-1 & 2 shows an example of Pattern III.
See Chapter 3 for a detailed description of Pattern III.

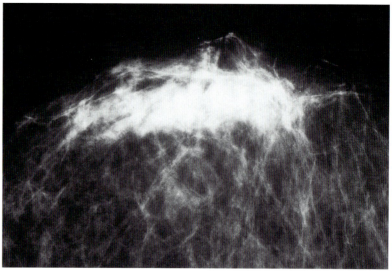

I.53-1

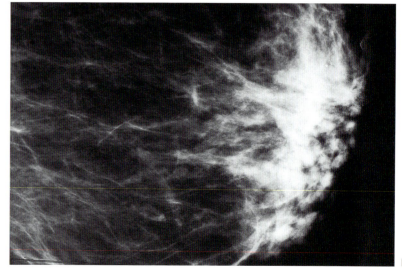

I.53-2

■ Mammographic Parenchymal Pattern IV

Mammographic parenchymal Pattern IV is dominated by prominent nodular and linear densities. Their presence often makes perception of pathological lesions difficult. Also, this pattern appears to be resistant to the process of involution (Fig. **I.54**-1 to 4).

See Chapter 4 for a detailed description of Pattern IV.

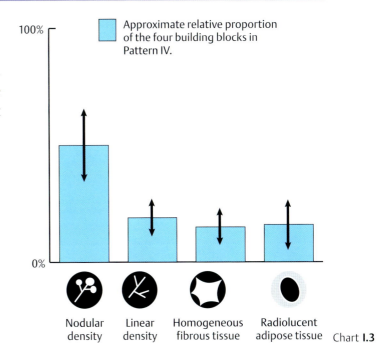

Approximate relative proportion of the four building blocks in Pattern IV.

Nodular density Linear density Homogeneous fibrous tissue Radiolucent adipose tissue

Chart **I.3**

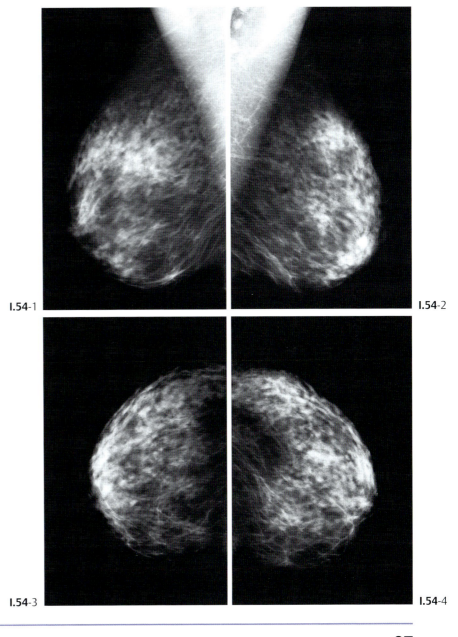

I.54-1

I.54-2

I.54-3

I.54-4

■ Mammographic Parenchymal Pattern V

Mammographic parenchymal Pattern V is dominated by extensive fibrosis. The overwhelming dominance of this homogeneous, structureless fibrous tissue limits the capabilities of mammography to demonstrate the details of normal anatomy and to reveal small pathological lesions (Fig. **I.54**-1 to 4).

See Chapter 5 for a detailed description of Pattern V.

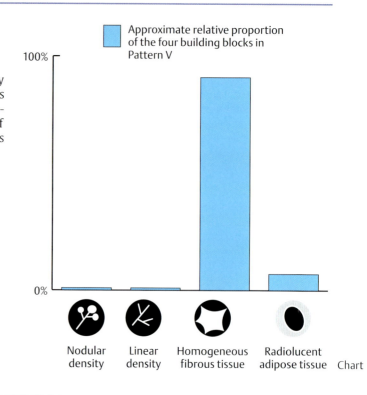

Approximate relative proportion of the four building blocks in Pattern V

| Nodular density | Linear density | Homogeneous fibrous tissue | Radiolucent adipose tissue | Chart |

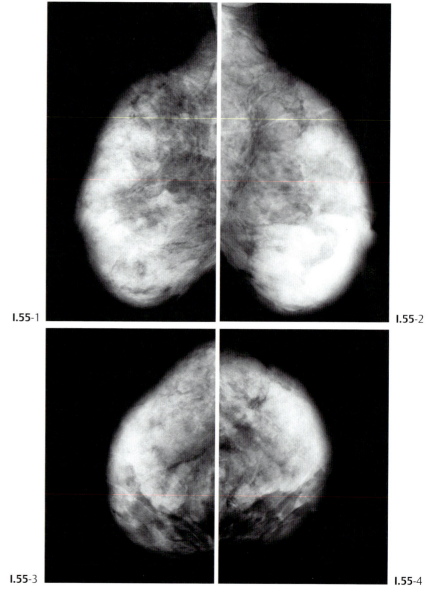

I.55-1

I.55-2

I.55-3

I.55-4

Chapter 1: Pattern I

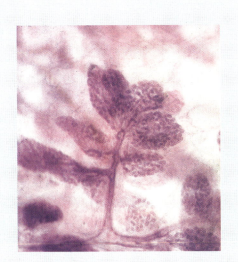 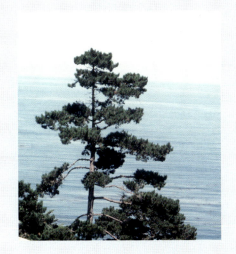

Characteristics of Pattern I

Pattern I is the mammographic image of normal fibroglandular tissue with partial fatty replacement. Although these breasts are "dense" radiologically, pathological changes can be fairly easily perceived in them.

The mammographic image is characterized by:

Radiopaque densities consisting of
    Nodular densities, evenly scattered, 1–2 mm in size
    Linear densities
    Fibrous tissue and Cooper's ligaments
Radiolucent areas

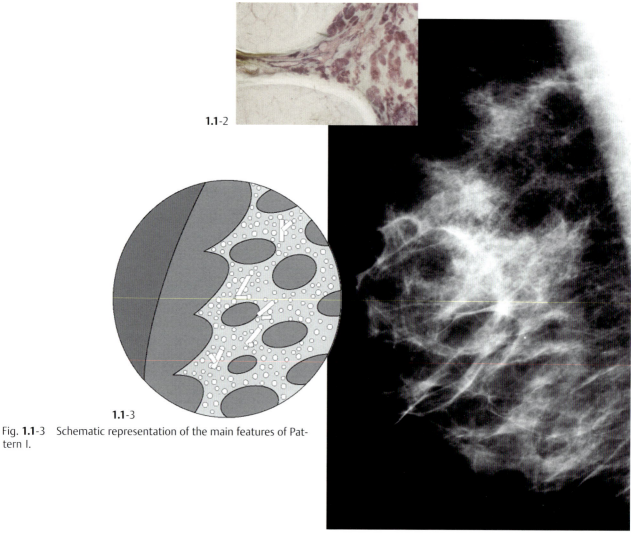

1.1-2

1.1-3

Fig. **1.1**-3   Schematic representation of the main features of Pattern I.

1.1-1

Fig. **1.1**-1   Characteristic mammographic image of a Pattern I breast with the four building blocks in approximately equal proportions. The insertion (**1.1**-2) shows a subgross histological image of a Cooper's ligament.

Fig. **1.2**-1 & 2   Mastectomy specimen slice with Cooper's ligaments, compared to the mediolateral projection on a mammogram.

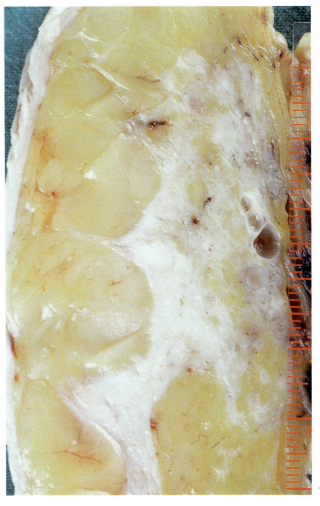

1.2-1

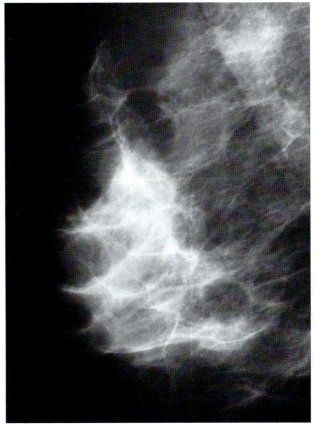

1.2-2

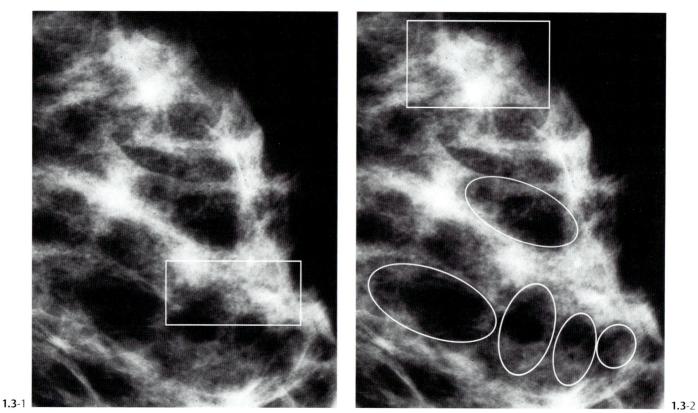

1.3-1   **1.3**-2

Fig. **1.3**-1 & 2   This detail image from an MLO projection demonstrates all three criteria characteristic of Pattern I: the Cooper's ligaments along the anterior contour, oval-shaped regions of fatty replacement, TDLUs surrounded by some fibrosis (squares).

Figures **1.3**-3 to 5 demonstrate the underlying histological details corresponding to the mammographic findings: the adipose tissue is encircled, corresponding to the oval-shaped radiolucent regions on the mammogram. The areas outlined by rectangles contain the TDLUs, ducts and their surrounding connective tissue, which results in concave contoured radiopaque densities on the mammogram.

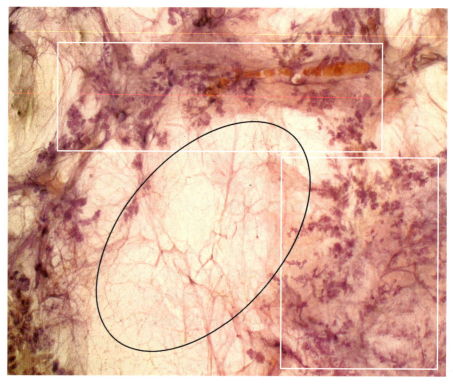

1.3-3

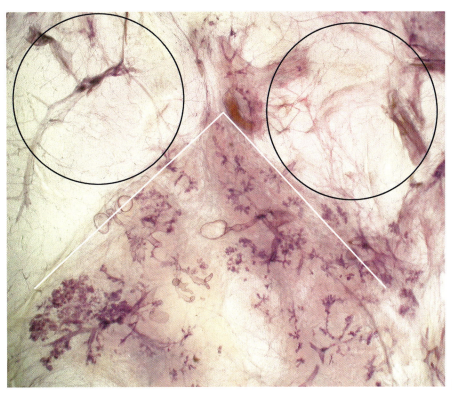

1.3-4

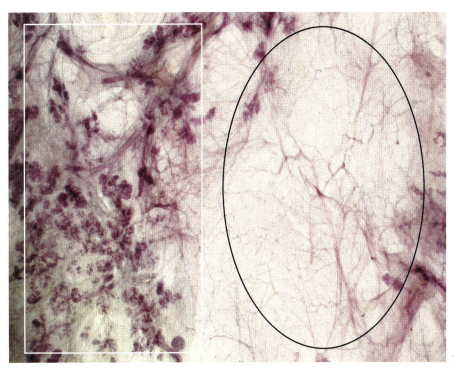

1.3-5

Fig. **1.4**-1 to 3   Correlative mammographic (**1.4**-1), galactographic (**1.4**-2), and histological (**1.4**-3) images demonstrating numerous normal TDLUs and their associated ducts.

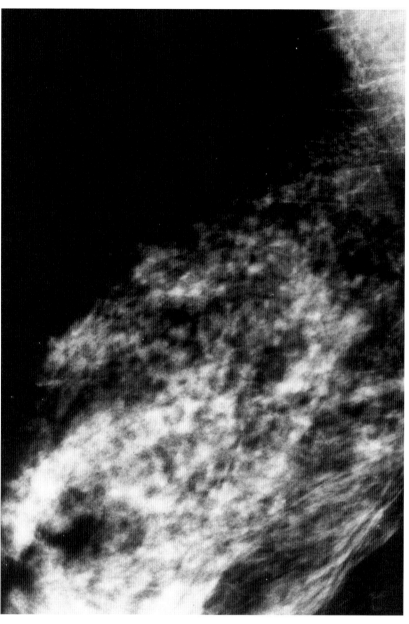

1.4-1

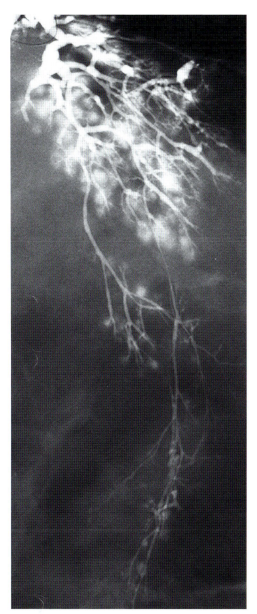

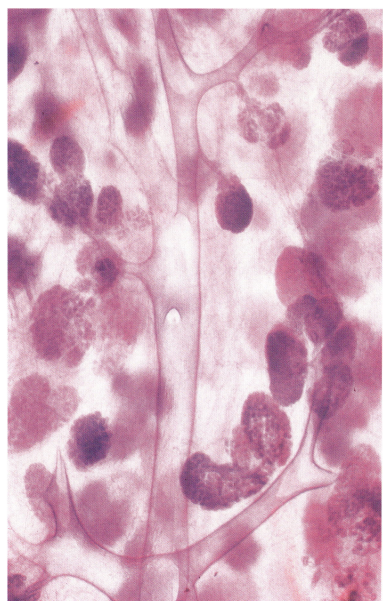

1.4-2

1.4-3

Radiopaque Densities

■ Nodular Densities

"The mature human female breast contains thousands of hormone-sensitive, potentially milk-producing micro-organs called lobules. A terminal duct attached to the main duct system drains each lobule. It is called the terminal ductal lobular unit (TDLU), which normally regresses at menopause. Most breast diseases except papillomas in major ducts arise in terminal ductal lobular units."[2]

The **radiopaque densities** seen on the mammogram of Pattern I are the radiological images of fibroglandular tissue, consisting of:

- 1–2 mm **nodular densities**, corresponding to terminal ductal lobular units
- **Linear densities**, images of ducts and their branches, fibrous strands, and blood vessels
- Dense **fibrous tissue**

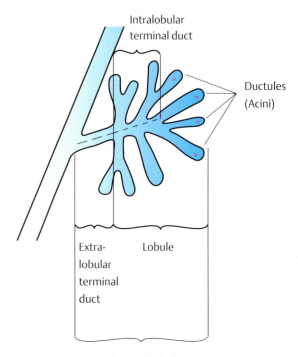

Fig. **1.5** Terminal ductal lobular unit (TDLU) (Adapted from Ref. 5).

1.5

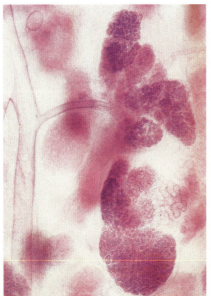

1.6-1

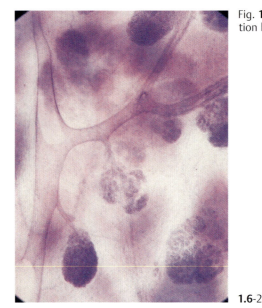

1.6-2

Fig. **1.6**-1 & 2 Subgross, thick-section histological images of TDLUs.

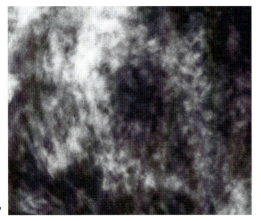

1.7

Fig. **1.7** Detail of a mammogram with Pattern I, demonstrating a large number of TDLUs. When the TDLUs and ducts are surrounded by adipose tissue, they are usually discernible; when they are surrounded by fibrous tissue, the individual TDLUs cannot be detected by mammography.

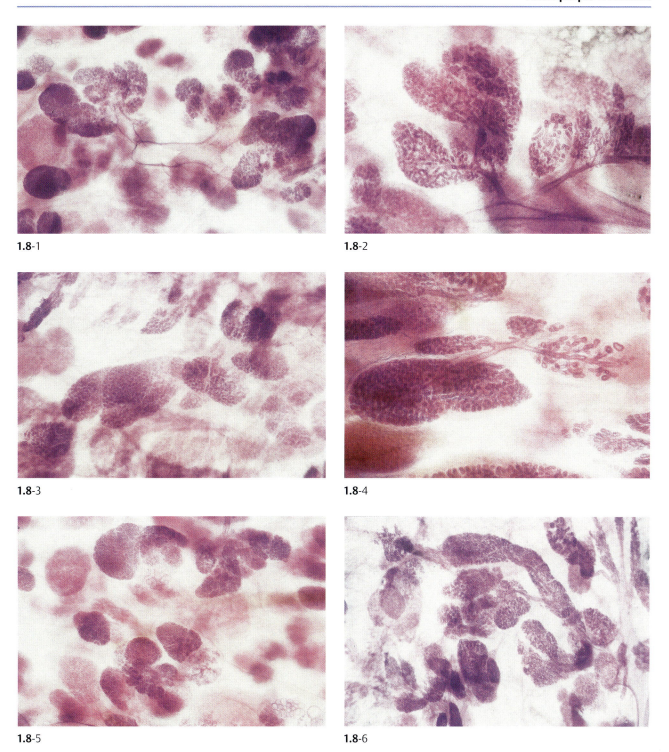

1.8-1

1.8-2

1.8-3

1.8-4

1.8-5

1.8-6

Fig. **1.8**-1 to 6   Subgross, thick-section histological demonstration of normal TDLUs and their associated ducts.

Nodular Densities

Fig. **1.9** The size and shape of the individual lobules vary, but most lobules are between 0.5 and **1.0** mm in diameter. The numerous acini within each lobule can be discerned and the associated terminal duct is easily visualized using subgross, thick-section histology.

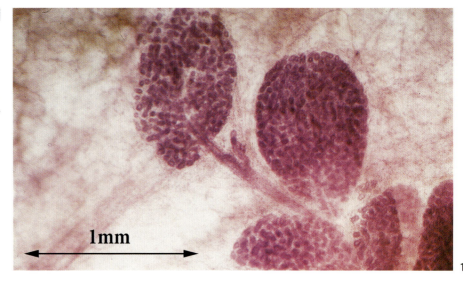

1.9

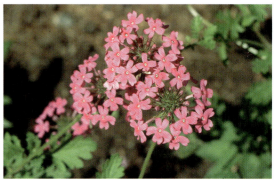

1.10-1

1.10-2

Fig. **1.10**-1 Conventional histology image of a lobule. The individual acini are surrounded by loose, intralobular connective tissue.

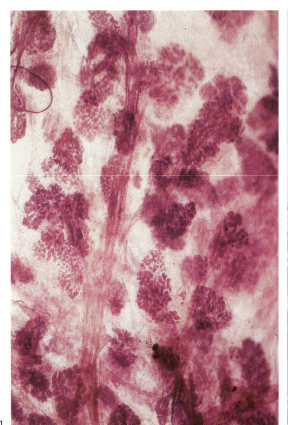

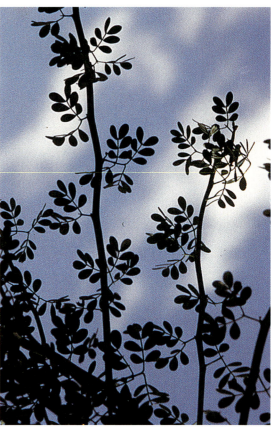

1.11-1

1.11-2

Fig. **1.11**-1 Subgross, thick-section histology image of a subsegmental duct and numerous TDLUs.

The hormone-sensitive, spherical lobules can be seen as circular/oval, approximately 1 mm radiopaque densities on a high-quality mammogram whenever they are outlined against a background of adipose tissue.

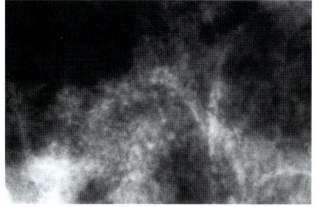

Fig. **1.12** Detail, craniocaudal projection. The numerous 1–2 mm nodular densities correspond to TDLUs surrounded by fat.

1.12

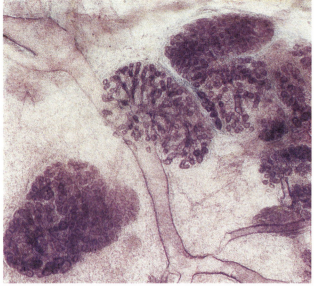

.13-1

Fig. **1.13**-1 Subgross, thick-section histology image of several lobules, the acini within the lobules, and the terminal duct.

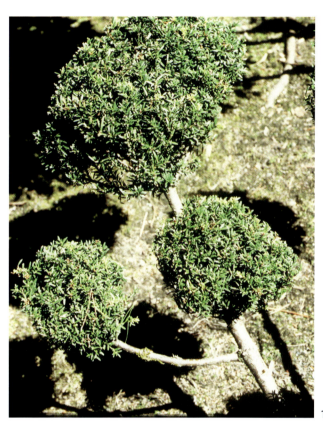

1.13-2

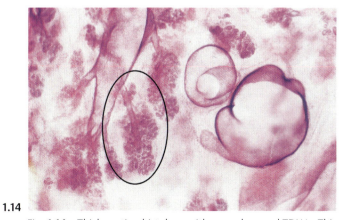

1.14

Fig. **1.14** Thick-section histology with several normal TDLUs. This image is comparable with that of the galactogram (Fig. **1.15**).

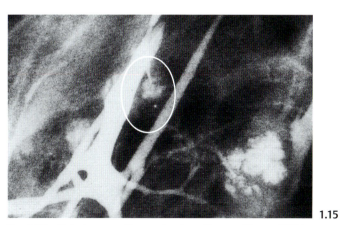

1.15

Fig. **1.15** Galactogram. The contrast medium outlines a TDLU.

49

Nodular Densities

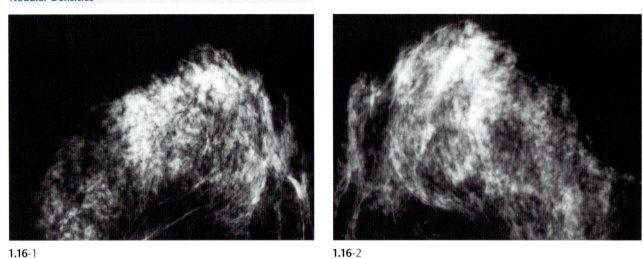

1.16-1   **1.16**-2

Fig. **1.16**-1 & 2   Mammograms of the right and left breasts in the craniocaudal projection showing a large number of TDLUs.

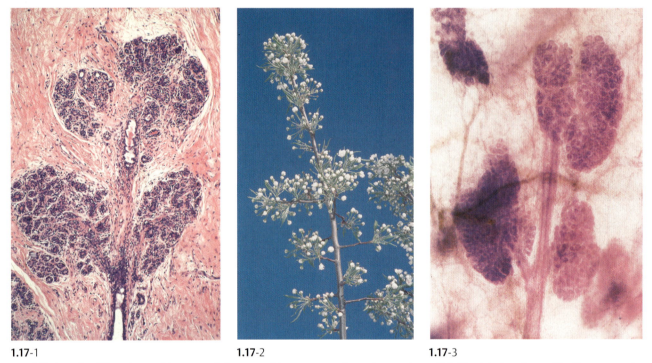

1.17-1   **1.17**-2   **1.17**-3

Fig. **1.17**-1 to 3   "The microarchitecture of the normal breast parenchyma is very beautiful. The lobules cluster like flowers on the branching duct tree."[2]

Fig. **1.18**-1   Subgross, thick-section histology of a subsegmental duct with several cystically dilated TDLUs.

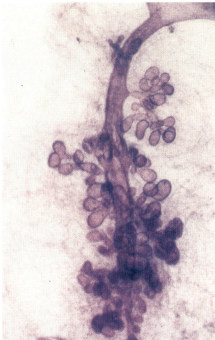

1.18-1

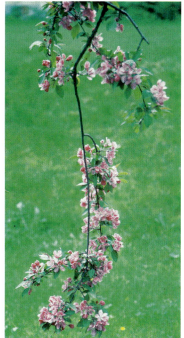

1.18-2

Fig. **1.19**-1   Thick-section histology of a subsegmental duct with several TDLUs.

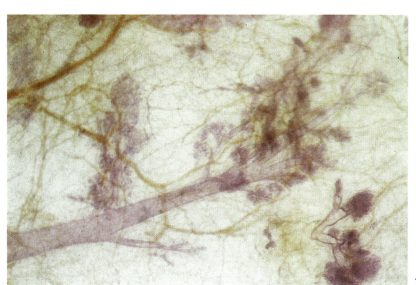

1.19-1

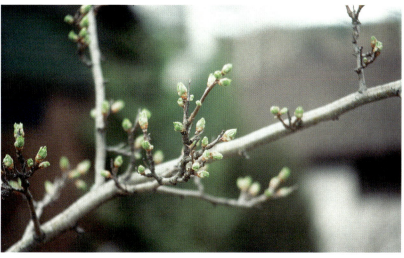

1.19-2

Nodular Densities

The average size of the individual lobule and the mean number of acini within individual lobules in the breast of an adult, premenopausal nonpregnant woman will change during the phases of the menstrual cycle.[4]

"There is a complex coexistence of proliferation and regression of the lobules during the menstrual cycle. Beginning a few days before ovulation in each menstrual cycle, clusters of cells bud from the smaller ducts, form lumens and grow rapidly into fully developed lobules and clusters. If pregnancy does not supervene, the newly formed structures atrophy over several months. Throughout menstrual life, there is almost continuous production and loss of tissue. A single biopsy of the breast may show budding lobules and mature lobules in various stages of regression. In the event of pregnancy, lobule formation and proliferation is intensified and becomes widespread throughout the breast."[1]

Fig. **1.20** Lobule size variation during phases of the menstrual cycle.

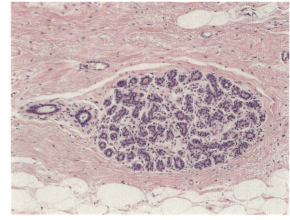

1.20-

1.20-1   Proliferative phase.

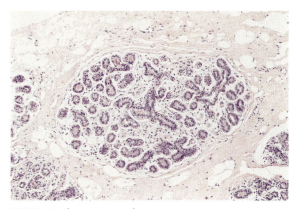

1.20-

1.20-2   Early secretory phase.

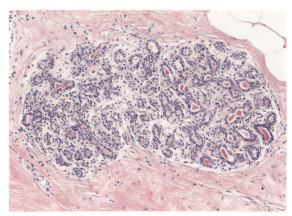

1.20-

1.20-3   Late secretory phase.

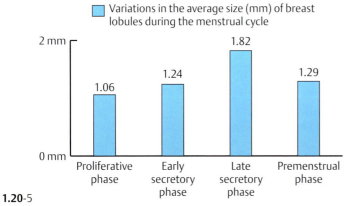

1.20-5

Fig. **1.20**-5   Variations in the average size (mm) of breast lobules during the menstrual cycle. (Adapted from Ref. 4)

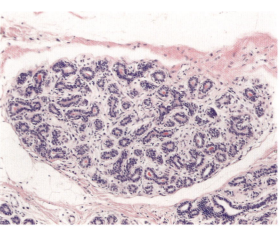

1.20-

1.20-4   Premenstrual phase.

In most cases these delicate physiological changes—however, well demonstrated **histologically**—are difficult or impossible to demonstrate **mammographically**. In some women the extensive proliferation and fluid retention will increase the volume of the breast during the secretory phase of the menstrual cycle. Compression of the breast during mammography will cause more pain in these women. Less compression and an increased amount of fluid and tissue will result in suboptimal image quality. Optimally, the mammographic examination should be performed shortly after the beginning of the menstrual cycle.

Fig. **1.21** Changes in the acini within a single lobule during phases of the menstrual cycle.

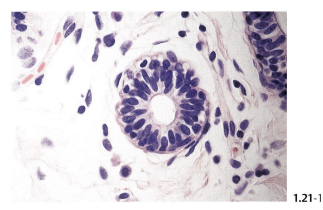

1.21-1

1.**21**-1 Proliferative phase.

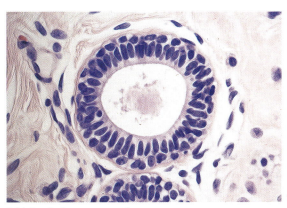

1.21-2

1.**21**-2 Early secretory phase.

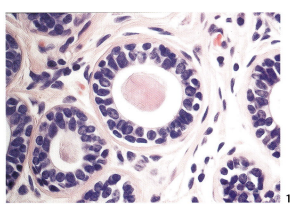

1.21-3

1.**21**-3 Late secretory phase.

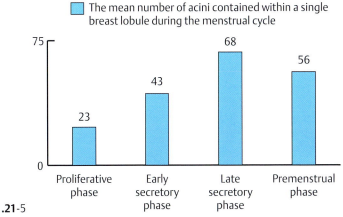

The mean number of acini contained within a single breast lobule during the menstrual cycle

```
75 ┐                         68
   │                              56
   │                   43
   │         23
 0 └───────────────────────────────────
    Proliferative  Early    Late    Premenstrual
      phase      secretory secretory  phase
                  phase     phase
```

.21-5

Fig. **1.21**-5 Mean number of acini contained within a single breast lobule during the menstrual cycle. (Adapted from Ref. 3)

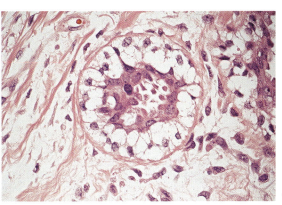

1.21-4

1.**21**-4 Premenstrual phase.

■ Fibrous Tissue

Figures **1.22** and **1.23** show two examples of Pattern I with dense fibrosis. The dense fibrous tissue obscures the delicate details of the nodular and linear densities, especially in younger women with Pattern I.

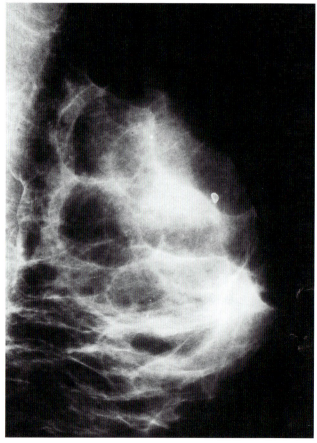

1.22-1

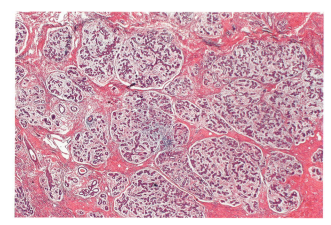

1.22-2

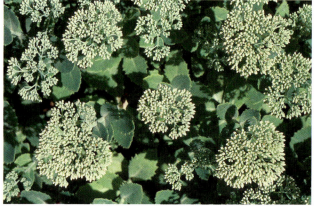

1.22-3

Fig. **1.23**-1   Although there is more fatty replacement in this case, the fibrosis still tends to obscure the TDLUs.

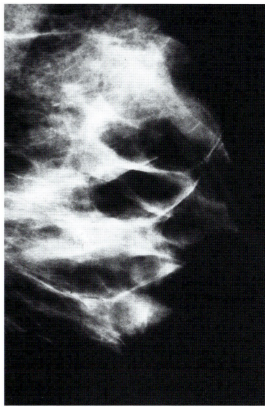

1.23-1

Fig. **1.23**-2   The histological image reveals the TDLUs within the surrounding fibrous tissue. The inability of mammography to discern the lobules when embedded in fibrous tissue explains the limitation of the method.

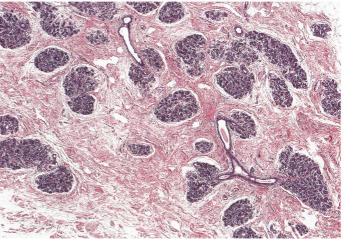

1.23-2

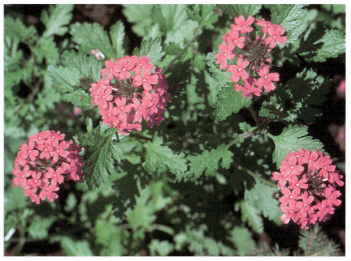

1.23-3

■ The Parenchymal Contour

The **parenchymal contour** in Pattern I forms a characteristic, scalloped border. The radiopaque, triangular projections, the so-called Cooper's ligaments, are in actuality normal breast parenchyma with the surrounding fibrosis.

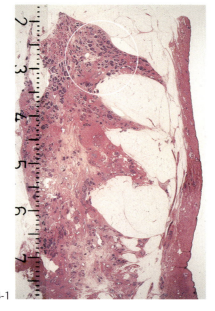

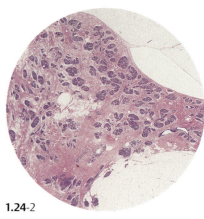

1.24-2

Fig. **1.24**-1 & 2   Large-section histology of a mastectomy specimen. There are large numbers of normal lobules within the dense fibrous tissue.   **1.24**-1

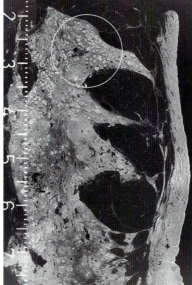

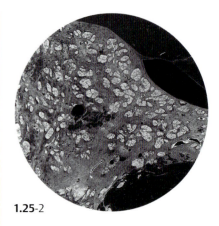

1.25-2

Fig. **1.25**-1 & 2   Negative mode, black-and-white copy of the histology images showing what we might expect a mammogram to demonstrate.   **1.25**-1

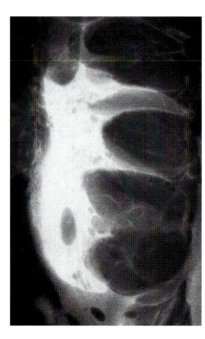

Fig. **1.26**   The specimen radiograph, unlike the histology specimen, fails to demonstrate the fine details of the glandular tissue contained within the homogeneous, structureless fibrosis.   **1.26**

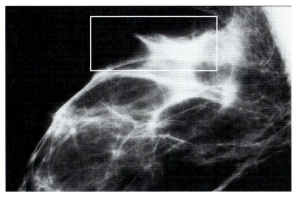

1.27-1

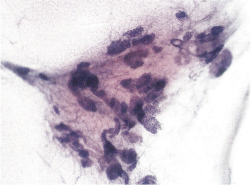

1.27-2

Figs. **1.27** and **1.28**   Two cases with mammographic–histological comparison of Cooper's ligaments. Thick-section histology demonstrates the large number of TDLUs and smaller ducts surrounded by dense connective tissue.

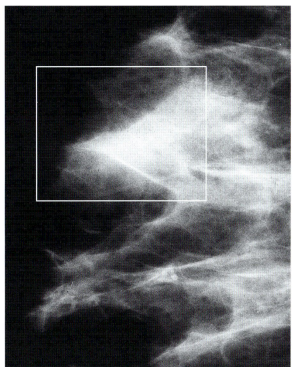

1.28-1

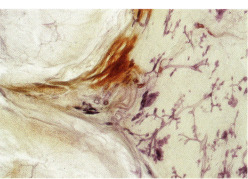

1.28-2

The Parenchymal Contour

Fig. **1.29**-1 & 2 Mammographic–histological correlation of a Cooper's ligament in a Pattern I breast.

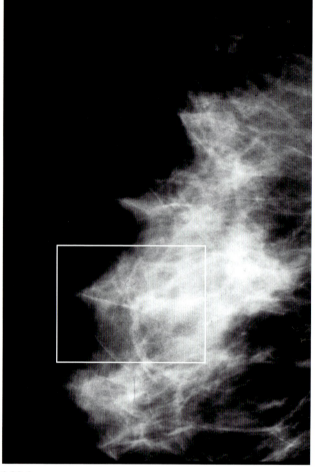

1.29-1

Fig. **1.29**-2 Subgross histological image corresponding to the rectangle on **1.29**-1.

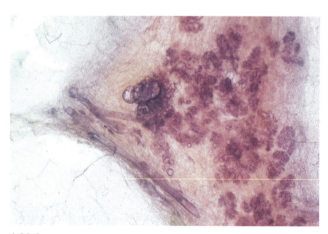

1.29-2

Fig. **1.29**-3 to 5 These subgross, thick-section histology images demonstrate some of the pathological abnormalities that the Cooper's ligaments may contain. Figs. **1.29**-4 to 5 are magnifications of the areas within the rectangles on Fig. **1.29**-3, containing mammographically occult cysts and dilated ducts.

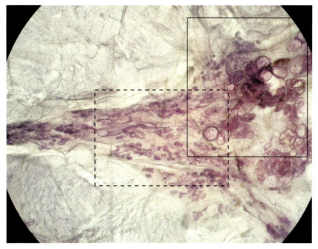

1.29-3

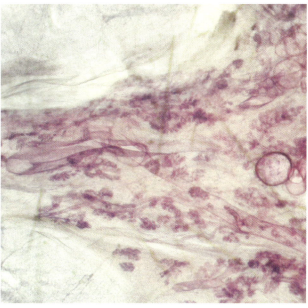

1.29-4

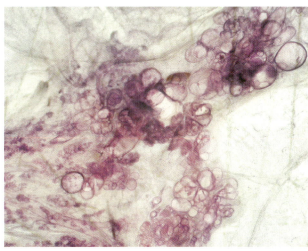

1.29-5

The Parenchymal Contour

Fig. **1.30**-1 to 4   Specimen radiograph (**1.30**-1) and large-section histology (**1.30**-2) of a large invasive lobular carcinoma invading Cooper's ligaments. The area enclosed by the rectangle is shown in **1.30**-3. Further magnification is seen in **1.30**-4.

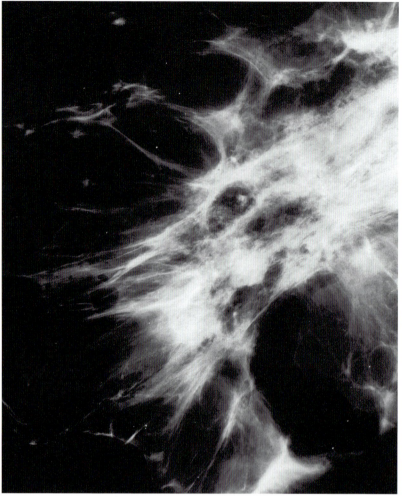

1.30-1

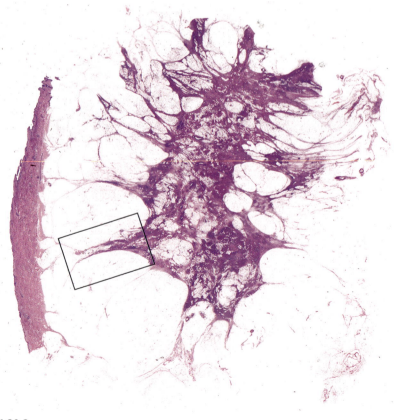

1.30-2

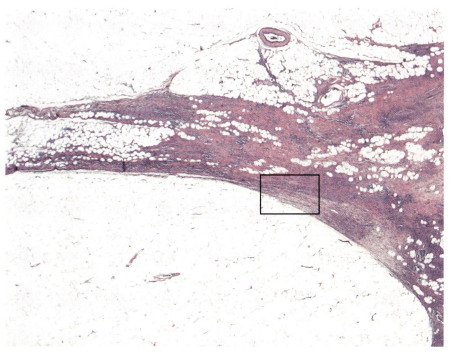

1.30-3

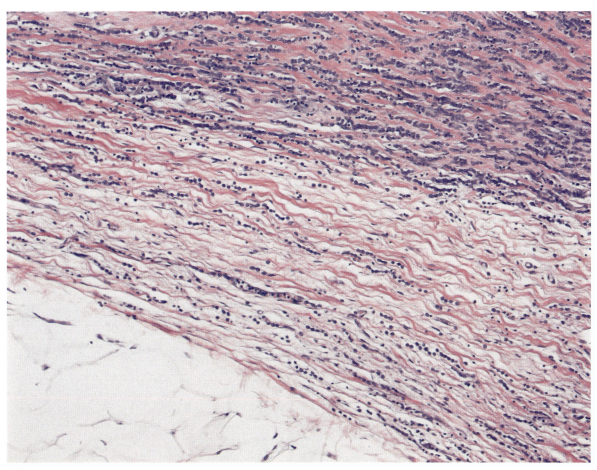

1.30-4

Radiolucent Areas

Ovoid radiolucent areas distributed throughout the breast correspond to fatty replacement.

As the adipose tissue outlines the concave contours of the anterior projections of the fibroglandular tissue (Cooper's ligaments), a similar phenomenon is seen in the interior of the breast undergoing involution. The persisting fibroglandular tissue has concave surfaces surrounded by spheres of adipose tissue. The **radiolucent areas** correspond to the structureless fat, while the **radiopaque regions** contain varying amounts of viable TDLUs embedded within fibrous tissue.

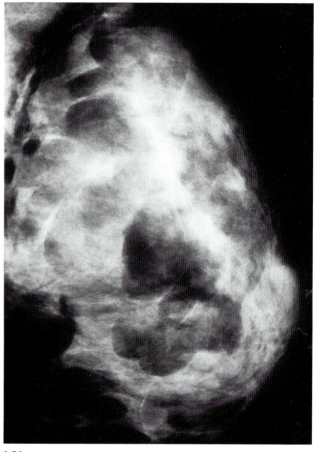

Figs. **1.31** and **1.32**-1 & 2 show two cases with Pattern I mammograms having varying degrees of fatty replacement.

1.31

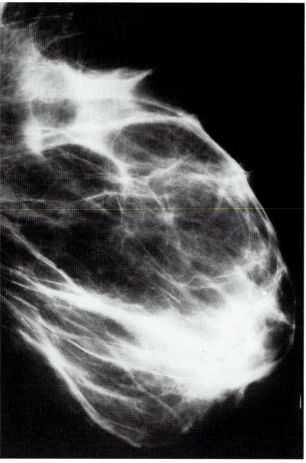

1.32-1

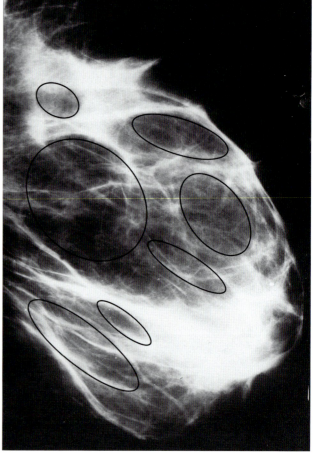

1.32-2

Figs. **1.33** and **1.35** Radiographs of mastectomy specimen slices demonstrating regions of fatty replacement surrounded by residual fibroglandular tissue. The pathological lesions, originating within the radiopaque fibroglandular tissue, will grow at the expense of the radiolucent adipose tissue, and thus become visible on the mammogram. Therefore, when reading mammograms, attention should be focused on the radiolucent areas in order to rule out or detect the presence of abnormalities encroaching upon the adipose tissue.

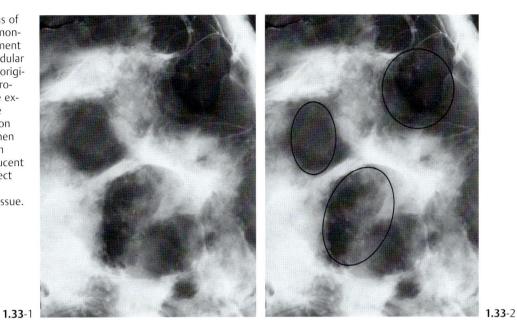

1.33-1

1.33-2

Fig. **1.34**-1 & 2 Corresponding subgross, thick-section histological image.

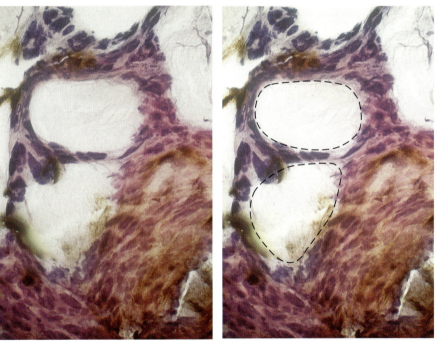

1.34-1

1.34-2

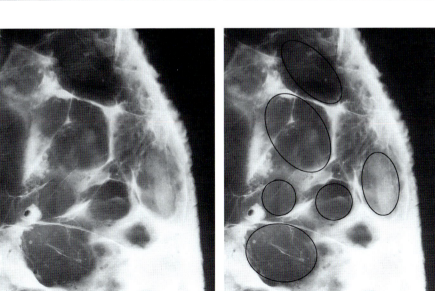

1.35-1

1.35-2

63

The presence of many ovoid radiolucent areas of fat inter-mingled with the radiopaque fibroglandular tissue is an important characteristic mammographic feature of Pattern I. The interface between the ovoid adipose tissue and the surrounding fibroglandular tissue is imaged as a curvilinear border. This gives us the harmonious image of the normal, most frequently occurring mammographic parenchymal pattern.

Example 1.1

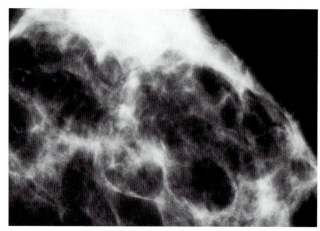

Ex **1.1**-1

Ex. **1.1**-1   Mammogram, detail of craniocaudal projection shows Pattern I with ovoid radiolucent areas. The radiopaque density is nearly structureless.

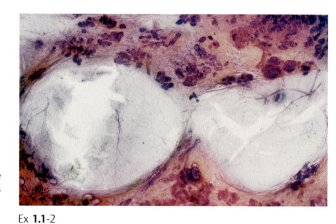

Ex **1.1**-2

Ex. **1.1**-2   Subgross, thick-section histology shows ovoid adipose tissue, but also shows the details in the surrounding dense fibrous tissue containing numerous TDLUs.

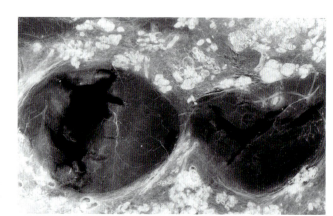

Ex **1.1**-3

Ex. **1.1**-3   Negative mode, black-and-white copy of the histological image demonstrates what we might expect to see on the specimen radiograph.

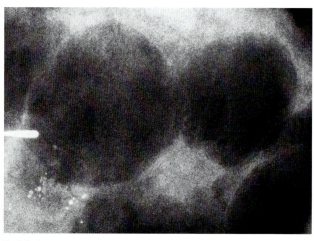

Ex **1.1**-4

Ex. **1.1**-4   However, the specimen radiograph shows only struc-tureless fibrosis with concave contours. The dense fibrous tissue obscures the delicate details of the nodular and linear densities.

Example 1.2

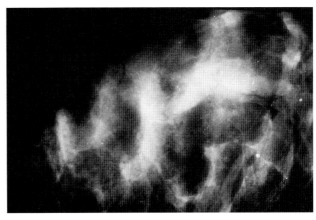

Ex. **1.2**-1   Mammogram showing oval-shaped regions with radiolucent adipose tissue surrounded by radiopaque density with concave contours.

Ex. **1.2**-1

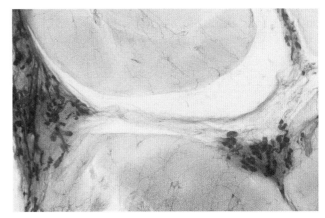

Ex. **1.2**-2 Subgross, thick-section histology demonstrates spheres of adipose tissue and persisting fibroglandular tissue (fibrosis, ducts, and TDLUs) with concave surfaces.

Ex. **1.2**-2

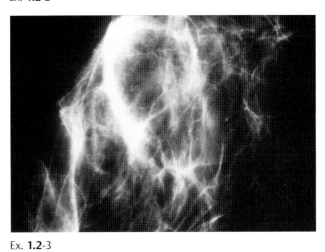

Ex. **1.2**-3 & 4   Mammogram and galactogram: the many branches of the ductal system interconnect the remaining parenchyma.

Ex. **1.2**-3

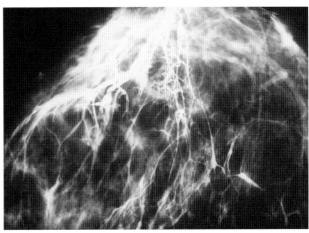

Ex. **1.2**-4

Involution

The dynamic nature of Pattern I can be described as a constant proliferation and regression of the terminal ductal lobular units and their supporting connective tissue.
Eventually, all Pattern I cases regress to either Pattern II or Pattern III. The rate at which this regression will occur is highly individual. Total fatty replacement (Pattern II) may occur in some women in their twenties and thirties, explaining the occasional mammograms of young women with essentially complete involution. More commonly, however, the transformation of Pattern I to Patterns II or III takes place gradually throughout menstrual life. Mammographic images taken at regular intervals, such as at periodic screening examinations, can document the inevitable transition from predominantly fibroglandular tissue to predominantly adipose tissue.

The process of involution includes both the TDLUs (nodular densities on the mammogram) and their supporting intralobular and extralobular connective tissue (homogeneous density on the mammogram). This is not an irreversible process; the best example is pregnancy when both the glandular and connective tissues proliferate to their extreme. Hormone replacement therapy induces a similar but less pronounced process in the menopause.

Fig. **1.36** Histological image of a single lobule showing partial fatty replacement. The number and size of acini gradually decrease, while adipose tissue simultaneously replaces the intralobular connective tissue and acini.

Fig. **1.37** Histological image of a single TDLU showing partial fatty replacement of the acini.

Fig. **1.38**-1 Histological image of a lobule stained for estrogen receptors. Note the uneven distribution of the positively stained (dark) nuclei among the acini. The acini without receptors will be less stimulated by the hormones, and will thus tend to atrophy.

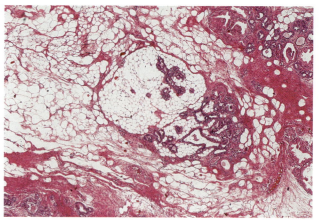

1.36

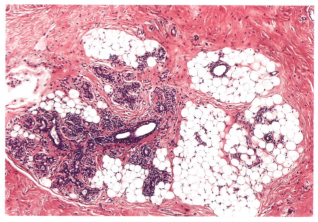

1.37

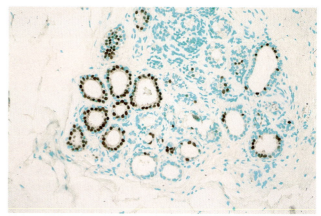

1.38-1

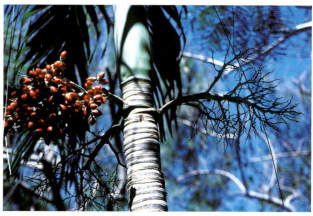

1.38-2

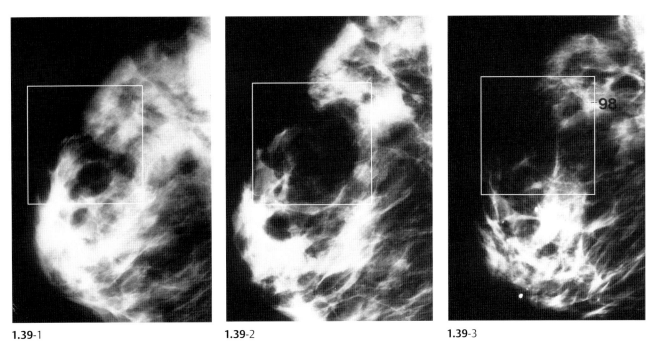

1.39-1   **1.39**-2   **1.39**-3

Fig. **1.39**-1 to 3   Three mammograms of the same woman taken during a period of 11 years. There is gradual replacement of the fibro-glandular tissue by adipose tissue.

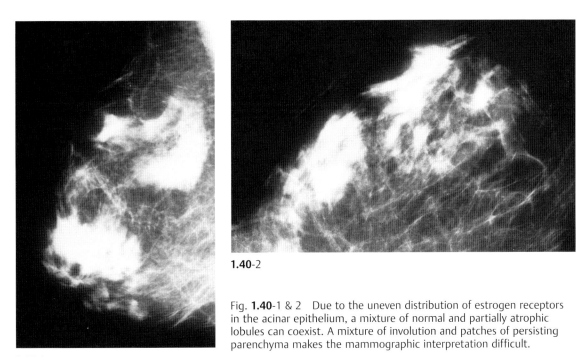

1.40-2

1.40-1

Fig. **1.40**-1 & 2   Due to the uneven distribution of estrogen receptors in the acinar epithelium, a mixture of normal and partially atrophic lobules can coexist. A mixture of involution and patches of persisting parenchyma makes the mammographic interpretation difficult.

Pattern I

Figures **1.41** and **1.42** demonstrate the transition of entirely fatty replaced (Pattern II) breasts to Pattern I type breasts as a result of hormone replacement therapy (HRT). There is mammographic evidence that a sudden proliferation of the fibroglandular tissue may also happen in the absence of HRT in perimenopausal women.

Fig. **1.41**-1 to 4   Images prior to HRT.

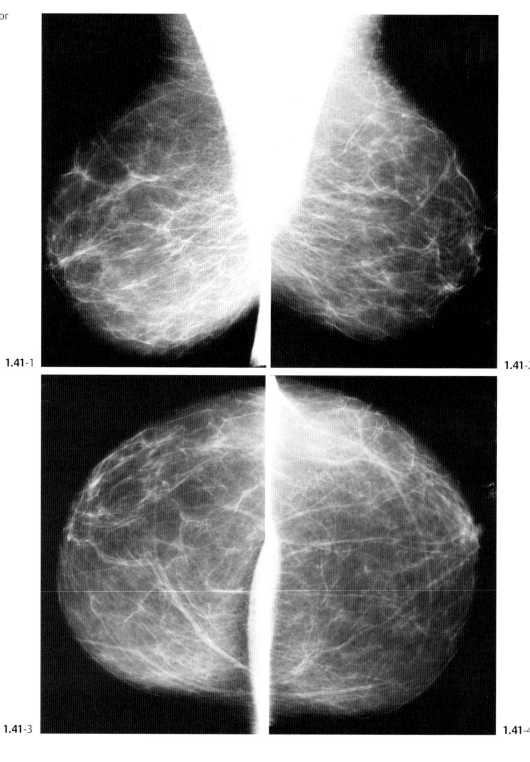

1.41-1

1.41-2

1.41-3

1.41-4

Fig. **1.42**-1 to 4 Images
following one year of HRT.

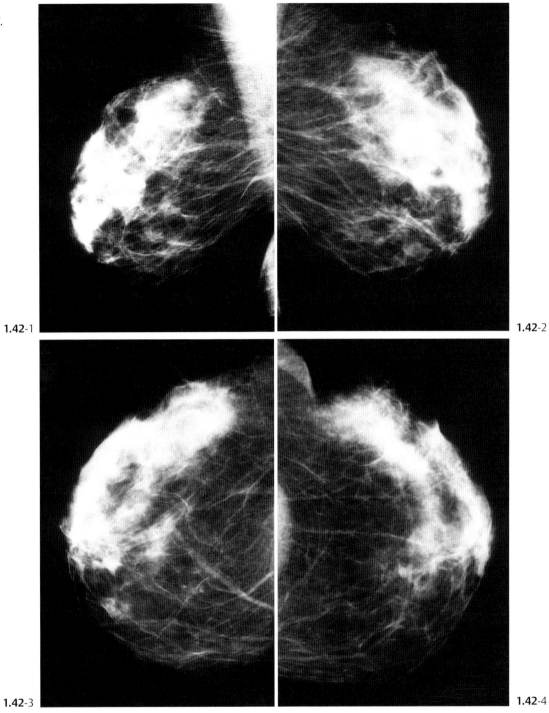

1.42-1

1.42-2

1.42-3

1.42-4

Pathological Lesions in Pattern I Type Breasts

■ How Do the Pathological Lesions Change the Mammographic Image of Pattern I Type Breasts and How Can We Perceive Them?

Attention should be focused on the radiolucent areas of the mammogram in order to better appreciate the radiopaque abnormalities that will grow at the expense of the adipose tissue.

All mass lesions developing in the breast, whether benign or malignant, will displace the normal parenchyma and fat. The contour of the normal tissue is concave, while the pathological lesion(s) represent an excess amount of tissue or accumulation of fluid. Consequently, the abnormalities will have **convex contours** (cysts, fibroadenoma, medullary cancer, etc.) or will cause **architectural distortion**.

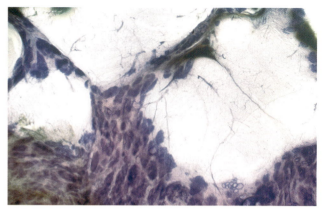

1.43

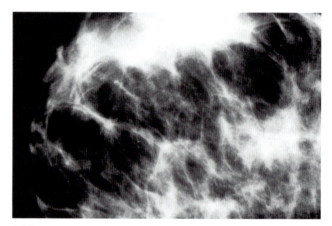

1.44

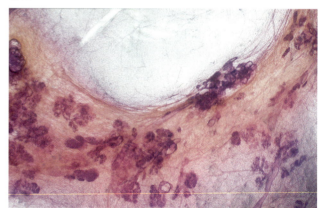

1.45

Figs. **1.43–1.46** Mammogram (Fig. **1.44**) and subgross histology images (Figs. **1.43**, **1.45**, **1.46**), demonstrating the normal concave contours of the fibroglandular tissue outlined by adipose tissue.

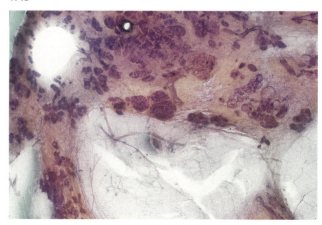

1.46

■ Lesions with Convex Radiopaque Contours

The TDLU will be distended by pathological processes early on. The ability to visualize a developing mass lesion on the mammogram will depend on whether or not it is surrounded by fibrous tissue or fat.

To be detectable on the mammogram, the abnormal lesions must:

● have convex radiopaque contours (cysts, fibroadenoma, medullary cancer, etc.), or
● cause architectural distortion (spiculated tumors, radial scar, surgical scars), or
● produce calcifications.

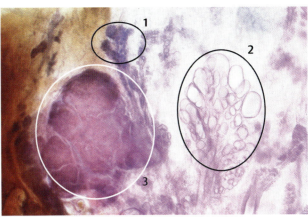

1.47

Fig. **1.47** Subgross, thick-section histology showing normal TDLUs (1) next to a cystically dilated TDLU (2) with a convex contour and carcinoma in situ distending a TDLU (3), also having a convex contour.

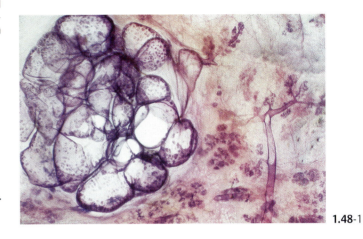

1.48-1

Fig. **1.48**-1 Thick-section histology of a cystically dilated TDLU. The contour is convex.

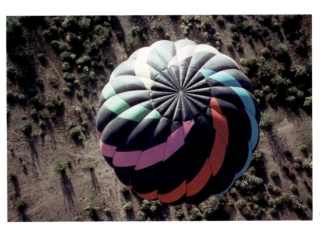

1.48-2

Fig. **1.49** Breast ultrasound image of a simple cyst.

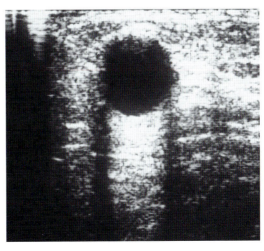

1.49

71

Lesions with Convex Radiopaque Contours

The accumulation of fluid distends and distorts both the TDLUs and the associated ducts and their branches. This distension results in spherical/ovoid balloon-like structures—fluid-filled cysts—easily visible on breast ultrasound and operative specimen radiographs and often seen on the mammograms. Figures **1.50–1.54** demonstrate cystically dilated TDLUs and distended ducts.

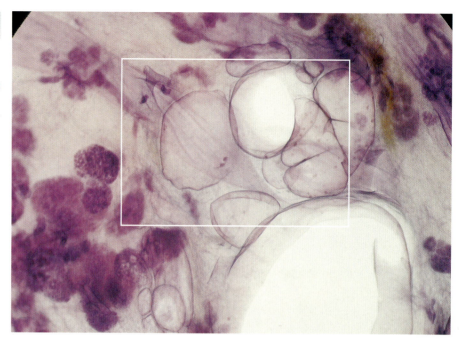

1.50

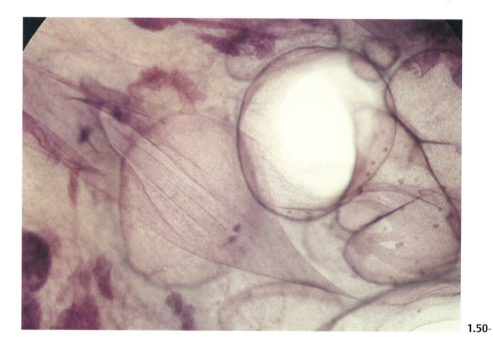

Fig. **1.50**-2 Detail from **1.50**-1.

1.50-

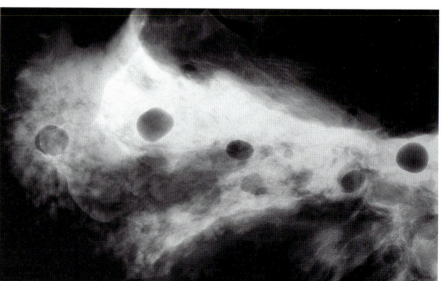

Fig. **1.50**-3 Radiograph of a sliced specimen containing several small cysts.

1.50-

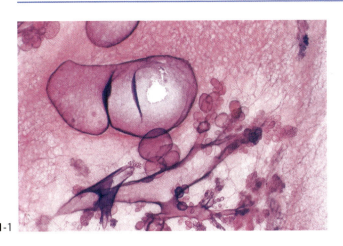

1.51-1

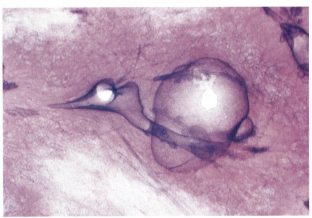

1.51-2

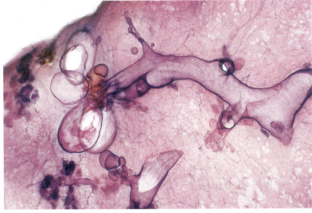

1.51-3

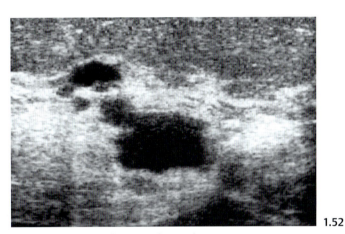

1.52

Fig. **1.51**-1 to 3   Subgross, thick-section histology images of cystically dilated TDLUs and distended ducts.

Fig. **1.52**   Ultrasound image of several cysts.

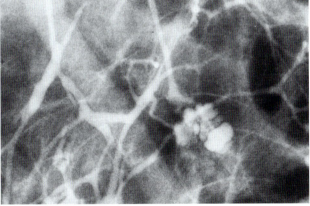

1.53

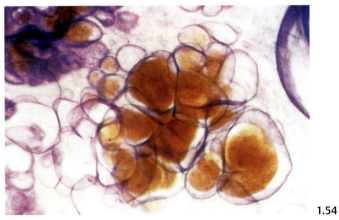

1.54

Fig. **1.53**   Galactogram showing focal cystic change with dilated ducts.

Fig.**1.54**   Subgross histological image of focal cystic change showing uneven cystic dilatation of the acini within a TDLU.

Lesions with Convex Radiopaque Contours

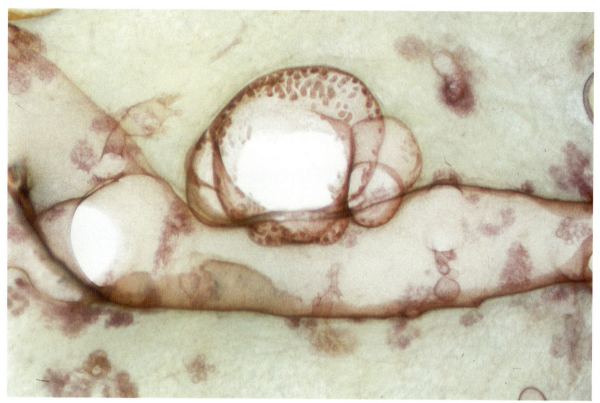

1.55

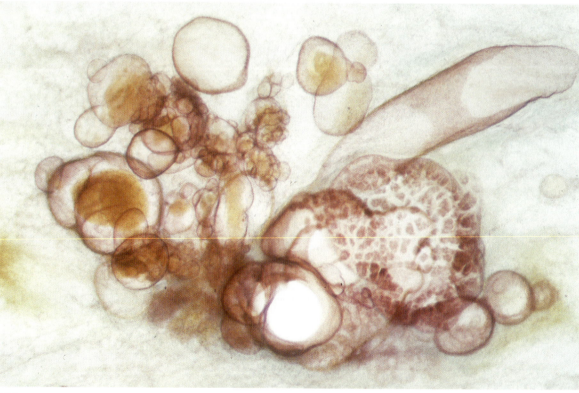

1.56

Figs. **1.55–1.62** Additional subgross, thick-section histology images showing the wide variations of changes caused by increased fluid production and accumulation in the breast glandular tissue. These images graphically demonstrate the underlying pathophysiology of fibrocystic change, helping to explain the clinical symptoms as well as the imaging findings.

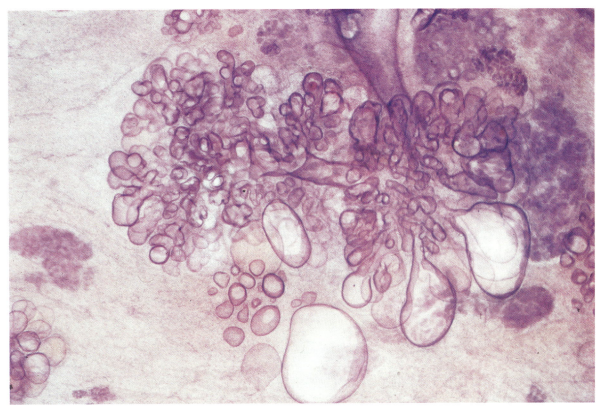

1.57

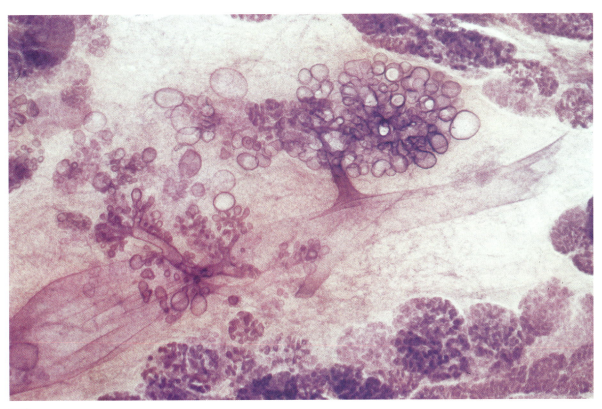

1.58

Lesions with Convex Radiopaque Contours

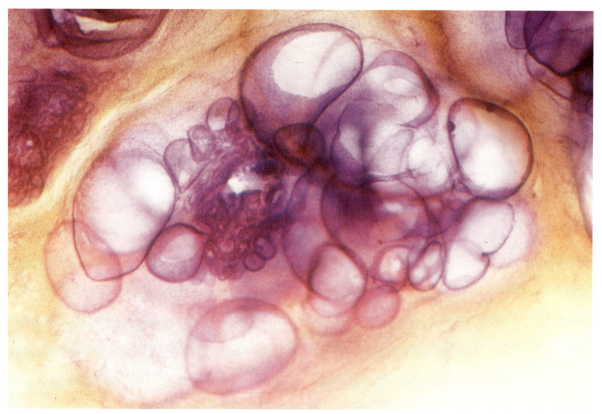

1.59

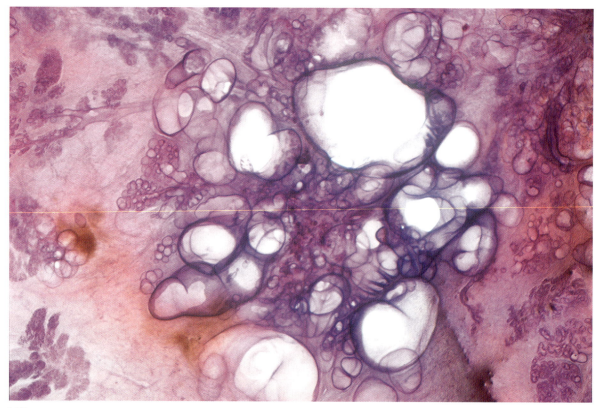

1.60

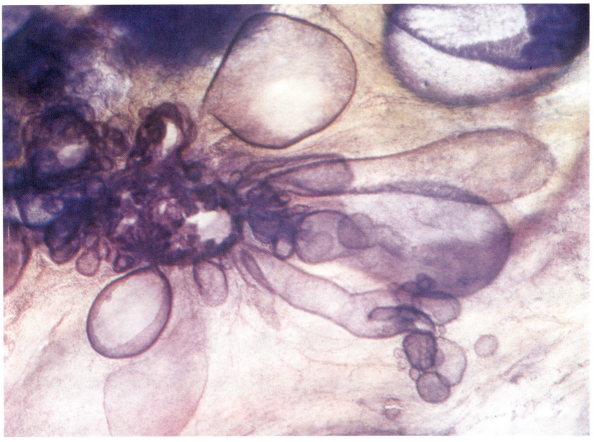

1.61

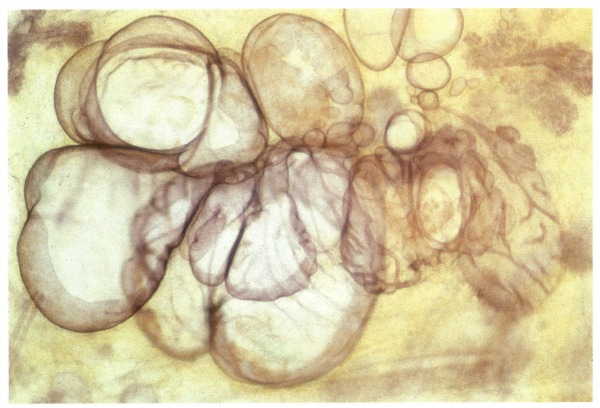

1.62

Example 1.3

A 45-year-old woman with a palpable lump in the right breast.

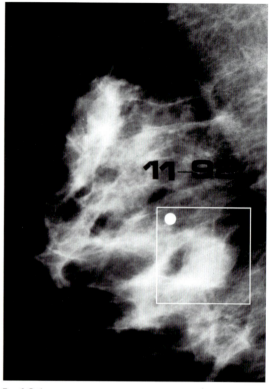

Ex. **1.3**-1   Pattern I mammogram with concave contours of the glandular tissue. The palpable abnormality with its convex contour stands out in contrast.

Ex. **1.3**-1

Ex. **1.3**-2   The palpable lesion is hidden by the dense parenchyma in the craniocaudal projection.

Ex. **1.3**-3   Breast ultrasound reveals a lobulated, solid tumor.

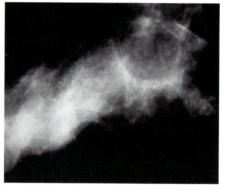

Ex. **1.3**-2

Ex. **1.3**-3

Ex. **1.3**-4   Thick-section histology image of the medullary carcinoma surrounded by tumor vessels and normal TDLUs.

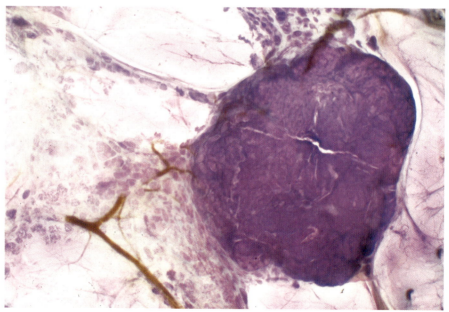

Ex. **1.3**-4

Lesions with Convex Radiopaque Contours

Example 1.4

32-year-old woman with a palpable lump in the upper inner quadrant of the right breast.

Ex. **1.4**-1   Mammogram, Pattern I. The concave contour of the normal parenchyma is outlined by fat. The convex contour of the abnormal lesion (fibroadenoma) facilitates its perception.

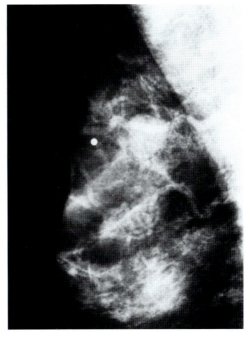

Ex.**1.4**-1

Ex. **1.4**-2   The convex contour of the radiopaque abnormality is in stark contrast with the concave contour of the normal parenchyma, which is outlined by radiolucent adipose tissue.

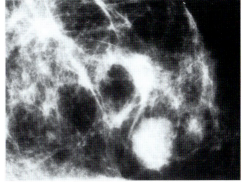

Ex.**1.4**-2

Ex. **1.4**-3   Breast ultrasound of the abnormality in Ex. **1.4**-1 and Ex. **1.4**-2.

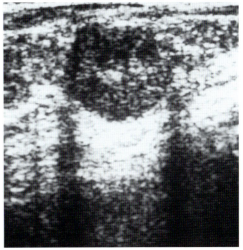

Ex.**1.4**-3

Ex. **1.4**-4   Large-section histology: benign fibroadenoma.

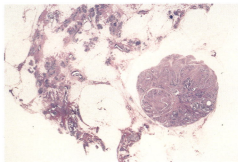

Ex.**1.4**-4

■ Lesions with Architectural Distortion

In addition to contour changes caused by pathological lesions, the harmonious image of Pattern I may also be disturbed by architectural distortion due to radiating structures, characteristically by **invasive malignant tumors**, occasionally by **radial scars**.

Example 1.5

Left-sided mastectomy for breast cancer.

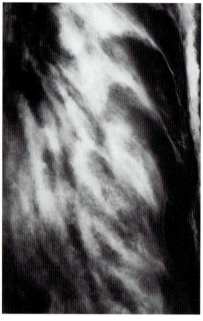

Ex. **1.5**-1

Ex. **1.5**-1   Radiograph of a mastectomy specimen slice: a regular, harmonious pattern is seen with Cooper's ligaments and prominent ducts outlined by adipose tissue. There is no pathological finding in this slice.

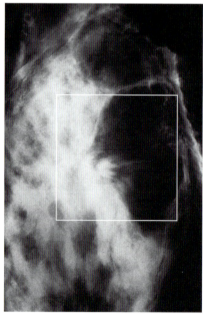

Ex. **1.5**-2

Ex. **1.5**-2   Radiograph of the adjacent specimen slice shows invasive ductal carcinoma causing architectural distortion (rectangle).

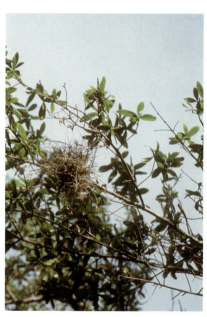

Ex. **1.5**-3

Lesions with Architectural Distortion

Example 1.6

Asymptomatic woman, screening examination. Called back for further examination because of mammographically detected architectural distortion in the central portion of the left breast.

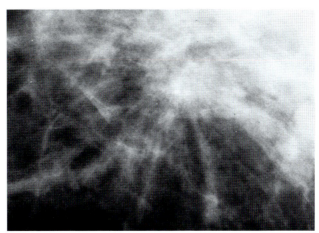

Ex. **1.6**-1

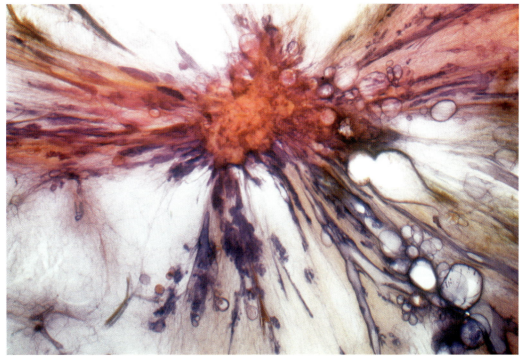

Ex. **1.6**-2

Ex. **1.6**-1 & 2   In this case the architectural distortion demonstrated on the microfocus magnification radiograph was caused by a radial scar. The subgross, thick-section histology reveals that the radiating structure corresponds to proliferating ducts. These ducts are arranged in a radiating fashion and are associated with a small central, fibroelastic core. An alternate term, sclerosing duct proliferation, expresses the underlying disease process more accurately.

■ The Evolution of a Tiny Spiculated Tumor

Example 1.7

A 50-year-old asymptomatic woman, first screening examination.

This case emphasizes the importance of perceiving subtle parenchymal contour changes in a Pattern I type breast. The subtle change is graphically demonstrated on the facing page.

Ex. **1.7**-1 & 2   Right and left axillary tails. Small densities with concave contours are seen bilaterally.

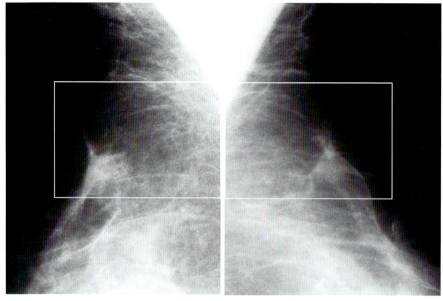

Ex. **1.7**-1   Ex. **1.7**-2

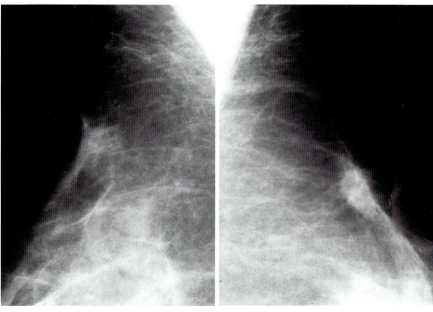

Ex. **1.7**-3 & 4   Second screening examination. A subtle change has developed since the first examination (see facing page for explanation).

Ex. **1.7**-3   Ex. **1.7**-4

Ex. **1.7**-5 & 6   The remaining fibro-glandular tissue has concave contours corresponding to normal breast parenchyma.

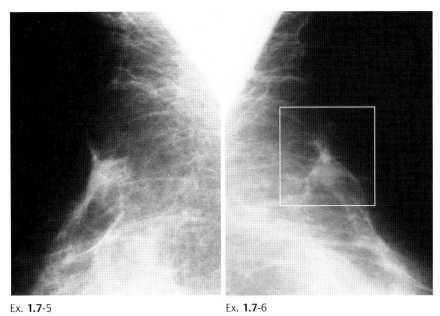

Ex. **1.7**-5

Ex. **1.7**-6

Ex. **1.7**-7 & 8   At the second screening examination the density in the right breast retains its concave borders, while the density in the left breast has now developed convex borders.

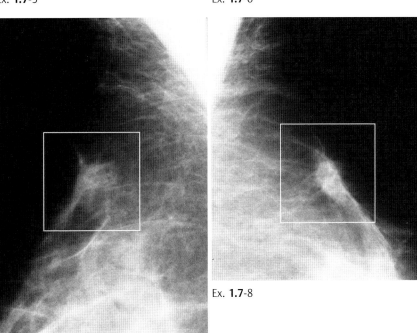

Ex. **1.7**-8

Ex. **1.7**-7

Ex. **1.7**-9 & 10 Spot compression microfocus magnification images in the CC and MLO projections show a 10 mm × 11 mm spiculated, mammographically malignant tumor.

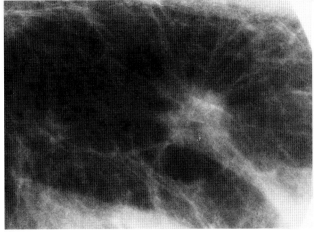

Ex. **1.7**-9

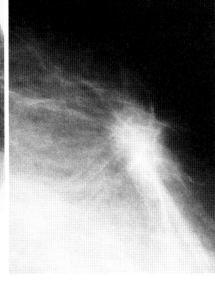

Histology: invasive ductal carcinoma.

Ex. **1.7**-10

■ Calcifications in a Pattern I Type Breast

Pathological lesions containing calcifications can be detected against the parenchymal background and are not as great a perception problem as noncalcified mass lesions or architectural distortion.

Example 1.8

A 49-year-old asymptomatic woman, screening examination.

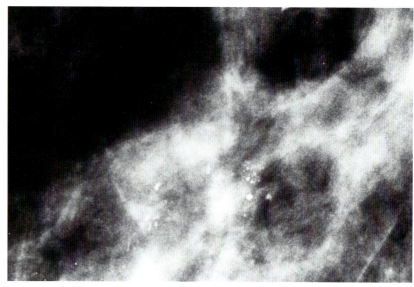

Ex. **1.8**-1

Ex. **1.8**-1 & 2   Both powdery (indistinct) and crushed stone–like (granular) calcifications are seen. There is no associated tumor mass.

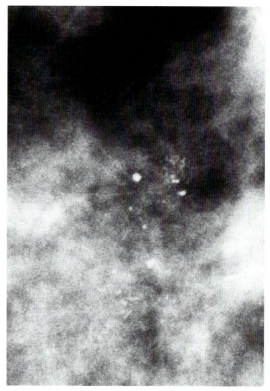

Ex. **1.8**-2

Ex. **1.8**-3 Specimen radiograph, microfocus magnification. Both the coarse, crushed stone-like and the indistinct calcifications can be distinguished through the dense, Pattern I type fibroglandular tissue.

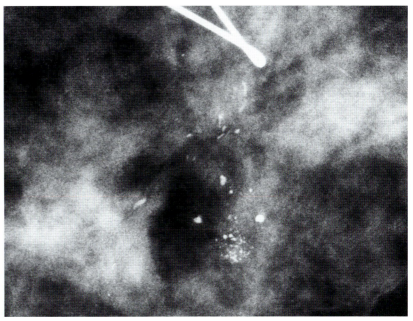

Ex. **1.8**-3

Ex. **1.8**-4 Corresponding to the coarser calcifications, histology shows necrosis (1) and coarse amorphous calcifications (2) surrounded by a thin layer containing a few viable cancer cells (3).

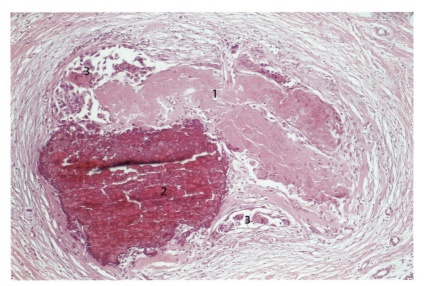

Ex. **1.8**-4

Ex. **1.8**-5 Corresponding to the powdery calcifications, histology shows tiny psammoma body–like calcifications in benign structures (normal and dilated acini).

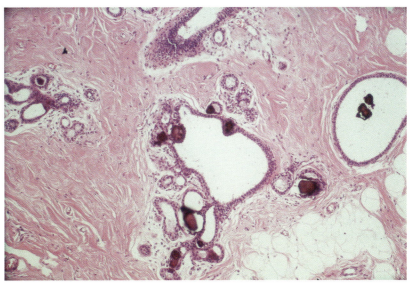

Ex. **1.8**-5

■ Mammographically Occult Lesions in Pattern I

Abnormal lesions that
- are not associated with calcifications or
- do not cause architectural distortion and
- do not protrude into the adipose tissue

are mammographically occult. In these cases the pathological lesions will not be detected unless they are palpable, or unless they are detected incidentally by adjunctive imaging methods such as breast ultrasound.

Example 1.9

A 33-year-old woman who completed nursing six months earlier and has now felt a lump in the lower half of her right breast, close to the chest wall.

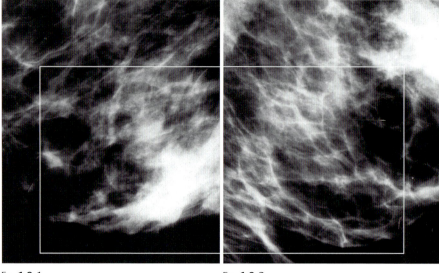

Ex. **1.9**-1 Ex. **1.9**-2

Ex. **1.9**-1 & 2   Details, right and left mediolateral oblique projections. Pattern I. A nonspecific asymmetric density with concave contours is seen along the lower border of the right breast corresponding to the palpable tumor. No architectural distortion or calcifications are present.

Ex. **1.9**-3 & 4   No distinct tumor mass is seen on the right or left craniocaudal projections. The palpable tumor is marked with a lead pellet (rectangle).

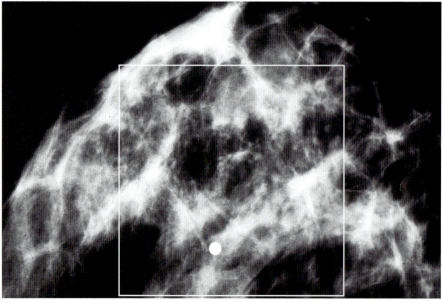

Ex. 1.

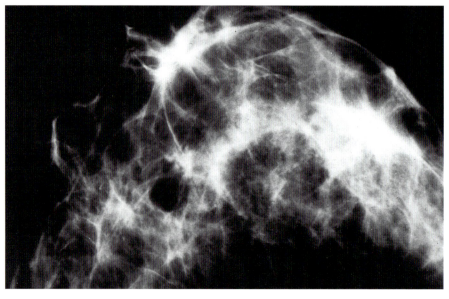

Ex. 1.

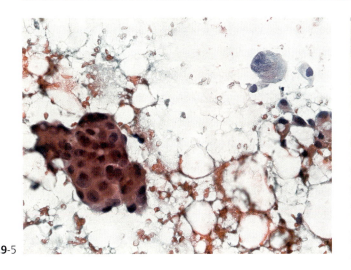

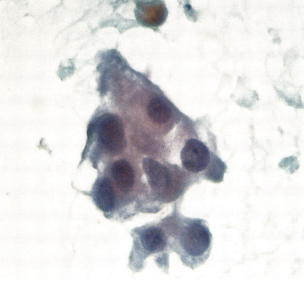

Ex. **1.9**-5 & 6   Fine-needle aspiration biopsy shows papillary cell groups with obvious cellular atypia.

Ex. **1.9**-6

Ex. **1.9**-7   14-gauge large-core needle biopsy demonstrates micropapillary carcinoma in situ.

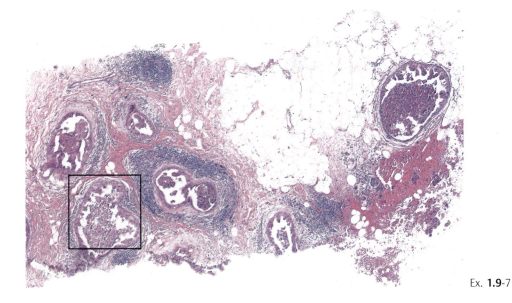

Ex. **1.9**-7

Ex. **1.9**-8   High-power image from Ex. **1.9**-7 (rectangle). Histological diagnosis: high-grade micropapillary carcinoma in situ with necrosis, but without microcalcifications.

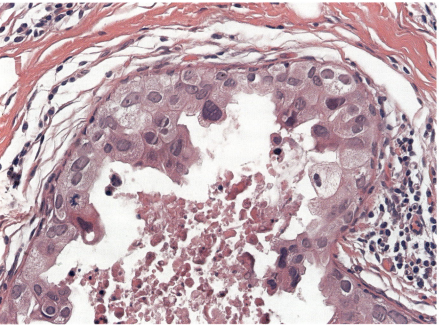

Ex. **1.9**-8

Ex. **1.9**-9   Specimen radiograph of the intact surgical specimen. There is no dominant mass nor any calcification.

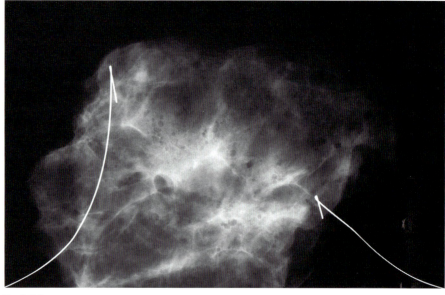

Ex. **1.9**-9

Ex. **1.9**-10   Large-section histology showing part of a 7.0 cm high-grade micropapillary ductal carcinoma in situ (DCIS).

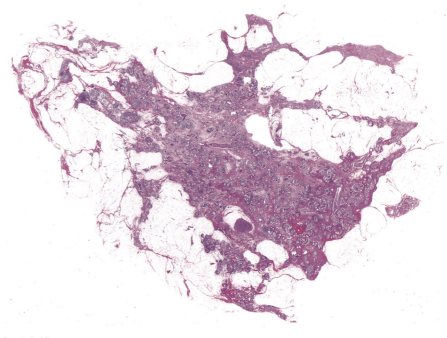

Ex. **1.9**-10

Ex. **1.9**-11 to 13   Histology of the excised tumor shows high-grade DCIS extending from the chest wall to the nipple. There was no evidence of invasion. Ex. **1.9**-11 and **1.9**-12 are subgross, thick-section histology images.

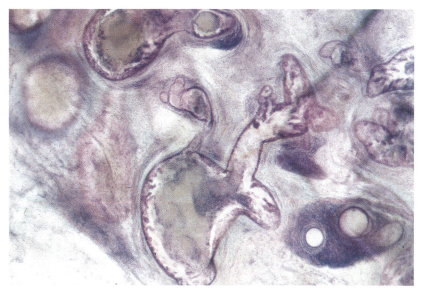

Ex. **1.9**-11

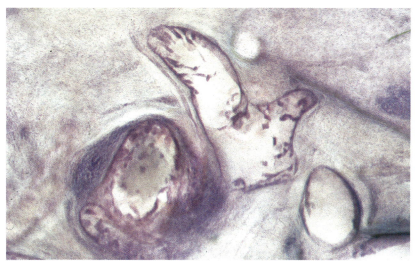

Ex. **1.9**-12

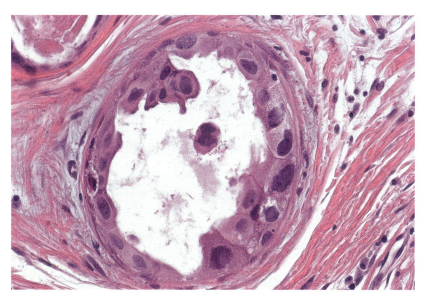

Ex. **1.9**-13

**Mammographically Occult Lesions in
Pattern I—Example 1.9**

Ex. **1.9**-14 & 15   The mastectomy
specimen still contains residual tumor
(larger rectangle). The region within
the smaller rectangle in **1.9**-14 is
magnified in **1.9**-15.

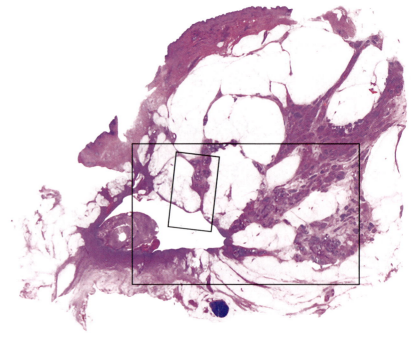

Ex. **1**

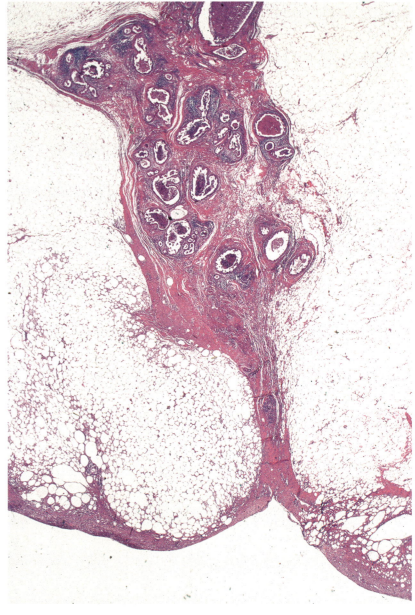

Ex. **1**

Ex. **1.9**-16 to 19   Subgross, thick-section histology images from the palpable tumor showing high-grade intraductal carcinoma (**1.9**-17 and **1.9**-18). This pathological process remained mammographically occult since it did not form a convex contour with the adipose tissue, nor did it calcify. Tumor detection was initiated through palpation. Note that the contours of the tissue containing cancer are concave, similar to the normal fibroglandular tissue in **1.9**-16 and **1.9**-19.

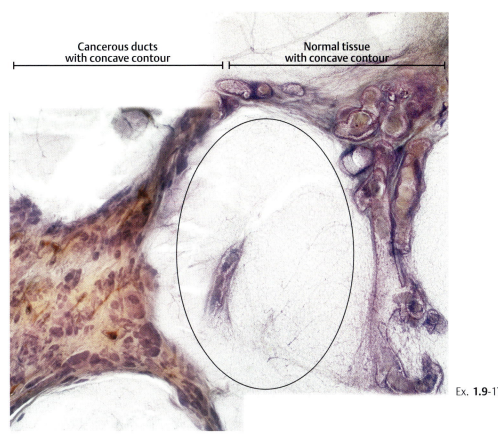

Ex. **1.9**-17

Ex. **1.9**-16

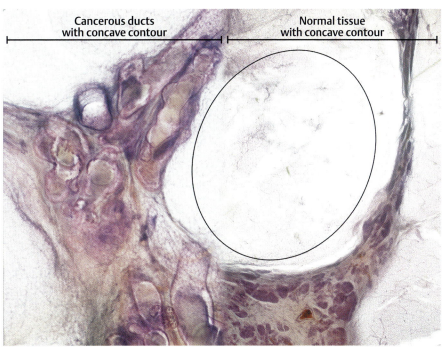

Ex. **1.9**-18

Ex. **1.9**-19

Follow up: The patient is alive and well 10 years after treatment.

Chapter 2: Pattern II

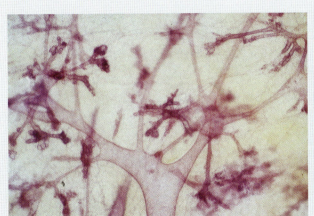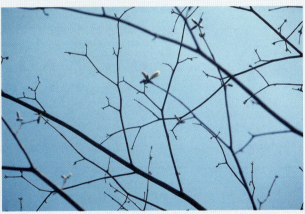

Characteristics of Pattern II

The mammographic image of Pattern II is characterized by the overrepresentation of *radiolucent adipose tissue*, one of the four structural components.

The radiolucent fatty tissue provides an excellent background for the visualization of any disease process. **Linear densities** are the second most dominant feature in Pattern II. These consist of:

1 Ducts (pages 95–108)
2 Fibrous strands (pages 109–111)
3 Blood vessels (pages 112, 113)

Although not seen on the mammogram, there are also dormant, persistent lobules (see page 95).

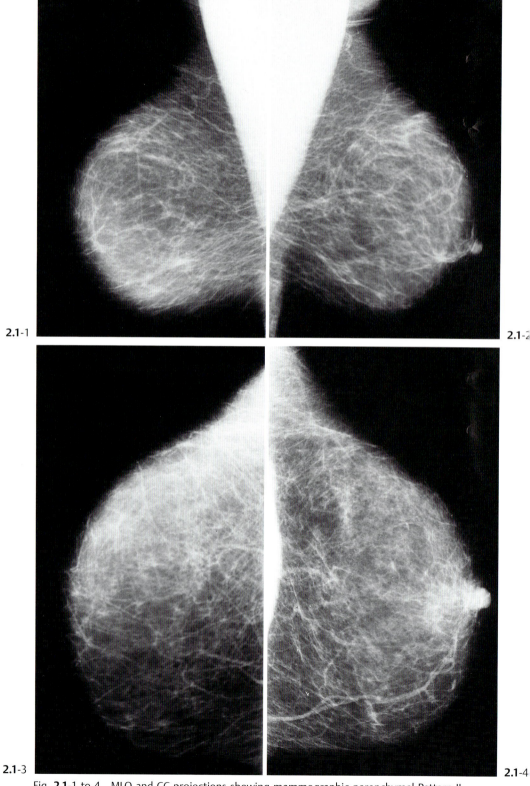

2.1-1

2.1-2

2.1-3

2.1-4

Fig. **2.1**-1 to 4   MLO and CC projections showing mammographic parenchymal Pattern II.

Linear Densities in Pattern II

■ Ducts

Atrophic Ducts and Their Branches

The **atrophic ducts** and their branches account for most of the fine, linear densities that make up the harmonious network seen on the mammogram.

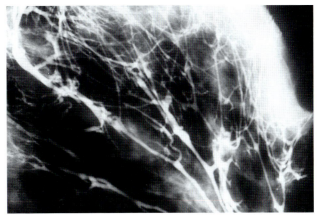

2.2

Fig. **2.2** Galactography can demonstrate that many of the fine linear densities are actually ducts in the resting state.

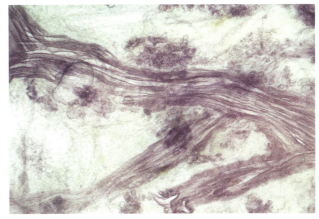

2.3

Fig. **2.3** Thick-section histology image of the atrophic ducts, which are pleated when not distended.

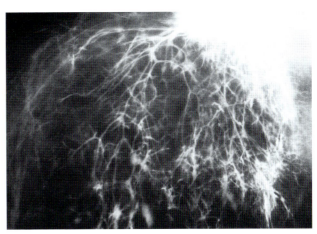

2.4-1

Fig. **2.4**-1 & 2 Galactography and thick-section histology image of atrophic ducts and dormant TDLUs.

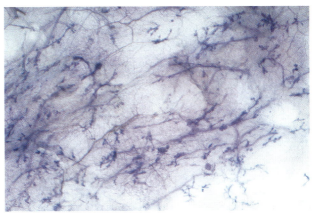

2.4-2

Ducts—Atrophic Ducts and Their Branches

Fig. **2.5** When discharge is present and galactography is performed, we can demonstrate which linear densities correspond to atrophic ducts, distinguishing them from the nearby fibrous strands.

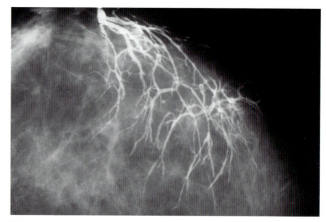

2.5

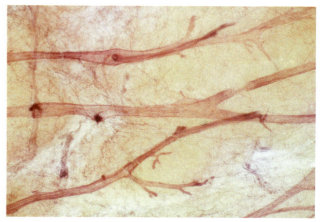

Fig. **2.6** Thick-section histology image of atrophic ducts and their branches.

2.6

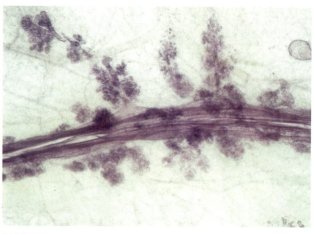

Fig. **2.7**-1 & 2 Subgross histology can demonstrate persistent lobules adjacent to pleated ducts. These lobules are often mammographically occult.

2.7-1

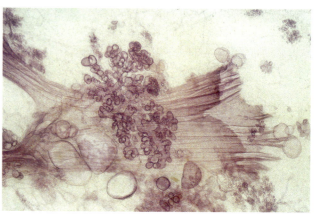

2.7-2

Persistent Lobules in Pattern II

During the process of involution, when Pattern I is transformed to Patterns II and III, the number and size of terminal ductal lobular units (TDLUs) decrease considerably. The nodular densities on the mammogram decrease correspondingly. Although no longer demonstrable mammographically, many TDLUs still exist as **persistent lobules**. They are demonstrable both on conventional and on thick-section histological examination. The persistent, atrophic lobules may be fairly evenly distributed, or may remain as tiny islands of parenchyma squeezed among large balls of fat.

Fig. **2.8**-1 Thick-section histology image of a Pattern II breast with persistent lobules. These are the sites in which pathological lesions may arise.

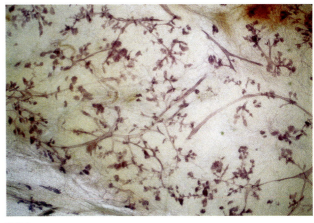

2.8-1

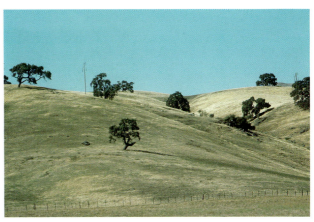

2.8-2

Fig. **2.9**-1 Thick-section histology image of a persistent lobule. (Image courtesy of Dr. Sefton R. Wellings, Davis, CA, USA)

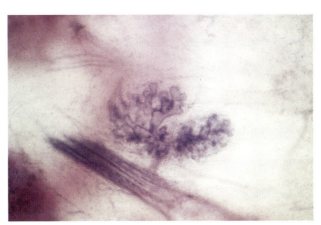

2.9-1

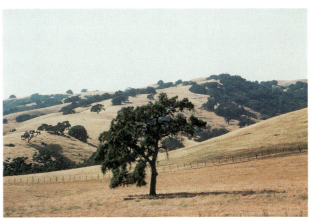

2.9-2

Normal Ducts

The **normal ducts** in a nonlactating breast are linearly pleated.

Fig. **2.10**-1   Thick-section histology of a branching milk duct in longitudinal section. The pleated structure enables the duct to greatly expand its diameter and store large volumes of fluid. The pleats of the saguaro cactus have a similar role in fluid storage.

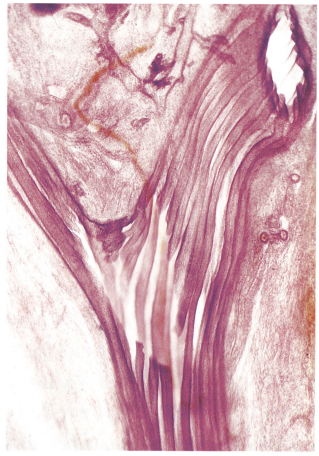

2.10-

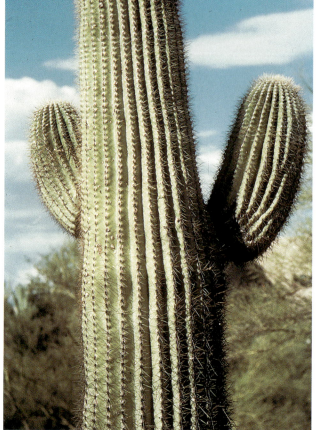

2.10-

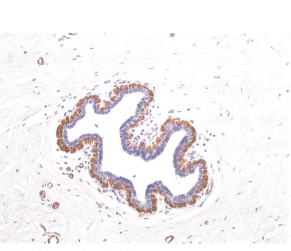

2.11

Fig. **2.11**   Cross section of a duct.

Ducts

Ductectasia

Ductectasia, dilatation of the duct, may be caused by:
- Increased fluid production by the TDLUs
- Fluid associated with papillomas
- High nuclear grade cancer in situ, when cancer cells and associated debris, including calcium or mucous material secreted by the cancer cells, fill the lumen

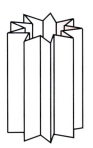
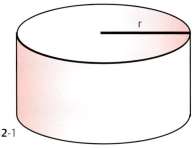

Fig. **2.12**-1 & 2 Diagrammatic illustration of the considerable expansion (increase in effective radius) of the milk duct. The volume v of a cylinder of length l is proportional to the square of its radius r: $v = l \times \pi r^2$.

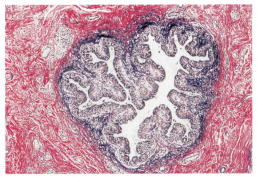
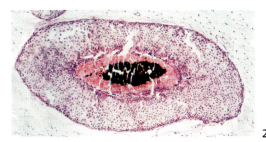

Fig. **2.13**-1 & 2 Cross section of a normal pleated duct compared with a duct distended by carcinoma in situ with necrosis and calcification.

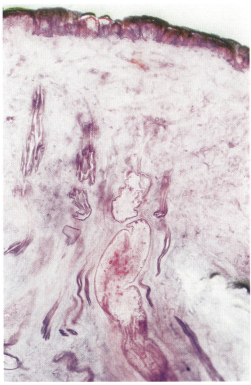
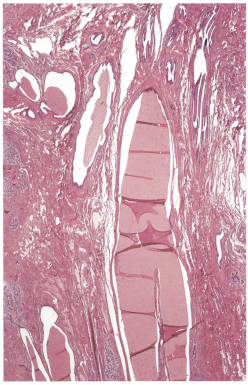

Fig. **2.14** One duct distended by DCIS, surrounded by normal pleated ducts. (Case courtesy of Dr. Melissa Trekell, Knoxville, TN, USA)

Fig. **2.15** Histology image of a duct distended by inspissated fluid, surrounded by normal pleated ducts.

Ductectasia Caused by Fluid

The most frequent and physiological cause of ductal distention is **lactation**, when the lobules and ducts become greatly dilated.

Fig. **2.16**-1   Lactating breast.

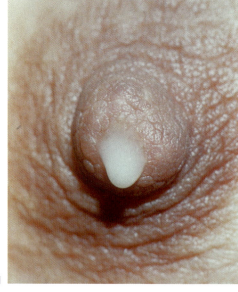

2.16-1

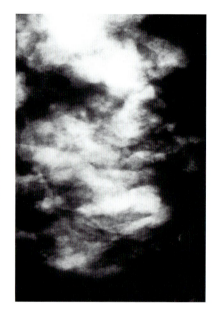

2.16-

Fig. **2.16**-2 & 3   Mammograms taken during lactation of this 31-year-old woman demonstrate the greatly dilated ducts and lobules.

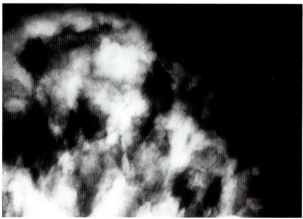

2.16-3

Fig. **2.17**   Histological picture of a lactating TDLU.

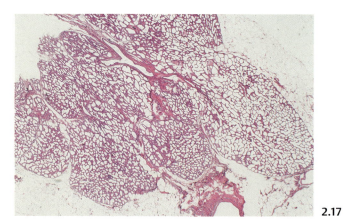

2.17

Fig. **2.18**   Subgross, thick-section histological image of fluid-filled ducts.

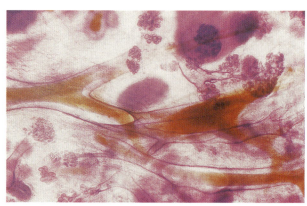

2.18

The lobules produce fluid throughout the fertile age, even in the absence of lactation. This proteinaceous, turbid fluid contains cellular debris. Fluid production peaks during the secretory phase of the menstrual cycle, contributing to premenstrual pain. This fluid is resorbed by the ductal system and rarely causes nipple discharge. Fluid resorption may not be complete, and debris may accumulate within the ducts, causing dilatation.

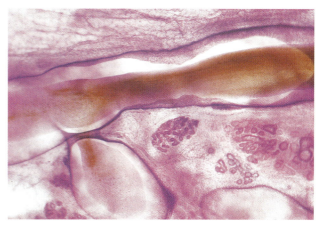

2.19

Fig. **2.19** Galactogram of a dilated duct.

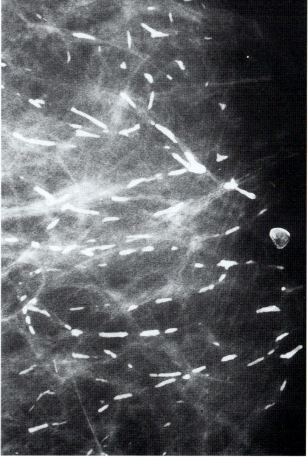

2.20

Fig. **2.20** Subgross, thick-section histological image of dilated ducts containing secretions.

Furthermore, there may be a build-up of calcifications within this alkaline environment. These calcifications fill in the dilated ducts, resulting in the characteristic mammographic image of "secretory disease" type, "plasma cell mastitis" type linear and branching calcifications.

Fig. **2.21** "Secretory disease" type, "plasma cell mastitis" type calcifications on a mammogram.

2.21

Ducts—Ductectasia

Fig. **2.22**-1 to 3   Subgross, thick-section histology images of fluid-filled ducts.

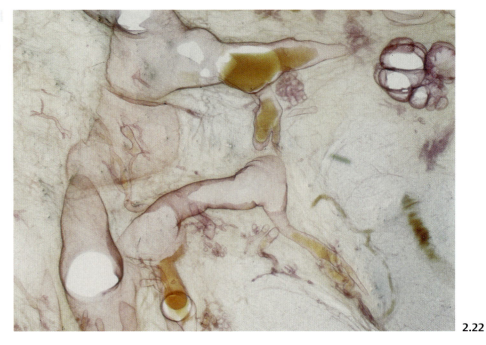

2.22

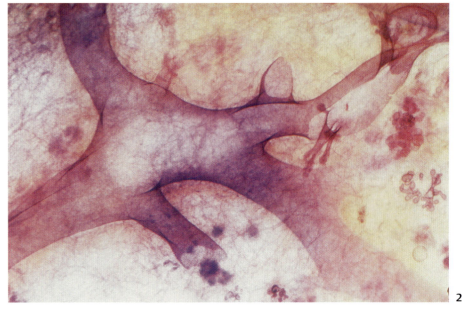

2.22

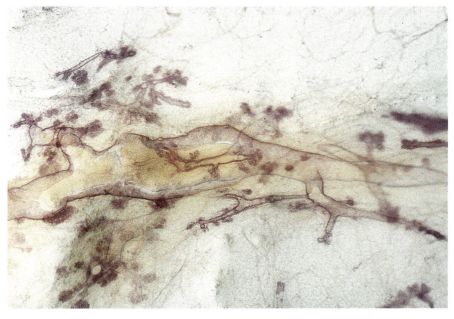

2.22

Fig. **2.23**-1 & 2 Microfocus magnification mammogram and subgross, thick-section histology of a portion of the left breast with postoperative scarring. The calcifications are caused by residual blood within dilated ducts and TDLUs, forming a cast of these cavities. The operation occurred 15 years earlier.

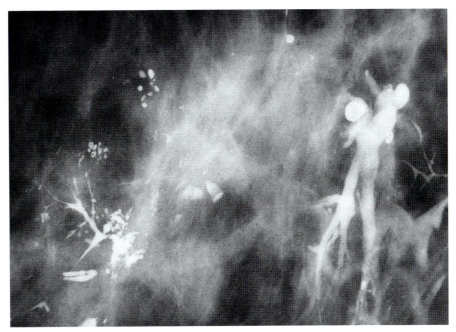

2.23-1

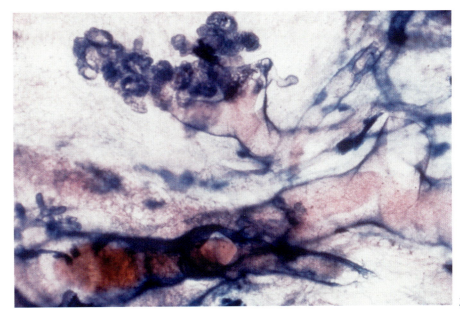

2.23-2

Ducts—Ductectasia

Ductectasia Caused by Solitary or Multiple Intraductal Papillomas

The duct and its branches become dilated with the excess fluid, often resulting in serous or bloody nipple discharge.

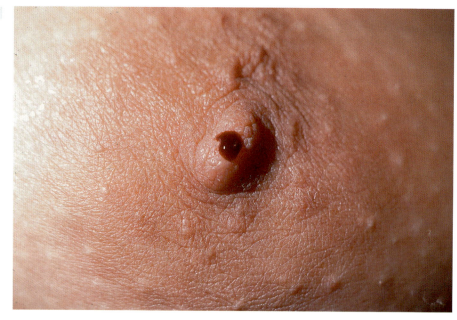

Fig. **2.24**-1   Bloody nipple discharge.

2.24

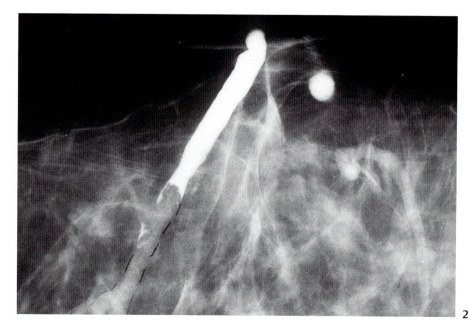

Fig. **2.24**-2   Galactography: the contrast media fills the dilated duct and outlines a filling defect.

2.24-

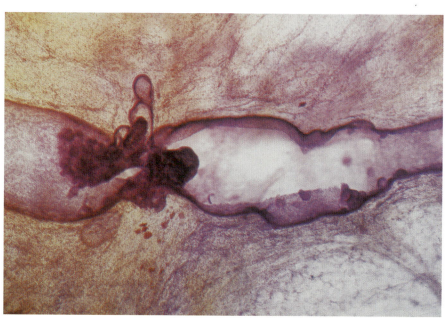

Fig. **2.24**-3   Thick-section histology shows multiple intraductal papillomas.

2.24-

Fig. **2.25**-1   Serous nipple discharge.

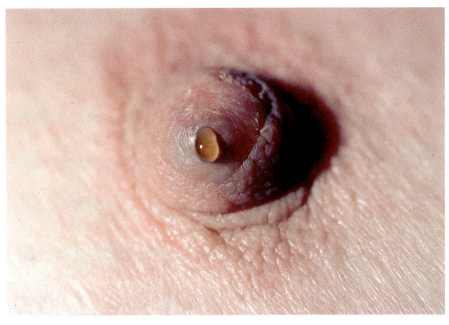

2.25-1

Fig. **2.25**-2   A solitary filling defect is seen on the galactogram.

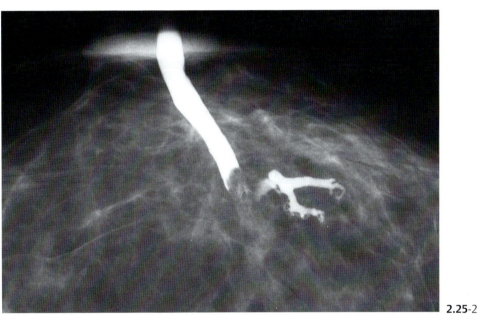

2.25-2

Fig. **2.25**-3   Corresponding thick-section histology shows an intraductal papilloma within the dilated duct.

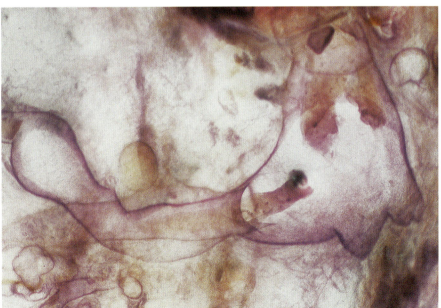

2.25-3

Duct Distention Caused by High Nuclear Grade DCIS with Micropapillary Cell Proliferation

High nuclear grade carcinoma in situ is the most frequent cause of extreme duct distention by a malignant process. This may affect most of the ductal tree within a single lobe. The presence of an unusually large number of ducts concentrated within a small area without associated TDLUs suggests that some of these ducts may actually be produced by neoductogenesis.

In high nuclear grade cancer in situ cases with predominantly **solid cell proliferation**, the duct lumen contains multiple layers of cancer cells. The innermost layer of the cells eventually becomes necrotic. The central portion of the lumen thus contains necrotic debris interspersed with amorphous calcifications. These fragmented calcifications appear on the mammogram as branching, fragmented casts of the ductal lumen, termed **casting-type calcifications**. This appearance is one of the most typical and reliable mammographic signs of malignancy, having a positive predictive value of 96%.

Fig. **2.26**-1 to 3   Mammographic and histological images of ducts distended by solid cell proliferation in high nuclear grade DCIS. The mammogram shows the casting-type calcifications associated with this malignant process.

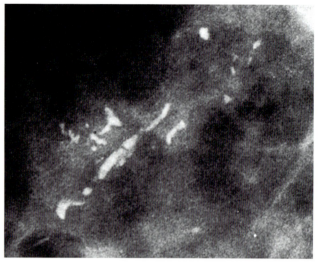

2.26-1

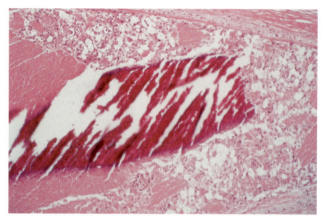

2.26-2

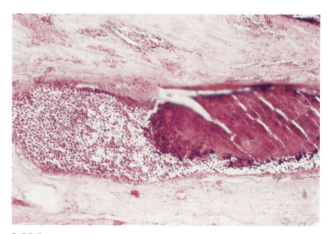

2.26-3

Ducts—Ductectasia

Duct Distention Caused by High Nuclear Grade DCIS with Micropapillary Cell Proliferation

When high nuclear grade cancer cells have **micropapillary architecture**, the duct lumen may be distended by necrosis, calcifications, and the mucin that the cancer cells secrete. The micropapillary protrusions may break off, undergo necrosis, and then calcify within the lumen. These calcifications form another typical pattern of casting-type calcifications, the so-called **dotted castings**. The lumen is filled with innumerable tiny, closely spaced calcified particles, giving the cast a dotted appearance. In most cases both the fragmented and dotted type calcifications will be seen, although usually one type will dominate the mammographic image.

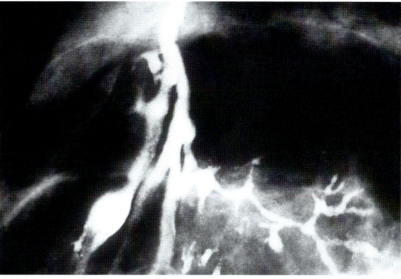

2.27-1

Fig. **2.27**-1   Mammogram (not galactogram!) showing innumerable calcium particles filling in and outlining the main duct and its branches within one lobe. (Case courtesy of Dr. Melissa Trekell, Knoxville, TN, USA)

Fig. **2.27**-2 & 3   Low-power and medium-power histological changes, H&E with von Kossa stains. Micropapillary carcinoma in situ. The calcium in the distended lumen stains black.

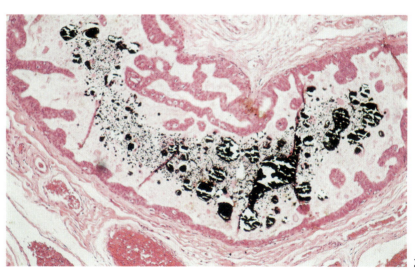

2.27-2

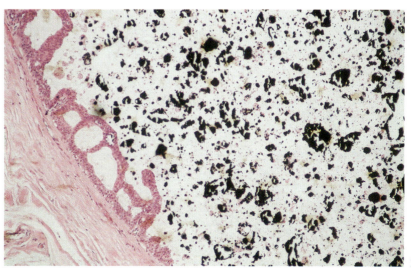

2.27-3

Ducts—Ductectasia

Duct Distention Caused By High Nuclear Grade DCIS with Micropapillary Cell Proliferation Associated with Mucin Secretion, but Lacking Calcification

High nuclear grade cancer cells with **micropapillary architecture** may secrete mucin, resulting in considerable ductectasia. In most of these cases there are no mammographically demonstrable calcifications. Although there may be serous nipple discharge, the galactogram will show dilated ducts with no filling defects. Thus, the diagnosis of extensive carcinoma in situ will often be a surprise.

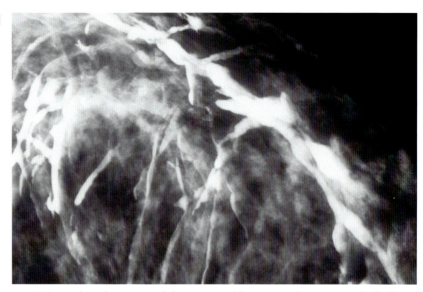

2.28

Fig. **2.28**-1   The galactogram of this 52-year-old woman with serous nipple discharge showed ductectasia without filling defects.

Fig. **2.28**-2 & 3   Subgross, thick-section and conventional histological images demonstrate micropapillary DCIS.

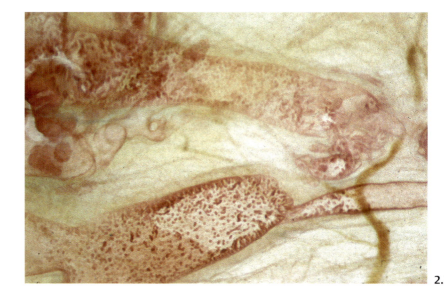

2.28

2.28

■ Fibrous Strands

Fibrous strands are composed of collagen fibers. Their mammographic appearance may be indistinguishable from that of atrophic ducts.

Fig. **2.29**-1 & 2   Details of the left mediolateral oblique projection, Pattern II. The fibrous strands form a very fine supporting framework outlined by the fat.

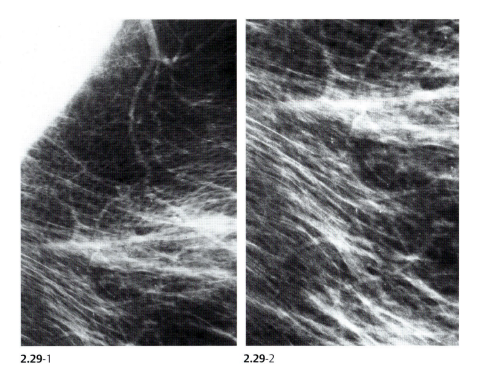

2.29-1   2.29-2

Fig. **2.30**   Histology of fibrous strands surrounded by fat cells.

Fig. **2.31**   Specimen radiographs show fine fibrous strands outlined by adipose tissue.

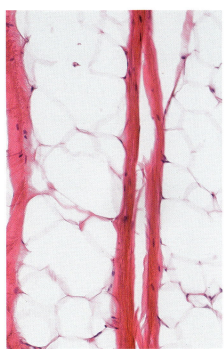

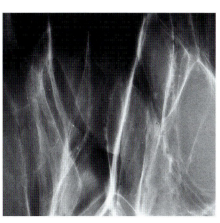

2.31

2.30

Fibrous Strands

Fig. **2.32**-1 to 3   The linear densities in the Pattern II mammogram, composed of atrophic ducts, fibrous strands and vessels, display a harmonious mammographic image.

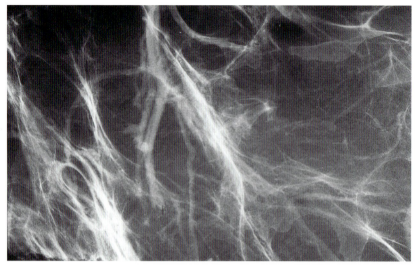

2.32-1

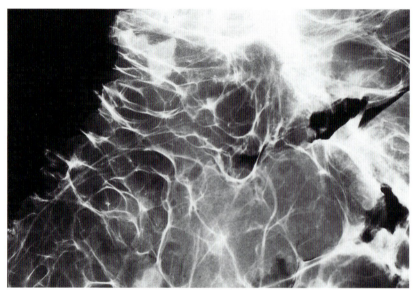

2.32-2

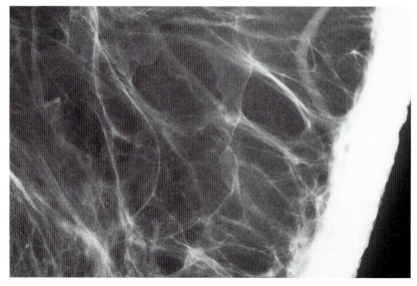

2.32-3

Fig. **2.33**-1 & 2   Mammograph in the CC projection and radiograph of the sliced specimen. The very fine linear architecture is distorted by the tiny oval-shaped, ill-defined mucinous carcinoma.

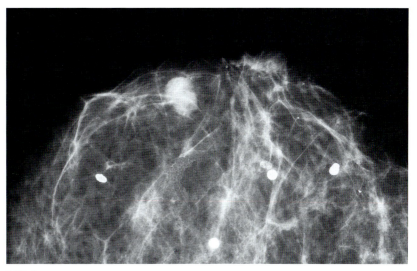

2.33-1

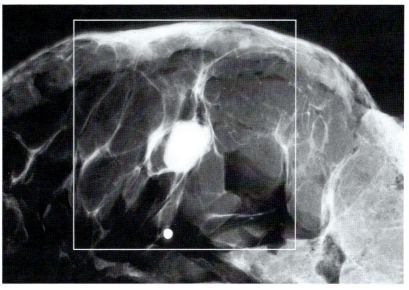

2.33-2

The harmonious image will be altered by pathological lesions, which will be seen as either circular/oval-shaped densities, stellate/spiculated lesions, or architectural distortion.

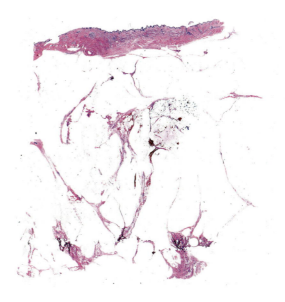

Fig. **2.33**-3   Large-section histology: colloid carcinoma.

2.33-3

■ Blood Vessels

The third type of linear density seen on the mammogram is composed of blood vessels, both veins and arteries.

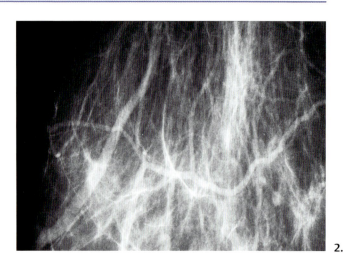

2.3

Fig. **2.34**-1 & 2 Details of Pattern II mammograms in the cranio-caudal projection. The mammograms show veins that are temporarily distended due to compression of the breast during mammography.

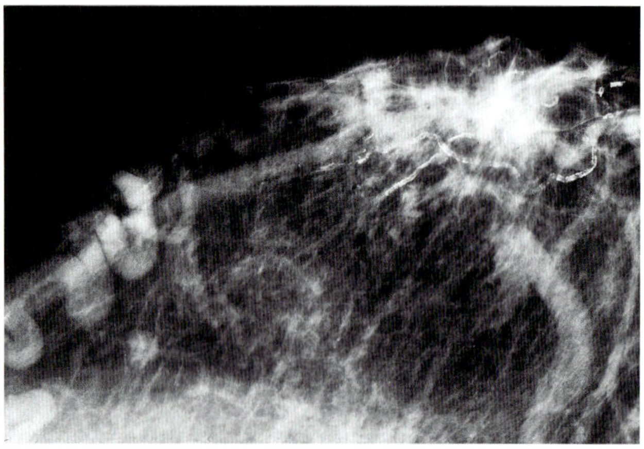

2.34

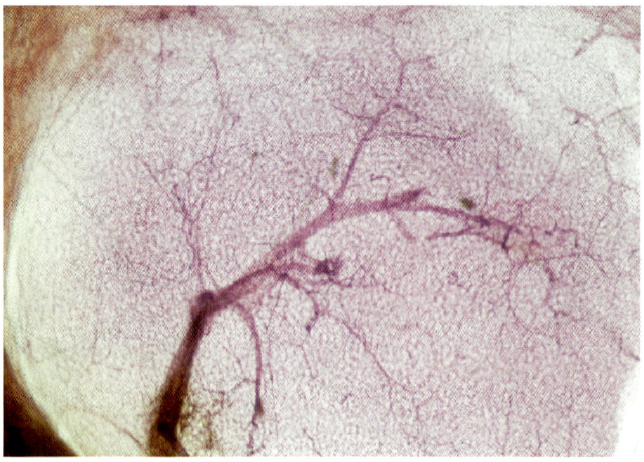

Fig. **2.35** Thick-section histology shows vessels outlined by adipose tissue.

2.35

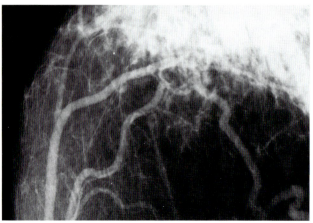

Fig. **2.36** Craniocaudal projection with prominent vessels.

2.36

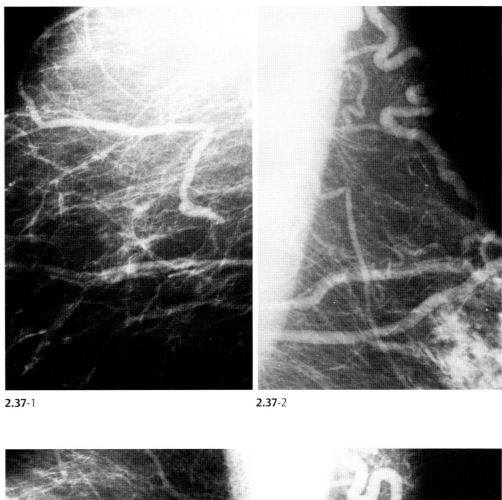

2.37-1   2.37-2

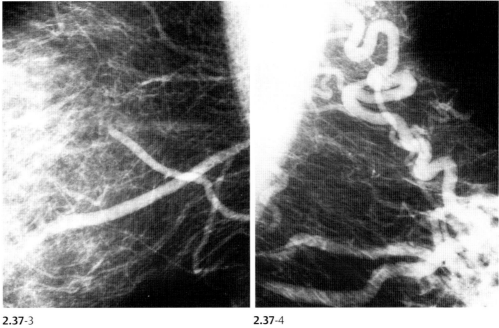

2.37-3   2.37-4

Fig. **2.37**-1 to 4   Some examples of blood vessels on the mammogram.

Pathological Lesions in Pattern II Breasts

■ Spiculated Invasive Ductal Carcinoma in a Pattern II Breast

Fig. **2.38**-1 & 2   Right breast, craniocaudal projection, of a breast undergoing involution. Screening mammogram (**2.38**-1) and microfocus magnification (**2.38**-2) show a solitary, <10 mm spiculated malignant tumor developing in the medial half of the breast.

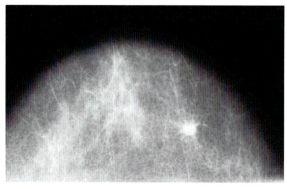

2.38-1

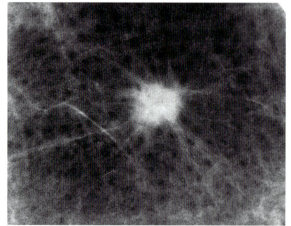

2.38-2

Fig. **2.38**-3   Subgross, thick-section histology image of a solitary invasive ductal carcinoma.

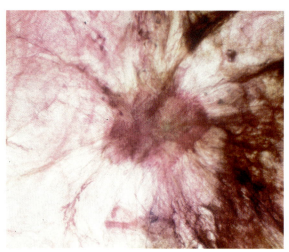

2.38-3

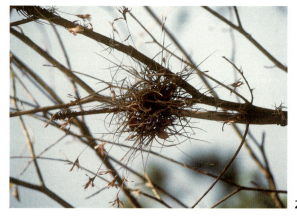

2.38-4

■ Microcalcifications in Pattern II Breasts

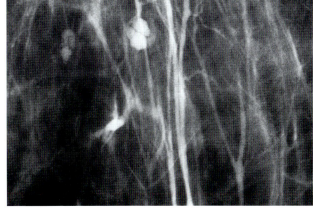

2.39-1

Fig. **2.39**-1   Galactography performed before breast reduction surgery shows a fluid-filled cystic dilatation of a solitary TDLU in a Pattern II breast.

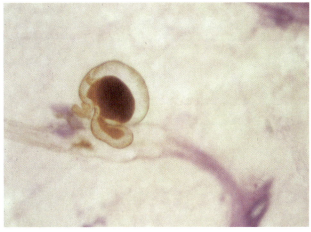

2.39-2

Fig. **2.39**-2   Thick-section histology demonstrates a cystic cavity containing "milk of calcium."

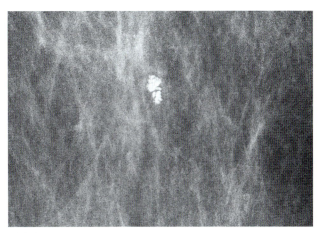

2.39-3

Fig. **2.39**-3   Calcification of cystic fluid may explain the presence of other solitary clusters of calcifications on the mammograms of Pattern II breasts.

■ Screening Findings in Asymptomatic Women with Pattern II Breasts

Example 2.1

A 59-year-old asymptomatic woman, screening case.

Ex. **2.1**-1   First screening, left breast, mediolateral oblique projection. No mammographic abnormality is seen.

Ex. **2.1**-2 & 3   Second screening, still asymptomatic. Left breast, MLO and CC projections. 5 cm deep to the nipple at the 12 o'clock position, there is a de novo solitary lesion with no associated microcalcifications. The preponderance of adipose tissue makes this tiny lesion easily detectable.

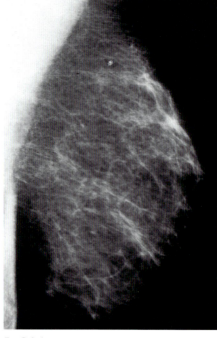
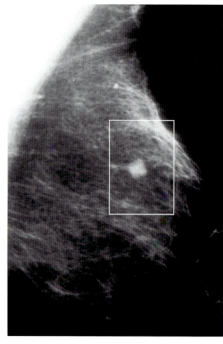

Ex. **2.1**-1

Ex. **2.1**-2

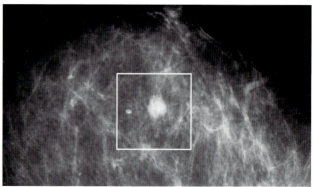

Ex. 2

Ex. **2.1**-4   Microfocus magnification demonstrates a lobulated, ill-defined, <10 mm, mammographically malignant tumor with no associated calcifications.

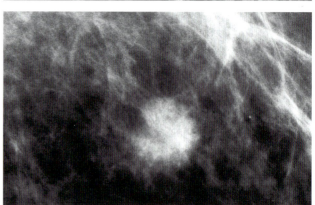

Ex. 2

Ex. **2.1**-5   Histological examination of 14-gauge large-core needle biopsy shows invasive ductal carcinoma.

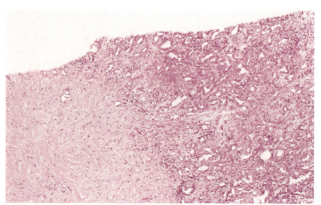

Ex. 2

Ex. **2.1**-6 Specimen radiograph. The lesion has been removed with wide margins.

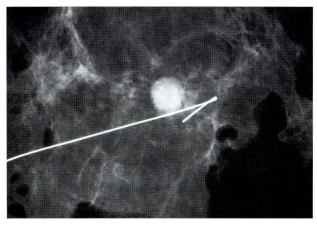

Ex. **2.1**-6

Ex. **2.1**-7–9 Large-section histology and low- and high-power magnification images of the 8-mm invasive carcinoma.

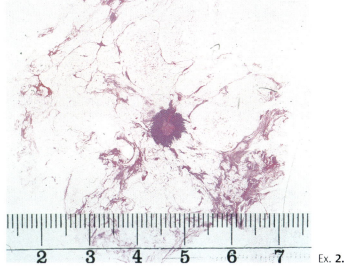

Ex. **2.1**-7

Ex. **2.1**-8 & 9 Low-power (Ex. **2.1**-8) and high-power (Ex. **2.1**-9) histology images show structures of a well-differentiated invasive carcinoma.

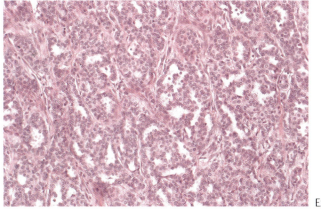

Ex. **2.1**-8

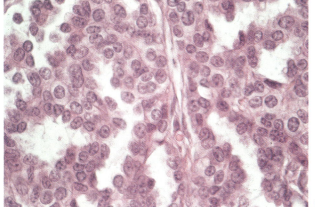

Ex. **2.1**-9

Chapter 3: Pattern III

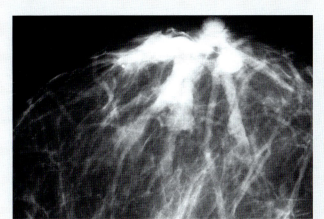 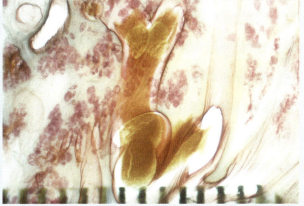

Characteristics of Pattern III

*Prominent Retroareolar Ducts
Surrounded by Adipose Tissue*

The mammographic image of parenchymal Pattern III is similar to Pattern II with the exception of prominent retroareolar ducts. Otherwise, neither of these patterns has nodular densities or diffuse fibrosis. There is an over-representation of adipose tissue, against which pathological lesions are generally easily detectable on the mammogram.
The prominent retroareolar linear densities may correspond to:

- Periductal connective tissue proliferation
- Distended, fluid-filled ducts

When the prominent duct pattern is caused by periductal connective tissue proliferation, the duct lumen is compressed instead of being dilated.
When the retroareolar ducts are prominent, a common cause is accumulation of fluid within the distended ducts.

Fig. **3.1**-1 Mammography of the right breast, detail, mediolateral oblique projection. There are prominent ducts in the retroareolar region. Histology showed a collar of periductal fibrosis/elastic tissue.

Fig. **3.1**-2 Special staining for elastic tissue demonstrates the relative amount of elastic (black) and collagen fibers (red) surrounding the duct.

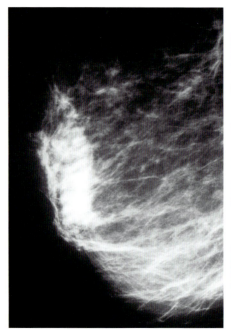

3.1-1

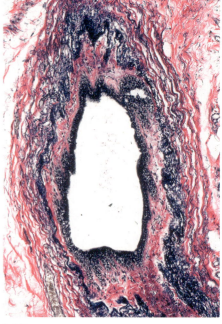

3.1-2

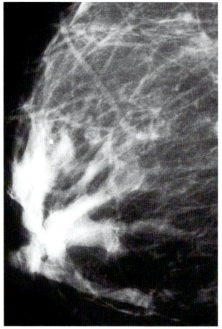

3.2-1

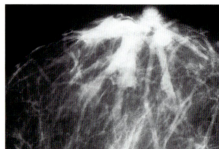

3.2-2

Fig. **3.2**-1 & 2 Mammography of right breast, mediolateral oblique (**3.2**-1) and craniocaudal (**3.2**-2) projections, Pattern III.

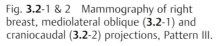

Fig. **3.2**-3 Large-section histology, mastectomy specimen. The retroareolar ducts are distended and fluid-filled.

3.2-3

In the presence of nipple discharge, a dilated duct can be demonstrated with galactography. In the absence of nipple discharge, ultrasound can demonstrate the fluid-filled duct.

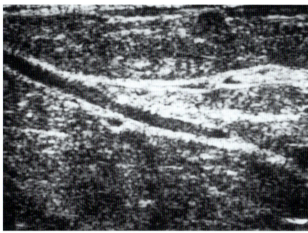

3.3-1

Fig. **3.3**-1 Galactogram demonstrating dilated retroareolar ducts.

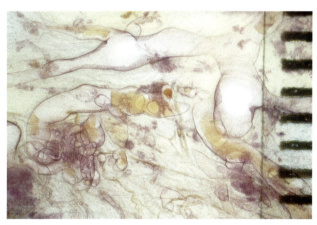

3.3-2

Fig. **3.3**-2 Ultrasound image of a dilated retroareolar duct.

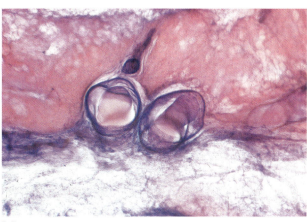

3.4

Fig. **3.4** Subgross, thick-section histology of retroareolar fluid-filled ducts. Note the millimeter scale.

Fig. **3.5** Subgross, thick-section histology of dilated fluid-filled ducts in cross section.

3.5

Chapter 4: Pattern IV

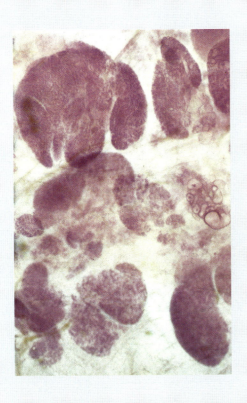

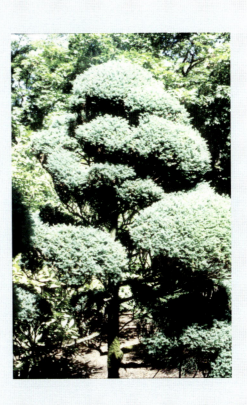

Characteristics of Pattern IV

Pattern IV is characterized by:
- Predominance of numerous, enlarged nodular densities
- Prominent linear densities caused by periductal fibrosis
- Fibrous connective tissue in varying amounts

Occurrence in the General Population

This characteristic pattern was found in about 12% of 27000 asymptomatic women attending their first mammography screening examination.[1, 3]
Unlike the other patterns, Pattern IV shows little change with age (Figs. **4.2** to **4.4**).
In this same population we found the prevalence of breast cancer to be more than twice as high in women with Pattern IV as it was in women with Patterns I–III.

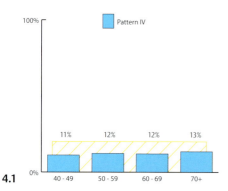

4.1

Fig. **4.1** The frequency of Pattern IV does not particularly change with age.[3]

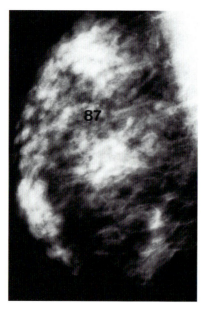

4.2-1

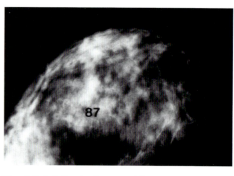

4.2-

Fig. **4.2**-1 & 2 A 43-year-old woman, first screening examination, mammographic Pattern IV.

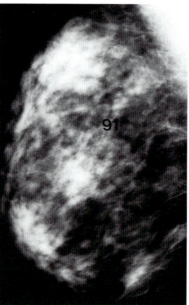

4.3-1

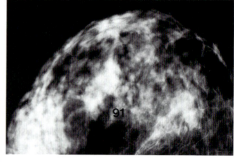

4.3-

Fig. **4.3**-1 & 2 Same woman, now age 47. Pattern unchanged.

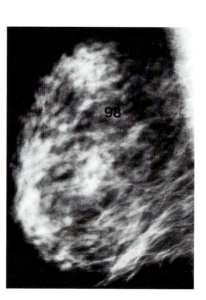

4.4-1

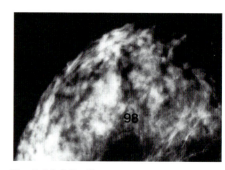

4.4-

Fig. **4.4**-1 & 2 Same woman, now age 54. Pattern unchanged.

The enlarged, 3–5 mm sized nodular densities seen on Pattern IV mammograms are the collective image of the enlarged lobules. The changes resulting in increased lobular size may be physiological, such as pregnancy and lactation, or aberrations of normal morphology. When a large number of lobules are affected, they give a characteristic mammographic image, Pattern IV. Many of the enlarged nodular densities seen on the mammogram, when examined histologically, correspond to a group of benign changes of the breast parenchyma termed by Hughes[2] **aberrations of normal development and involution** (**ANDI**):

- **Adenosis and its variations (sclerosing, microglandular, blunt duct)**
- **Papillomas and juvenile papillomatosis**
- **Fibroadenomatoid change and fibroadenomas**
- **Macrocysts and microcysts**
- **Lactation**
- **Lactational changes** in nonlactating women
- **Ductectasia/periductal mastitis**

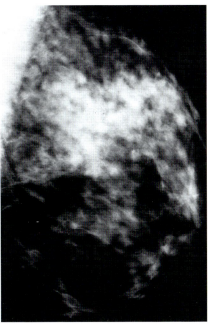
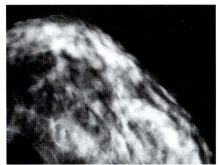

4.5-1   **4.5**-2

Fig. **4.5**-1 & 2   Mammograms of the left breast, mediolateral oblique and craniocaudal projections, parenchymal Pattern IV.

Adenosis

Adenosis is the hyperplasia and hypertrophy of the glandular elements. In this condition the number of acini is considerably increased and the lobules are correspondingly enlarged.

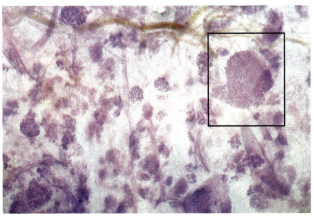

4.6

Fig. **4.6**   Thick-section histology. The lobules are mostly of normal size, with an enlarged lobule (adenosis) seen on the right of the image (in rectangle).

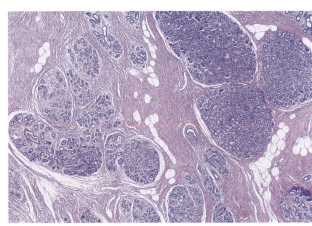

4.7

Fig. **4.7**   Histology, H&E stain. A mixture of normal lobules and adenosis is seen surrounded by interlobular fibrosis.

Adenosis

Fig. **4.8** Mammogram, craniocaudal projection. Pattern IV with prominent nodular and linear densities.

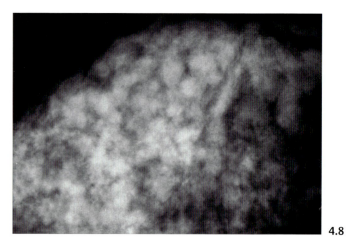

4.8

Fig. **4.9**-1 to 3 Thick-section histology images showing lobules of varying size. The larger lobules represent adenosis. The millimeter scale demonstrates the size of the adenosis nodules relative to normal TDLUs.

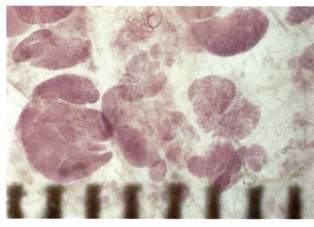

4.9-

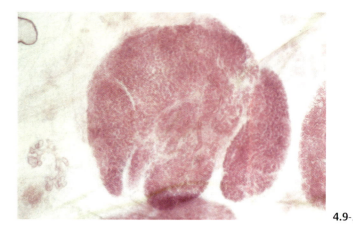

4.9-

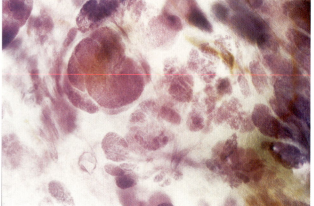

4.9-

Adenosis is often associated with various cellular changes such as apocrine metaplasia with or without atypia, columnar cell change, etc.

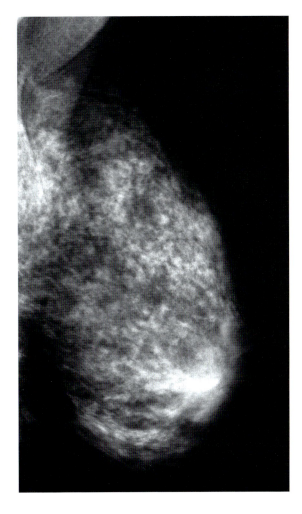

Fig. **4.10** Mammogram, MLO projection. Pattern IV.

4.10

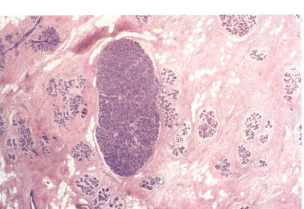

Fig. **4.11** Large-section histology image of a large hyperplastic TDLU (simple adenosis) surrounded by normal lobules and fibrosis.

4.11

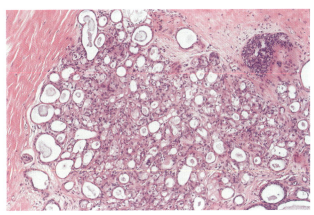

Fig. **4.12** Histological image of a distended TDLU with apocrine adenosis.

4.12

Sclerosing Adenosis

There are several histological subtypes of adenosis (sclerosing, blunt duct, microglandular, etc.), of which **sclerosing adenosis** is the most relevant for the radiologist, since it may be associated with calcifications that cause differential diagnostic problems. Sclerosing adenosis cannot be detected on the mammogram in the absence of microcalcifications.

When psammoma body–like calcifications develop, the summation of many particles results in multiple clusters of powdery, indistinct, cotton ball–like calcifications. These are too small to be individually visualized on the mammogram.

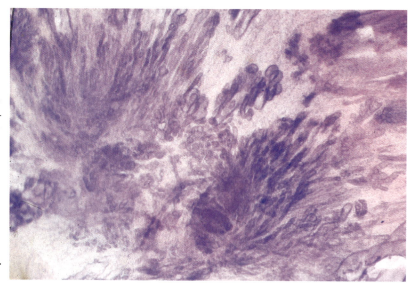

4.13

Fig. **4.13**-1 & 3   Subgross histology image of sclerosing adenosis without calcifications.

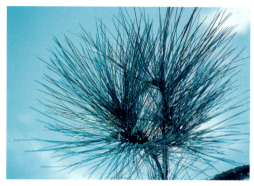

4.13-2

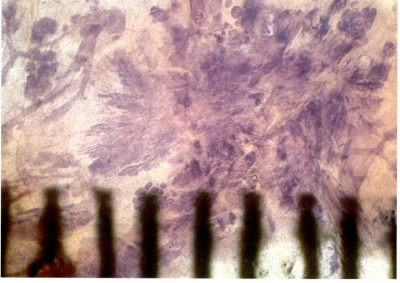

4.13

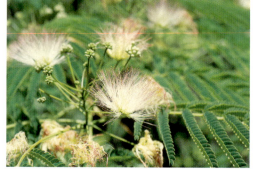

4.13-4

Mammographic–Histological Correlation of Sclerosing Adenosis with Calcifications

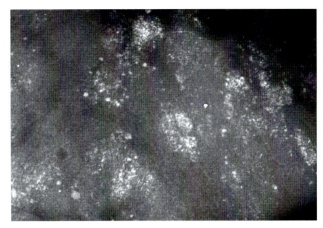

Fig. **4.14**-1   Specimen radiograph. Note that the individual calcifications cannot be distinguished on the mammographic image. The result is a cotton ball–like appearance.

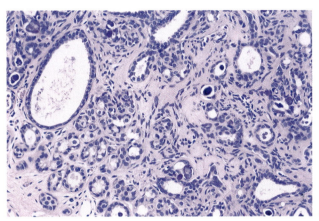

Fig. **4.14**-2   Histological image of sclerosing adenosis with psammoma body–like calcifications.

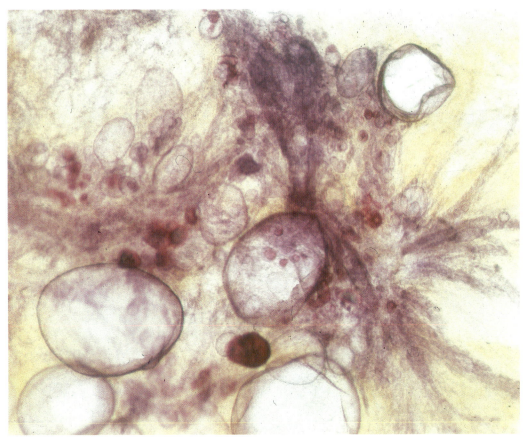

Fig. **4.14**-3   Subgross, thick-section histology of sclerosing adenosis with psammoma body–like calcifications and fibrocystic change.

Sclerosing Adenosis

Fig. **4.15** Specimen radiograph of multiple clusters of powdery calcifications. Note that the individual calcifications cannot be distinguished on the mammographic image. The result is a cotton ball–like appearance.

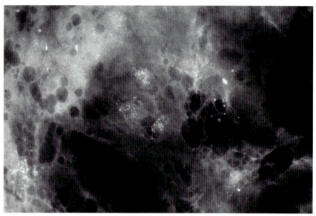

4.1

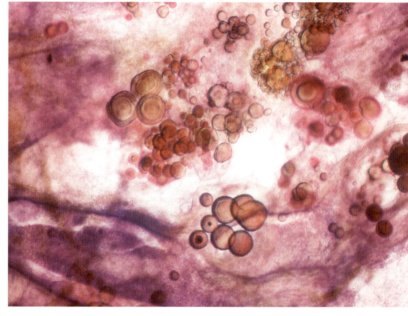

Fig. **4.16**-1 Thick-section histology image of sclerosing adenosis associated with multiple clusters of calcifications. The individual psammoma body–like calcifications are seen as laminated, spherical particles.

4.16

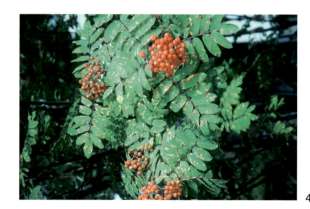

4.16-2

Fig. **4.17** Subgross, thick-section histological image of sclerosing adenosis with calcifications.

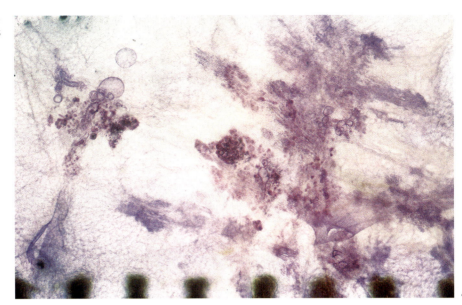

4.17

Fig. **4.18**-1 & 2   The individual psammoma body–like calcifications are seen at higher power magnification (subgross, thick-section and conventional histology). The same type of psammoma body–like calcifications occur in apocrine metaplasia (**4.18**-2), sclerosing adenosis (**4.17**), and Grade 1 DCIS.

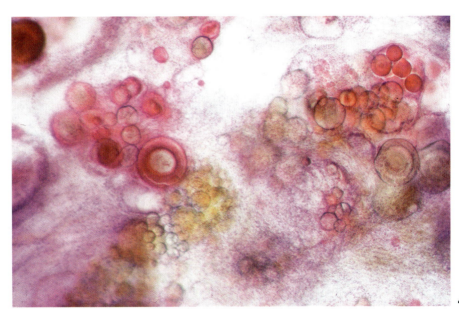

4.18-1

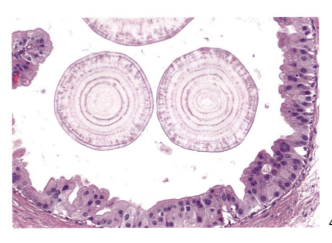

4.18-2

Fibroadenomatoid Change of the Lobule

When the intralobular connective tissue proliferates, the lobule enlarges. This is most often an incidental finding at histology with little, if any, mammographic relevance. When larger in size and recognizable mammographically or clinically, it is termed a fibroadenoma. Some of the enlarged nodular densities in Pattern IV mammograms correspond to fibroadenomatoid change.

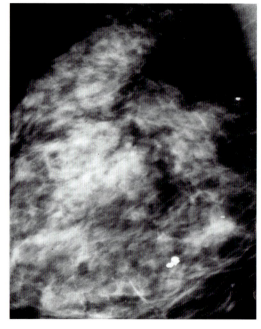

4.19

Fig. **4.19** Detail of a mammogram in the mediolateral oblique projection.

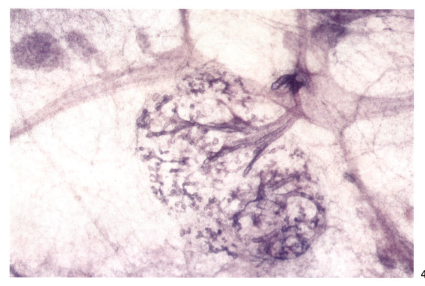

4.2

Fig. **4.20**-1 Thick-section histology image of fibroadenomatoid change.

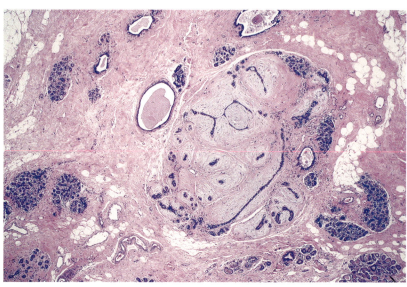

4.2

Fig. **4.20**-2 Histological image of an enlarged lobule with fibroadenomatoid change.

Patchy Fibrosis

In some cases the prominent nodular densities of Pattern IV may consist entirely of fibrous tissue. These nodules may often contain ductal remnants, indicating that they were once enlarged lobules.

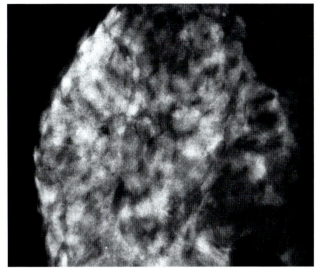

Fig. **4.21**-1 Specimen radiograph, prominent nodular pattern corresponding to Pattern IV.

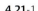

4.21-1

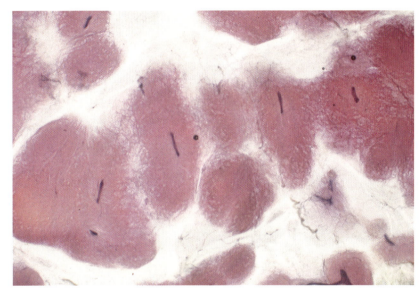

Fig. **4.21**-2 & 3 Subgross, thick-section histological images. The nodules consist of fibrous tissue containing ductal remnants.

4.21-2

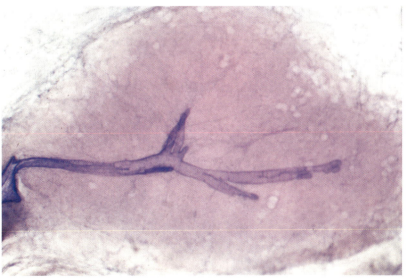

4.21-3

Pathological Lesions in Pattern IV Breasts

The degree to which a radiologist is able to detect small abnormalities on the mammogram is related to the relative proportion of adipose tissue in the breasts. Since breasts with a Pattern IV mammogram contain a large proportion of radiopaque structural elements at the expense of fatty tissue, noncalcified pathological lesions are easily obscured by the overlying radiopaque fibroglandular tissue in these "dense" breasts.

Example 4.1

A 61-year-old asymptomatic woman, screening examination.

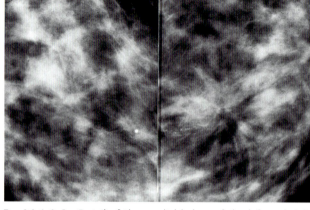

Ex. **4.1**-1

Ex. 4

Ex. **4.1**-1 & 2   Detail of the medial halves of the left and right breasts in the craniocaudal projection. Pattern IV with architectural distortion and associated calcifications in the right breast.

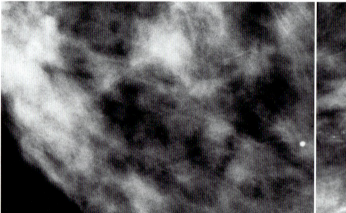

Ex. **4.1**-3

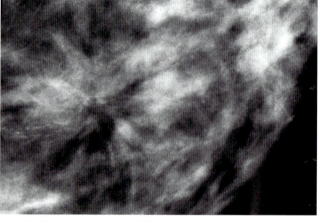

Ex. 4

Ex. **4.1**-3 & 4   Microfocus magnification image showing the architectural distortion and the calcifications.

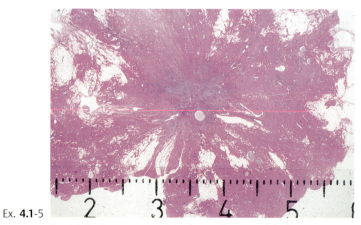

Ex. **4.1**-5

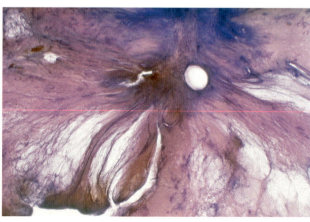

Ex. 4

Ex. **4.1**-5   Large-section histology of invasive lobular carcinoma.

Ex. **4.1**-6   Thick-section histology showing the architectural distortion caused by this carcinoma.

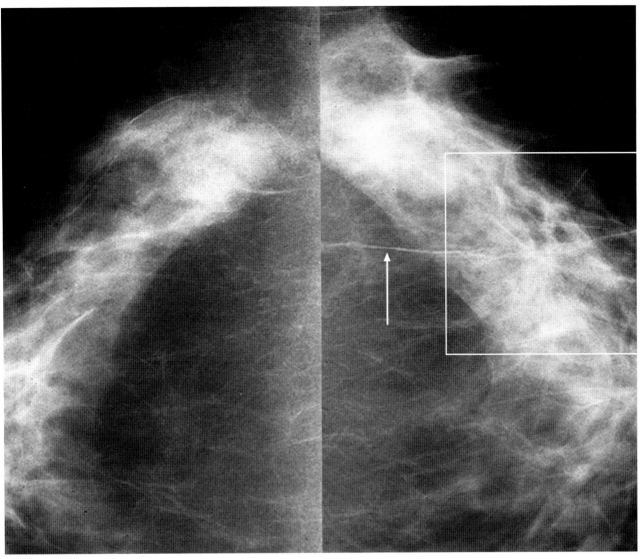

Ex. **4.2**-2

Ex. **4.2**-1 & 2   Right and left breast, details of the craniocaudal projections. The straight line in the retroglandular clear space (arrow) leads to the detection of the architectural distortion within the dense fibroglandular tissue.

Example 4.2

When a noncalcified invasive carcinoma develops in a Pattern IV type breast, the pathological lesion, shown as architectural distortion, spiculated or circular tumor, will have grown to a fairly large size before it can be detected mammographically. The lesion will often be obscured by the dense, overlying radiopaque fibroglandular tissue. Detection of abnormalities in Pattern IV type breasts requires the combined use of high-quality, well-penetrated mammographic images with ultrasound examination and palpation.

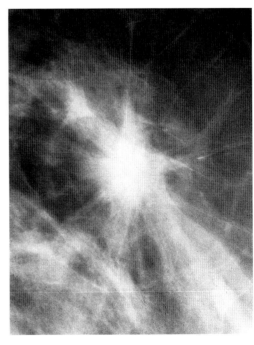

Ex. **4.2**-3   Spot microfocus magnification view demonstrates the stellate tumor.
Histology: invasive ductal carcinoma.

Ex. **4.2**-3

135

Example 4.3

A 70-year-old asymptomatic woman, screening examination. This case has Pattern IV type nodular densities, mainly in the upper outer quadrants.

This case demonstrates:

- How difficult it is to detect even large abnormalities in Pattern IV type breast tissue, especially when the lesion in question is an invasive lobular carcinoma.
- How much easier it is to detect a small tumor when it is surrounded by adipose tissue.

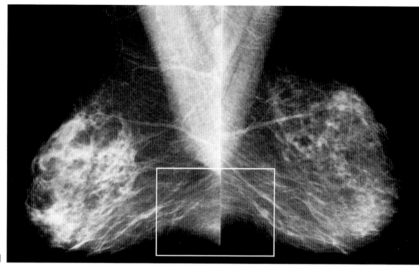

Ex. **4.3**-1

Ex. 4

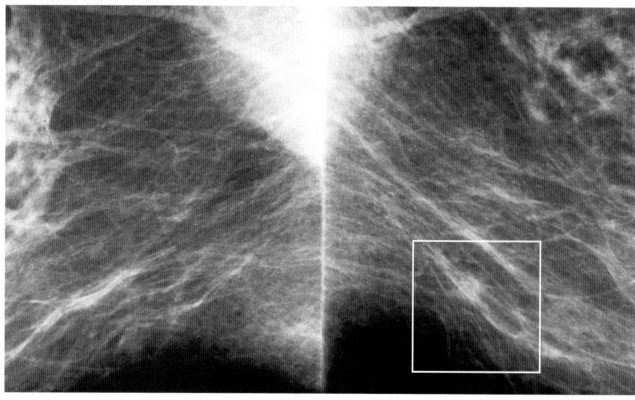

Ex. **4.3**-3

Ex. 4

Ex. **4.3**-1 & 2   A tiny asymmetric density can be found in the lower inner quadrant of the **left breast**.

Ex. **4.3**-3 & 4   The asymmetric lesion is more easily detected when comparison is made to the contralateral side. These images demonstrate the usefulness of the hand-held mammographic viewer.

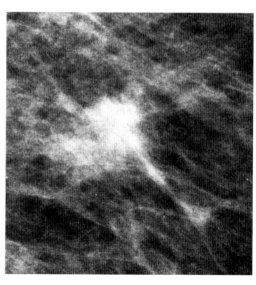

Ex. **4.3**-5   Microfocus magnification view shows a small spiculated lesion, mammographically malignant.

Ex. **4.3**-5

Ex. **4.3**-6 Craniocaudal projection with the tiny spiculated lesion in the medial half of the breast.

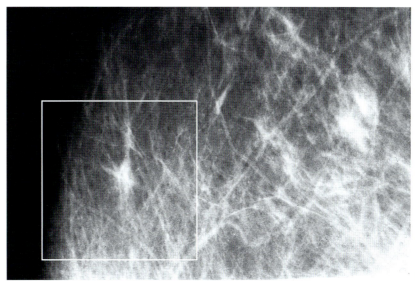

Ex. **4.3**-6

Ex. **4.3**-7 Specimen radiograph shows the tiny cancer with good margins.

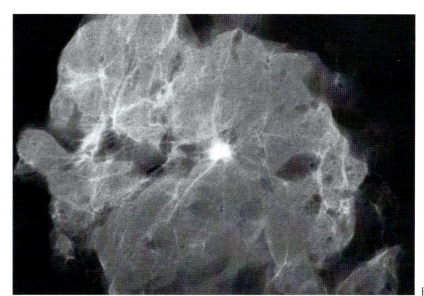

Ex. **4.3**-7

Ex. **4.3**-8 Large-section histology: Grade 2 ductal carcinoma < 10 mm.

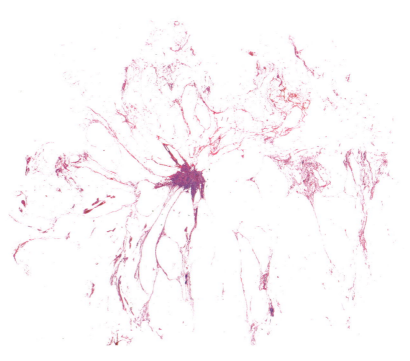

Ex. **4.3**-8

In addition to the small tumor in the lower inner quadrant of the **left breast**, architectural distortion is seen in the upper outer quadrant of the **right breast** (Ex. **4.3**-9 to 12).

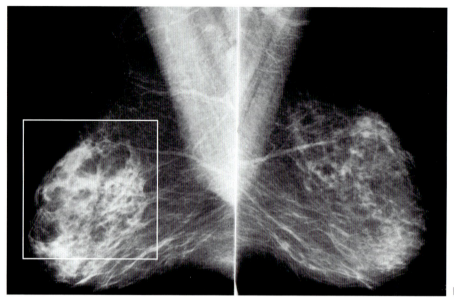

Ex. **4.3**-9
Ex.

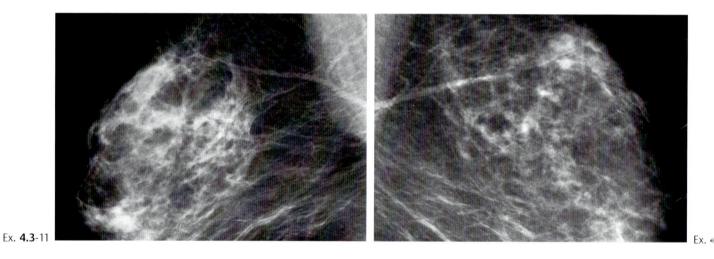

Ex. **4.3**-11
Ex.

Ex. **4.3**-13 & 14   The architectural distortion is more obvious on the CC projection, as is often the case with invasive lobular carcinoma.

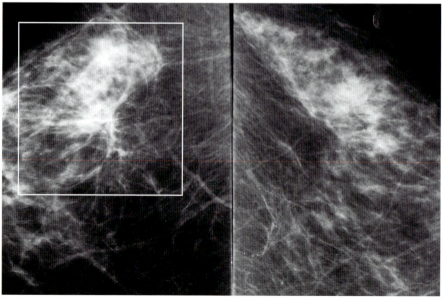

Ex. **4.3**-13
Ex.

Ex. **4.3**-15   Right breast. Microfocus magnification in the cranio-caudal projection emphasizes the extensive architectural distortion more clearly. There is no central tumor mass, nor are any calcifications seen.

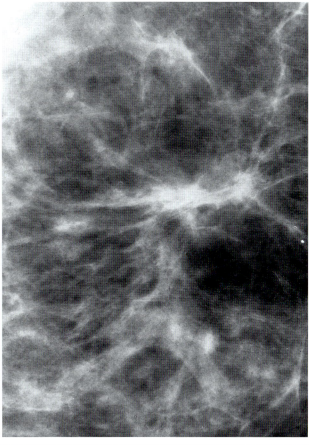

Ex. **4.3**-15

Ex. **4.3**-16   Specimen radiograph with the extensive architectural distortion.

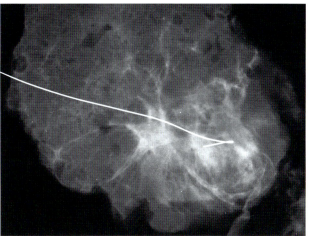

Ex. **4.3**-16

Ex. **4.3**-17   Histology shows a 20 × 20 mm invasive lobular carcinoma. There were no demonstrable metastases in 11 axillary nodes removed at surgery.

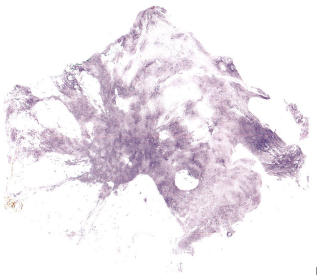

Ex. **4.3**-17

Chapter 5: Pattern V

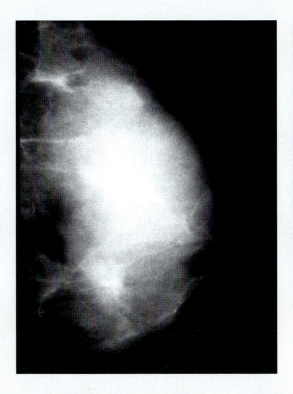

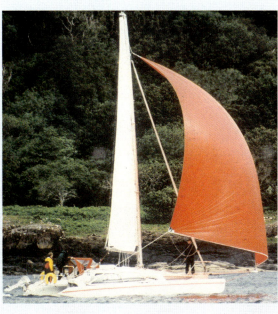

Characteristics of Pattern V

Pattern V is characterized by overrepresentation of fibrous connective tissue and the underrepresentation of adipose tissue, resulting in a nearly structureless radiopaque density involving most of the breast. The fine structural details are hidden within the homogeneous tissue, so that the extent to which the normal glandular tissue has undergone involution cannot be determined from the mammogram (Fig. **5.1**-1 & 2). There may be a large number of functioning terminal ductal lobular units (TDLUs) present (Fig. **5.2**) or all of them may have undergone involution (Fig. **5.3**). Therefore, the radiology report should not mention "dense fibroglandular tissue." Rather, it should state "extensive fibrosis," the only demonstrable feature.

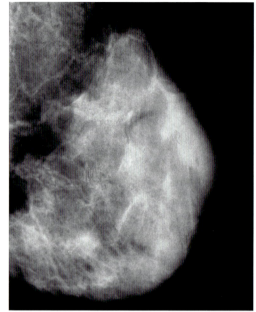

Fig. **5.1**-1 & 2 Mammograms of Pattern V, mediolateral and craniocaudal projections. Extensive, structureless fibrosis is seen with little subcutaneous adipose tissue.

5.1-1

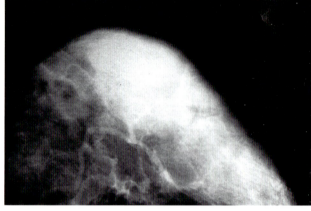

5.1-

Fig. **5.2** Histology may show a large number of normal TDLUs and ducts surrounded by extensive fibrosis.

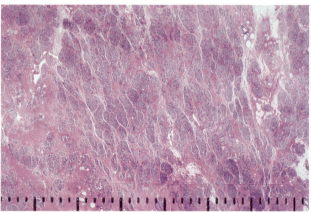

5.2

Fig. **5.3** Histology may demonstrate atrophy of the glandular elements hidden within extensive fibrosis. The mammograms of Figs. **5.2** and **5.3** may be identical.

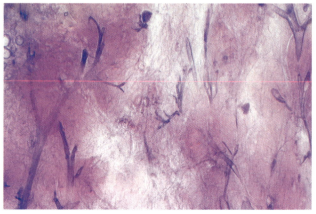

5.3

Pattern V shows very little, if any, change with age.

Figs. **5.4**, **5.5** and **5.6**   Mammograms of the left breast, mediolateral oblique and craniocaudal projections, in an asymptomatic woman at three different occasions over a nine-year period at ages 40, 43, and 49, respectively.

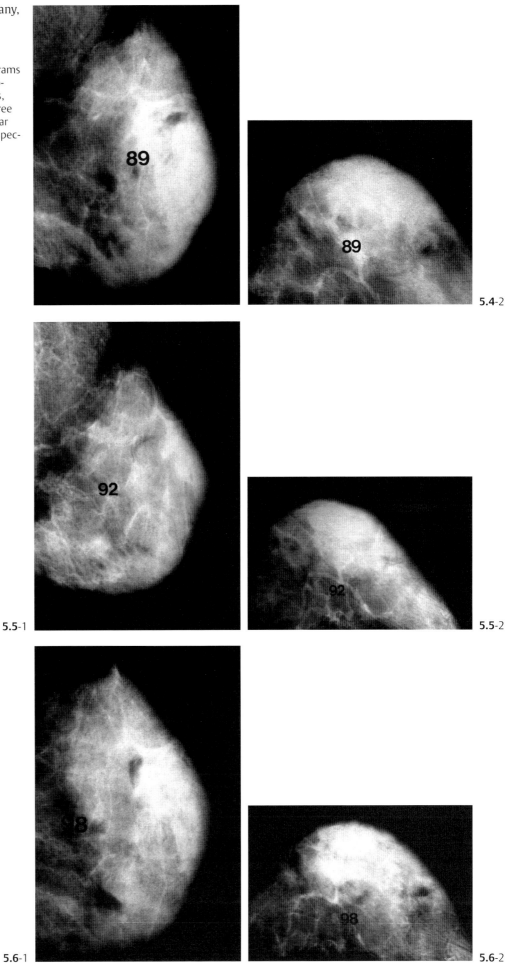

Involuting Lobule with Fibrous Replacement

When the TDLU **involutes**, it will most often be replaced by adipose tissue. However, in women with Pattern V breasts, fibrous tissue replaces the involuting acini. Several stages of this process are demonstrated in Fig. **5.7**-1 to 5.

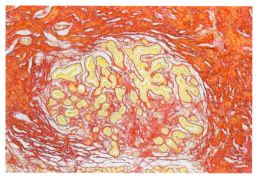

5.7-1

Fig. **5.7**-1   Normal lobule surrounded by extensive fibrous tissue.

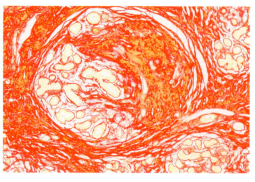

5.7-2

Fig. **5.7**-2 to 5   Connective tissue fills in the space vacated as the acini undergo atrophy. There will eventually be extensive, homogeneous fibrosis.

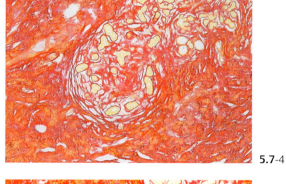

5.7-3

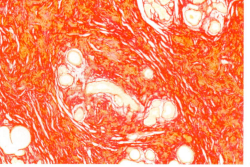

5.7-4

5.7-5

Calcifications in Pattern V Breasts

When pathological lesions on a Pattern V mammogram are associated with **calcifications**, they can be detected quite easily in spite of the dense fibrous tissue.

Example 5.1

A 49-year-old asymptomatic woman, screening examination.
Calcifications are seen bilaterally on the mammograms, within the dense fibrous tissue and with no associated tumor masses.

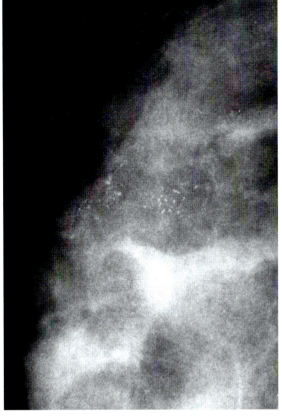

Ex. **5.1**-1

Ex. **5.1**-1 & 2   Detail of the right mediolateral oblique projection, as well as microfocus magnification image of the area with calcifications. The multiple clusters of calcifications are of the mammographically malignant type.

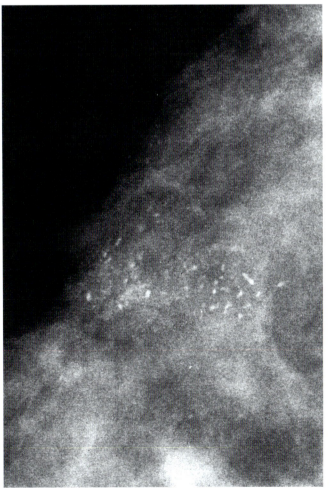

Ex. **5.1**-2

145

Example 5.1

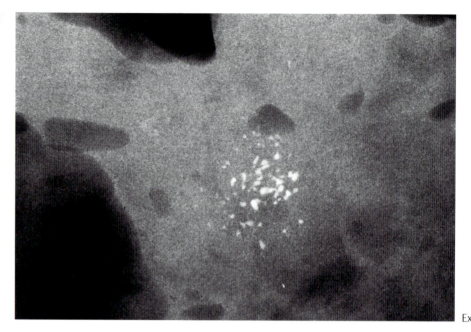

Ex. **5.1**-3 & 4   Radiographs of specimen slices, demonstrating that the microcalcifications are irregular in size, shape, and density and are distributed in multiple clusters.

Ex. **5**

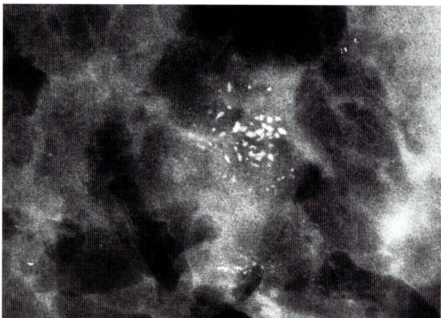

Ex. **5**

Ex. **5.1**-5   Histology shows extensive ductal carcinoma in situ with necrosis (H&E stain, low power). The area inside the rectangle is enlarged in Ex. **5.1**-6.

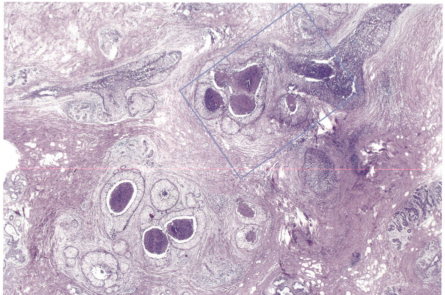

Ex. **5**

Ex. **5.1**-6 to 8   At progressively higher powers, the cellular details of this high-grade ductal carcinoma in situ with solid cell proliferation are better seen. The area inside the rectangle in Ex. **5.1**-7 is enlarged in Ex. **5.1**-8.

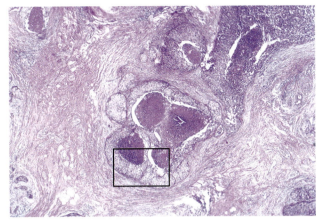

Ex. **5.1**-6

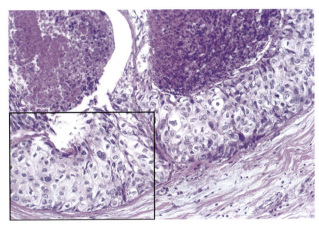

Ex. **5.1**-7

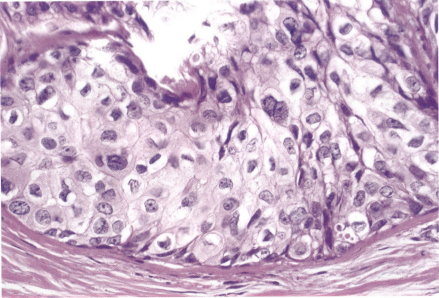

Ex. **5.1**-8

147

Example 5.1

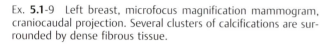

Case continued, demonstrating that not only malignant type, but also benign type calcifications will be demonstrable in Pattern V breasts.

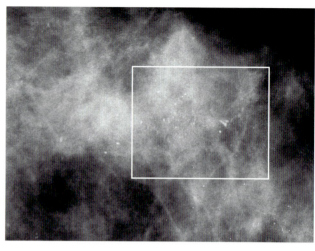

Ex.

Ex. **5.1**-9   Left breast, microfocus magnification mammogram, craniocaudal projection. Several clusters of calcifications are surrounded by dense fibrous tissue.

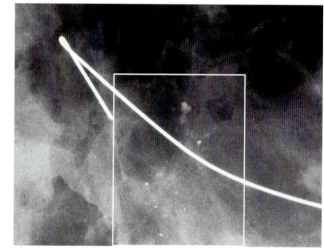

Ex. 5

Ex. **5.1**-10 & 11   Specimen radiograph containing the calcifications.

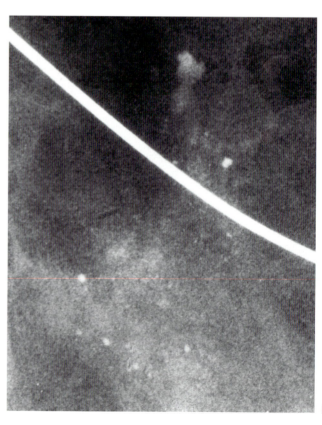

Ex. 5

Ex. **5.1**-12 Radiograph of specimen slice showing a cluster of smudgy calcifications surrounded by fibrosis.

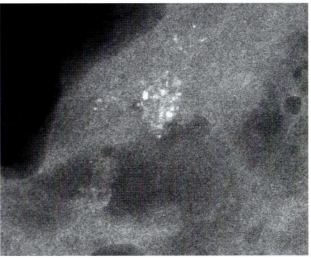

Ex. **5.1**-12

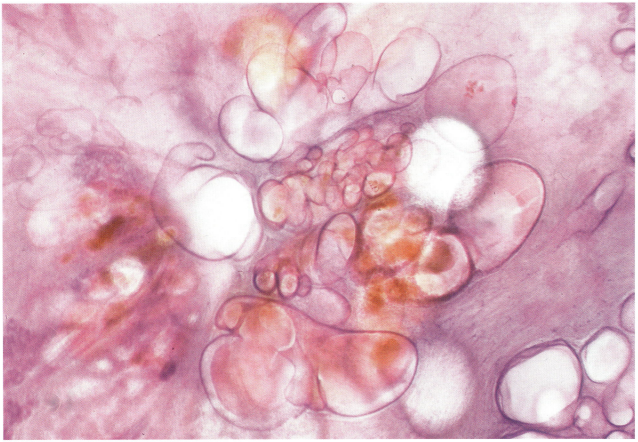

Ex. **5.1**-13

Ex. **5.1**-13 Subgross, thick-section histology of focal fibrocystic change with milk of calcium contained within the small cysts.

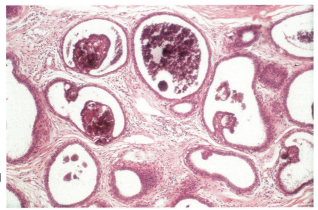

Ex. **5.1**-14 Histology demonstrates that the mammographically detected calcifications are localized in cystically dilated acini.

Ex. **5.1**-14

Calcifications in Pattern V Breasts— Example 5.1

Ex. **5.1**-15   Histology: fibrocystic change and normal TDLUs surrounded by fibrosis.

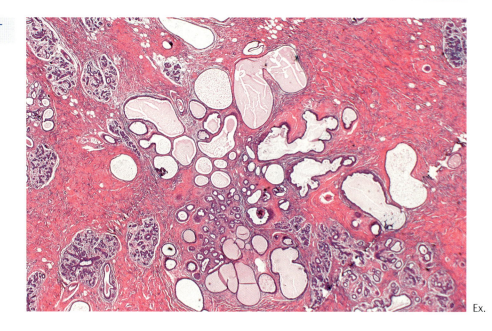

Ex.

Ex. **5.1**-16 & 17   Subgross, thick-section histology images demonstrating dilated ducts, TDLUs with cystic dilatations and interlobular fibrosis. The fine structural details of normal anatomy and pathology are obscured by the dense fibrous tissue, but only the calcifications are discernible on the mammogram.

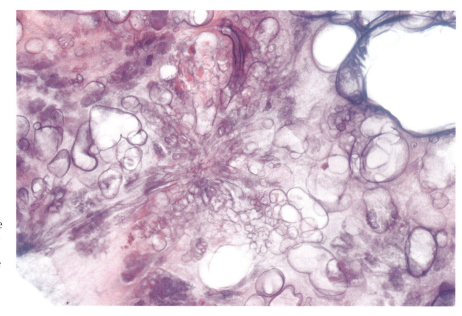

Ex.

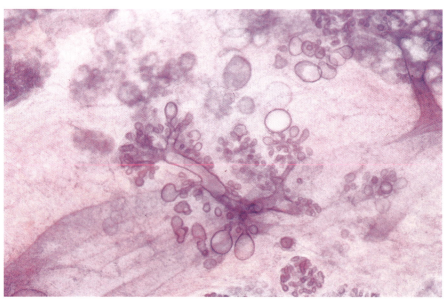

Ex.

Perception of Noncalcified Lesions in Pattern V Type Breasts

A more serious consequence of the overrepresentation of fibrous tissue is the limited ability of the mammogram to reveal many pathological changes. Additional imaging modalities may help compensate for this deficiency.

Abnormalities with a **convex contour** such as cysts, fibroadenomas, medullary cancer, or other circular/oval benign or malignant lesions may be detected mammographically if they protrude from the dense parenchymal contour into the subcutaneous fat. Such lesions may otherwise be mammographically occult even when they are palpable. Ultrasound examination is important in demonstrating these cases.

Stellate lesions or abnormalities with architectural distortion cause considerable perception problems when viewing mammographic Pattern V. These lesions may be detected by visualization of indirect signs, such as a subtle parenchymal contour retraction, an example being the tent sign. Stellate lesions may also remain undetected until they have become palpable.

Examples 5.2 and 5.3

Ex. **5.2**-1 & Ex. **5.3**-1 Spot compression and magnification images demonstrate the "tent-sign." Spot compression in two cases showing the "tent-sign" with corresponding histological images.

Ex. **5.2**-2 & Ex. **5.3**-2 The cancer causing the "tent-sign" is demonstrated on the histological images in both cases.

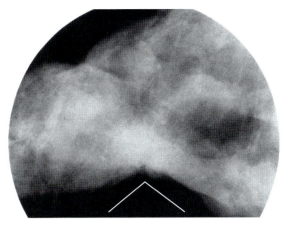

Ex. **5.2**-1

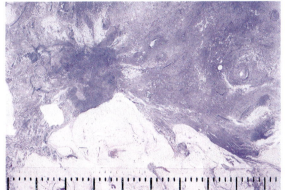

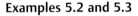

Ex. **5.2**-2

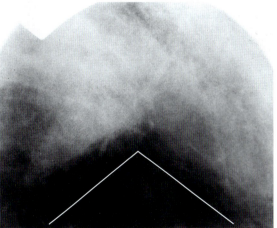

Ex. **5.3**-1

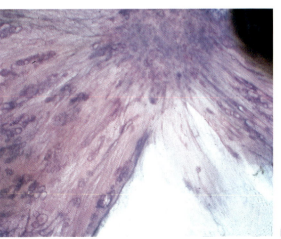

Ex. **5.3**-2

Example 5.4

Ex. **5.4**-1 to 4 demonstrate the value of searching for the "tent-sign," an indication that a pathological lesion may be hidden within the dense parenchyma near the peak of the tent. The arrows point to the carcinoma at the apex of the tent.

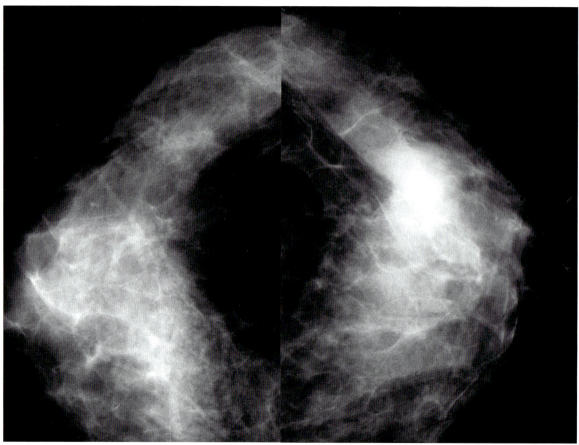

Ex. 5.4-1   Ex. **5.4**-2

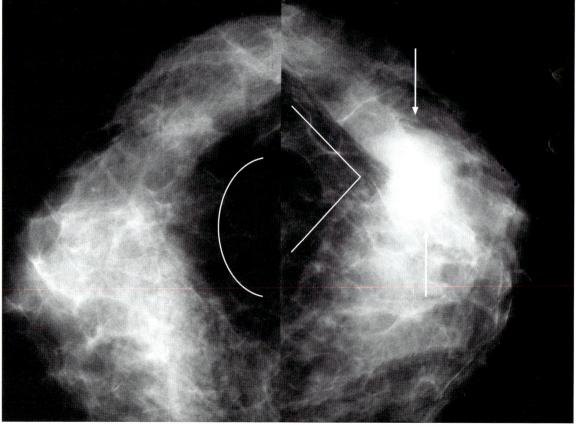

Ex. 5.4-3   Ex. **5.4**-4

Example 5.5

Ex. **5.5**-1 & 3   Correlation of this specimen radiograph with the corresponding large-section histological image demonstrates how most of the cancer is hidden within the extensive fibrosis of this Pattern V breast.

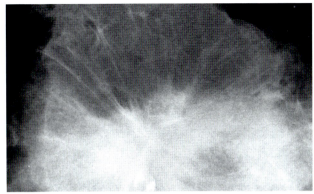

Ex. **5.5**-1

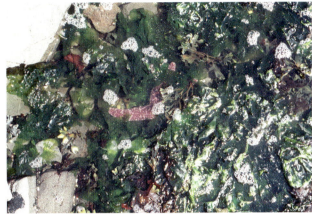

Ex. **5.5**-2

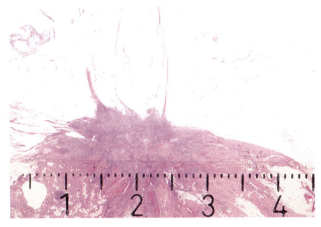

Ex. **5.5**-3

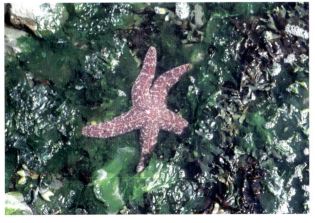

Ex. **5.5**-4

Example 5.6

Ex. **5.6**-1   Right breast, CC projection, and Pattern V type mammogram with parenchymal contour change along the posterior border.

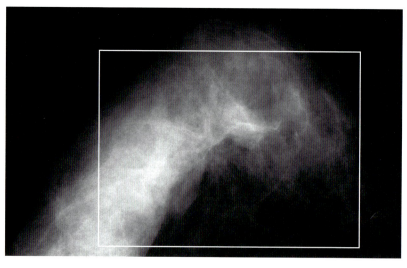

Ex.

Ex. **5.6**-2 & 3   Spot compression microfocus magnification mammograms showing an obvious spiculated lesion radiating into the retroglandular clear space.

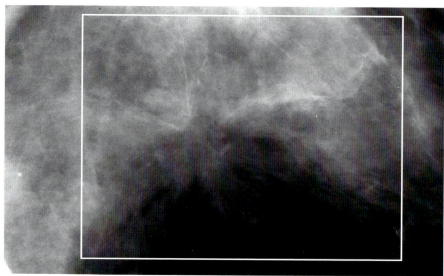

Ex. 5

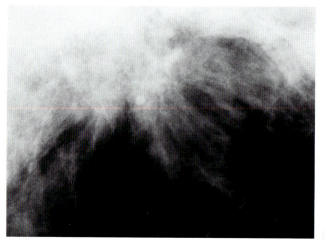

Ex. **5.6**-3

Ex. **5.6**-4   Specimen X-ray with the tumor in a central location.

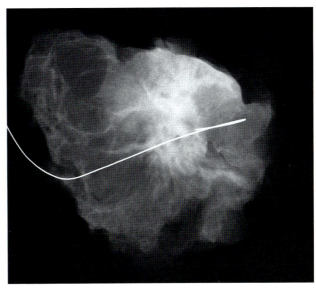

Ex. **5.6**-4

Ex. **5.6**-5   Detail of the large-section histology. Most of the invasive tumor is obscured by fibrosis. The small protruding part made mammographic detection possible.

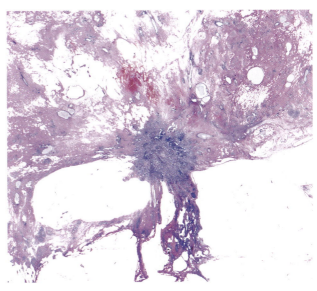

Ex. **5.6**-5

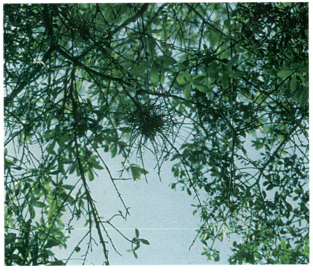

Ex. **5.6**-6

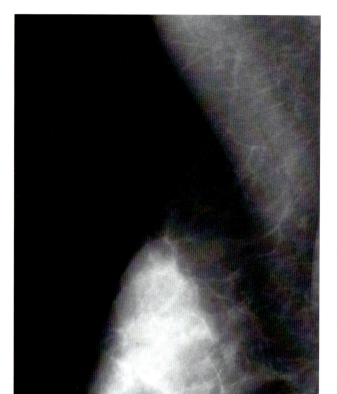

Example 5.7

A 50-year-old asymptomatic woman, routine screening examination. She was called back for evaluation of non-specific microcalcifications in the upper half of the right breast.

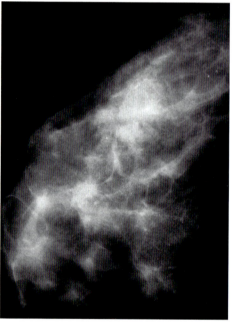

Ex. **5.7**-1

Ex. **5.7**-2

Ex. **5.7**-1 & 2   Extensive fibrosis, no tumor mass visible on the MLO and CC screening mammograms, but numerous nonspecific microcalcifications in the upper half of the breast prompted the call-back for further examination.

Ex. **5.7**-3   Microfocus magnification with spot compression in the CC projection shows very faint calcifications with no associated tumor mass.

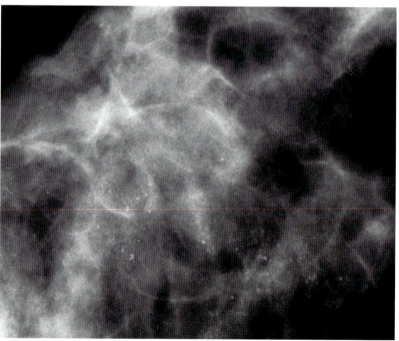

Ex. **5**

Fig. **5.7**-4 Microfocus magnification with spot compression in the MLO projection shows the calcifications more clearly. The presence of multiple clusters of calcifications and the surrounding dense fibrosis is an indication for using adjunctive examination methods, such as breast ultrasound and core needle biopsy.

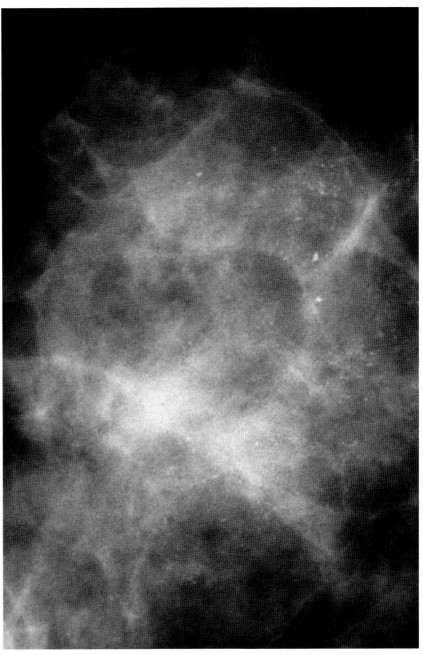

Ex. **5.7**-4

Ex. **5.7**-5 & 6 Breast ultrasound demonstrates a malignant tumor, possibly multifocal.

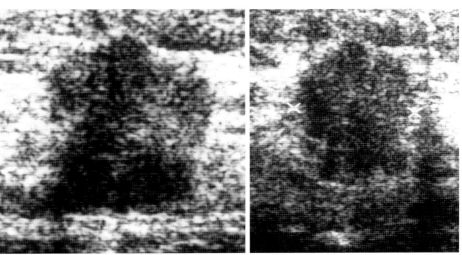

Ex. **5.7**-5

Ex. **5.7**-6

157

Example 5.7

Ex. **5.7**-7   Large-section histology of the mastectomy specimen demonstrating a 12 mm invasive micropapillary carcinoma surrounded by extensive fibrosis.

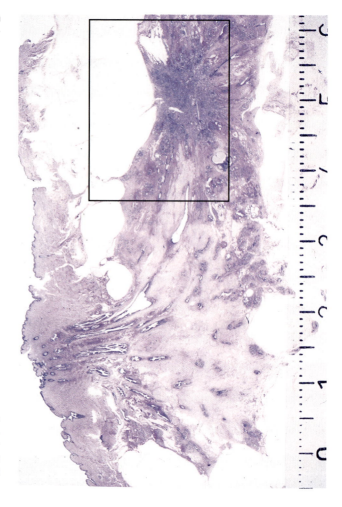

Ex. **5.7**-8 & 9   Detail of the large-section histology image and corresponding specimen radiograph. Most of the carcinoma is obscured by the surrounding fibrous tissue, explaining the difficulty in demonstrating it mammographically. The solitary spiculation and the parenchymal contour change led to the detection of the underlying tumor.

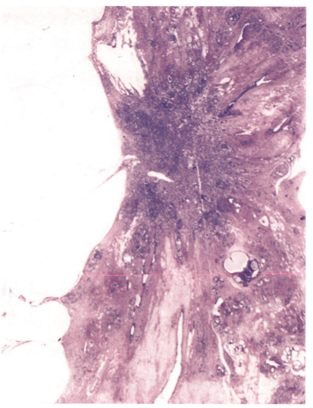

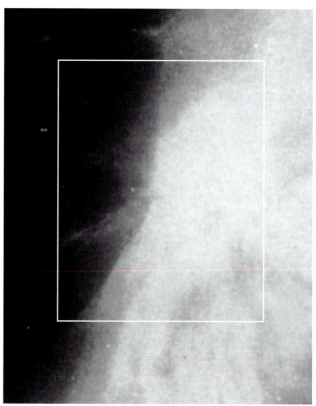

Ex. **5.7**-8

Ex. **5**

Ex. **5.7**-10 to 12   Low- and high-power microscopic magnification images showing structures of invasive micropapillary carcinoma embedded within dense, fibrous stroma.

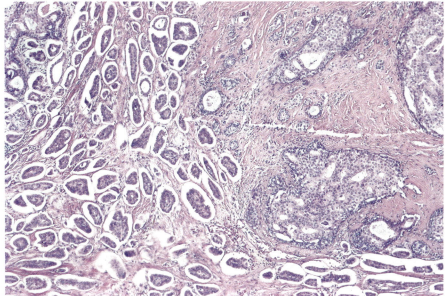

Ex. **5.7**-10

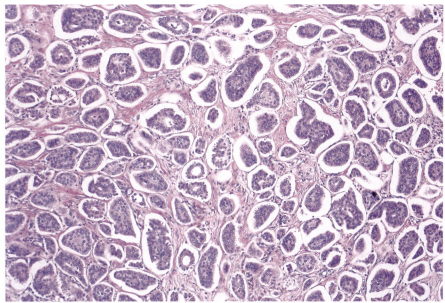

Ex. **5.7**-11

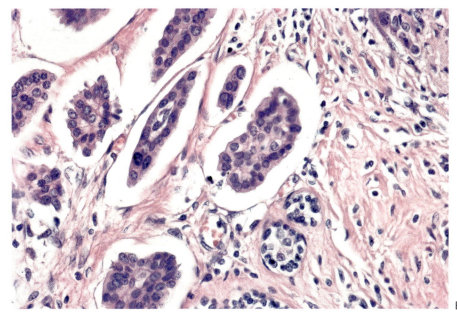

Ex. **5.7**-12

Relative Frequencies of the Mammographic Patterns in the General Population

In the population-based, randomized controlled mammographic screening trial in Kopparberg County, Sweden, a prospective classification of the mammographic parenchymal patterns was made on 27 000 consecutive women aged 40 years and older, and repeated on 9000 of these women several years later. This material gives a reliable representation of the female population over 40 years of age, since 92.4 % of those aged between 40 and 70 years actually came to the first screening examination when they were invited to do so. This study was performed prior to the introduction of hormone replacement therapy (HRT) in the county. The mammographic parenchymal patterns of an additional 1900 clinically referred women were also classified from their mammograms.[1]

The **effect of age** upon the relative frequency of mammographic parenchymal patterns is shown in Figures **5.8** to **5.11**[1] and can be summarized as follows:

- The most frequently occurring mammographic parenchymal pattern in women aged 40 and older is Pattern II (involution).
- The relative frequency of both Pattern II and Pattern III increases with age at the expense of Pattern I.
- The relative frequency of mammographic parenchymal Pattern IV is 10–12 % in an asymptomatic population (Table **5.1**) and in symptomatic, referred patient material (Table **5.2**), showing no change with age.
- Pattern V is even less common in women over 50 years of age, and its incidence is relatively stable in postmenopausal women.

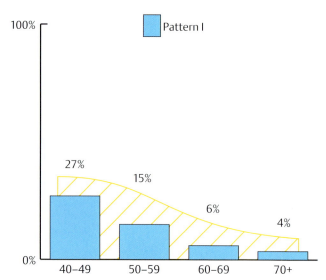

Fig. 5.8 The frequency of mammographic Pattern I decreases progressively with advancing age.

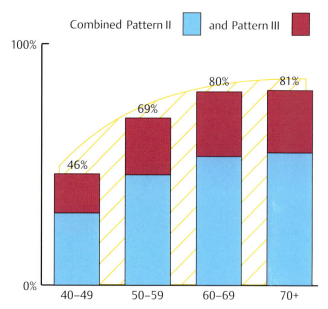

Fig. **5.9** More than 70 % of postmenopausal women in an asymptomatic population have breasts that are predominantly in involution (Patterns II and III). This figure exceeds 80 % in women over 60 years of age.

Table 5.**1** Distribution of Pattern IV according to age in asymptomatic screening material

| Age (years) | Number of women | | |
	Pattern IV	Total	%
40–49	769	5 947	11.9
50–59	872	7 425	11.7
60–69	688	7 629	9.0
70+	613	6 129	10.0
Total	2 682	27 157	10.6

Table 5.**2** Distribution of Pattern IV according to age in symptomatic, referred screening material

| Age (years) | Number of women | | |
	Pattern IV	Total	%
40–49	354	3 159	11.2
50–59	323	2 635	12.3
60–69	285	2 373	12.0
70+	110	816	13.5
Total	1 072	8 952	11.9

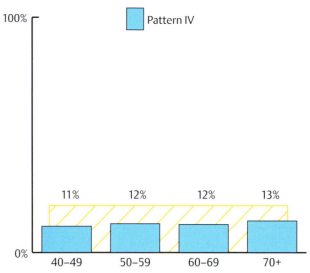

Fig. **5.10** About 10 % of women in an asymptomatic population will have mammographic Pattern IV. The frequency of this pattern shows no change with age.

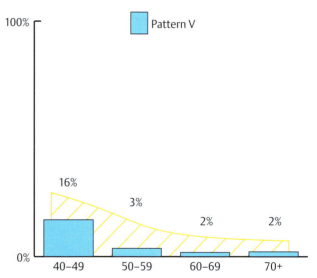

Fig. **5.11** Pattern V accounts for a small, stable percentage of the patterns in postmenopausal women. The higher frequency of this pattern in premenopausal women may result from the difficulty of differentiating between a true Pattern V and a very dense Pattern I on a mammogram.

Distribution of Mammographic Parenchymal Patterns by Age in a Screening Population versus Clinically Referred Women

When comparing the distribution of mammographic parenchymal patterns by age in an asymptomatic screening population with that of a clinically referred population, only small differences were observed, as shown in Figures **5.12** and **5.13**.[1]

In countries where mammography is not offered to all women in defined age groups, a large proportion of the women undergoing mammography will be self selected. The distribution of mammographic patterns may then be different from that described above, with a bias towards the more dense breasts.

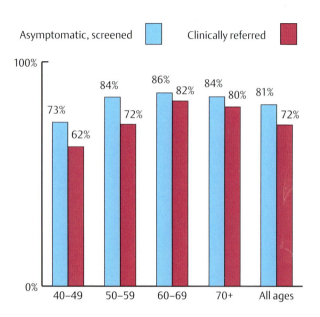

Fig. **5.12** 81% of the asymptomatic screened women had either mammographic Pattern I, II or III, while 72% of the clinically referred patients had these same mammographic patterns.

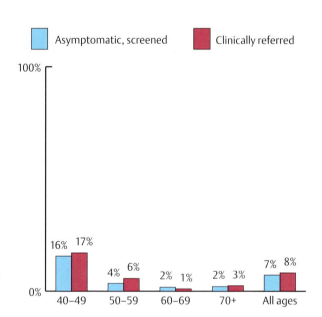

Fig. **5.13** The true Pattern V occurs infrequently. There is no apparent difference in the frequency of its occurrence in asymptomatic screened women versus clinically referred women.

The Prevalence of Breast Cancer According to Mammographic Parenchymal Pattern and Age

The cancer prevalence in women with combined patterns IV–V was higher in all age subgroups than it was in women with combined Patterns I–III. The breast cancer risk increased with age in both the lower (Patterns I–III) and higher (Patterns IV–V) risk groups.

Figure **5.15** shows that women aged 40–54 with Patterns IV–V had the same risk of developing breast cancer as did women aged 55–69 having Patterns I–III. Thus, it may take about 15 more years for women with Patterns I–III to arrive at the same cancer risk that women of the same age with Patterns IV–V already have.

When all age groups were combined, women with Patterns I–III had half the overall breast cancer prevalence of women with Patterns IV–V (Fig. **5.14**).

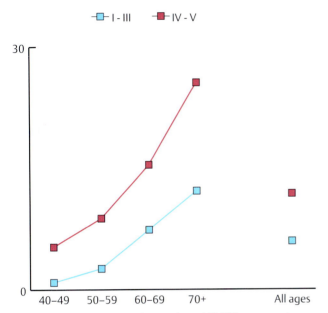

Fig. **5.14** Breast cancers detected per 100 000 women at prevalent screening, according to the mammographic pattern type and 10-year age groups.[1]

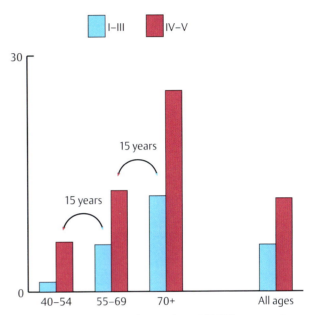

Fig. **5.15** Breast cancers detected per 100 000 women at prevalent screening, according to the mammographic pattern type and 15-year age groups.[1]

Summary

These small differences in the relative risk of developing breast cancer that are related to the mammographic parenchymal patterns are not of major importance in comparison to the ever-increasing risk every woman encounters as she ages. Furthermore, since the vast majority of women in an asymptomatic population will have mammographic Patterns I–III, most breast cancers will be found in this so-called low-risk group, as were 72 % of the breast cancers in the Kopparberg material.

Chapter 6: Finding Breast Cancer When It Is Still Small: Rationale and Scientific Evidence

A New Era in the Diagnosis and Treatment of Breast Cancer

■ Detection of Breast Cancer in the Preclinical Phase

Prevention of death from breast cancer is the primary goal of all physicians dealing with breast diseases. The approaches traditionally taken to accomplish this goal were doomed to limited success because, until quite recently the therapeutic regimens were applied to predominantly late-stage breast cancer. Advanced breast cancer is more likely associated with systemic disease at the time of diagnosis and treatment and is strongly associated with breast cancer death.

The outcome of women diagnosed with late-stage breast cancer has been poor regardless of the therapy given, as has been convincingly demonstrated by the NSABP trials.[15] However, **the most important finding of this study** was the considerably more favorable outcome of women with node-negative breast cancers as compared to node-positive cases, demonstrating the value of treating breast cancer at an earlier stage.[15]

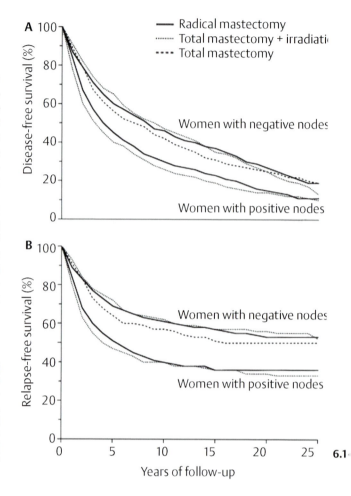

Fig. **6.1**-1   Disease-free survival **(A)** and relapse-free survival **(B)** during 25 years of follow-up after surgery among women with clinically negative axillary nodes and women with clinically positive axillary nodes. (Reprinted from Fisher B, Jeong JH, Anderson S, Bryant J, Fisher ER, Wolmark N. Twenty-five-year follow-up of a randomized trial comparing radical mastectomy, total mastectomy, and total mastectomy followed by irradiation. N Engl J Med 2002; 347: 567–575. Copyright © 2002 Massachusetts Medical Society. All rights reserved.)

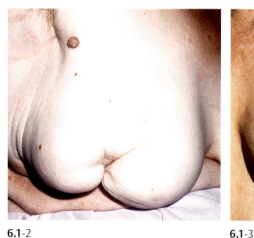

6.1-2

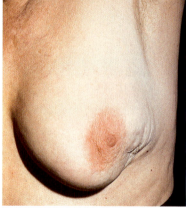

6.1-3

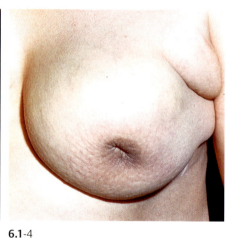

6.1-4

Fig. **6.1**-2 to 4   Examples of advanced breast cancers.

Furthermore, women with mammographically detected, nonpalpable breast cancer localized to the breast will have excellent survival, again irrespective of the mode of treatment.[38] (Fig. **6.2**). Figure **6.2**-1shows the results of 20-year follow-up of 852 invasive breast cancer cases from the Swedish Two-County randomized controlled mammographic screening trial. These cancers were all smaller than 15 mm at the time of operation. The prerequisite for this excellent long-term survival was early detection combined with surgical removal of the tumors. Such an outcome has never been accomplished by any combination of therapeutic regimens in the absence of early detection. We are led to the inescapable conclusion that **the outcome of each woman with breast cancer depends mostly upon whether the treatment is given early or late in the natural history of the disease, rather than upon the particular mode of treatment given.**

The challenge has been to develop and perfect a method for finding early breast cancer.

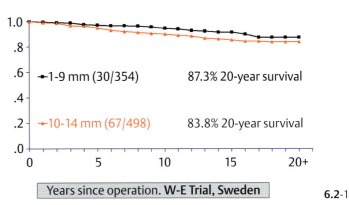

Fig. **6.2**-1   Twenty-year outcome of patients with 1–9 mm and 10–14 mm breast cancer. Data are from the Two-County (W-E) Swedish Trial.

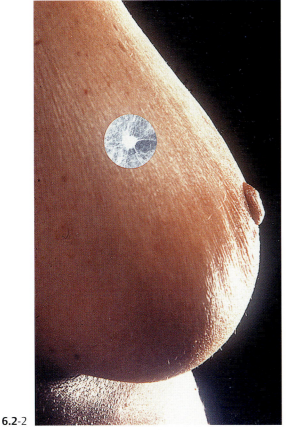

6.2-2

Fig. **6.2**-2   Artist's rendition of a nonpalpable but mammographically detectable breast cancer.

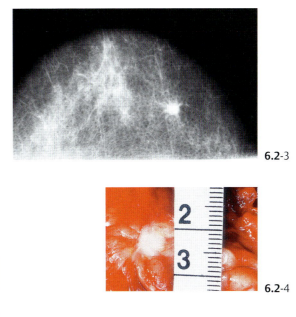

Fig. **6.2**-3 & 4   Mammographic image and specimen photograph of a nonpalpable breast cancer.

■ A New Paradigm: Prevent Breast Cancer from Growing to Advanced Stages

Removing a breast cancer early in its preclinical detectable phase, before it has developed viable metastases, gives promise for a major improvement in breast cancer control. Achieving the potential benefits of early detection required the development of an imaging method capable of finding tumors in an asymptomatic population long before they become palpable. It had become evident by the late 1970s that mammography was sufficiently developed to detect a high proportion of ductal carcinoma in situ (DCIS) and small, impalpable invasive breast cancers. The time difference between mammographic and clinical detectability is the so-called **sojourn time** (preclinical, but mammographically detectable phase) (Fig. **6.3**). This time difference, an expression of tumor growth, varies considerably according to tumor type and patient's age.[34, 35, 37, 41] Due to a number of potential biases, it was necessary to test the hypothesis that intervening at an earlier, preclinical stage in the natural history of the disease would indeed have a significant impact upon the mortality from breast cancer. The best investigative methodology—randomized controlled trials in a defined population with disease specific mortality as the end point—was used to answer this question. The results of these trials published during the 1980s and 1990s represented a breakthrough in the approach to controlling breast cancer. The trials demonstrated that the natural history of breast cancer could be significantly altered by early detection combined with effective therapy.[36, 40–49] A new era in the diagnosis and treatment of breast cancer was thus opened.

The first of these studies that successfully demonstrated a significant reduction in mortality from breast cancer achieved through mammographic screening, was the Swedish Two-County Trial[36] (Fig. **6.4**). The results clearly demonstrated that the prerequisite for decreasing mortality from the disease is a significant decrease in the incidence of advanced-stage breast cancer (Fig. **6.5**). Such a decrease can be accomplished by finding the high-risk breast cancer cases earlier in their natural history, before they have spread viable metastases. The striking association between the rate of advanced cancers and the subsequent mortality from breast cancer emphasizes the necessity of acting to prevent breast cancers from progressing to advanced stage (Figs. **6.4** and **6.5**).[43] Mammography screening that, for whatever reason, fails to decrease the rate of advanced breast cancer will subsequently fail to decrease breast cancer mortality.[21]

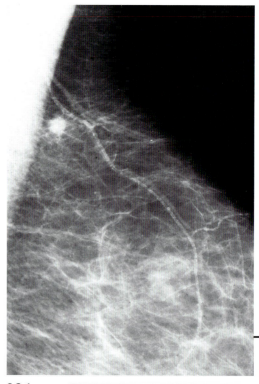

6.3-1

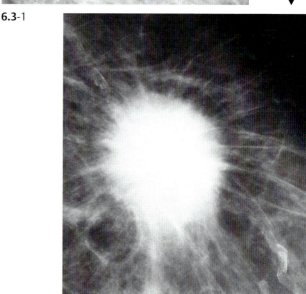

6.3

Fig. **6.3**　Screening with mammography can move the time of diagnosis of breast cancer from a palpable tumor to an earlier, nonpalpable stage.

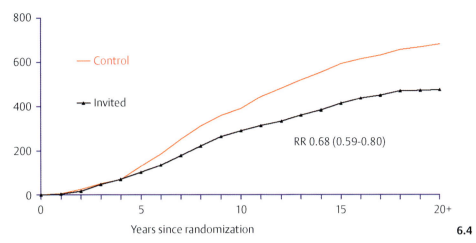

6.4

Fig. **6.4** Cumulative breast cancer deaths in women aged 40–74 at randomization. These data from the Two-County (W-E) Swedish Trial show a 32% significant reduction in breast cancer death among women invited to mammographic screening in comparison to those not invited. (RR = relative risk)

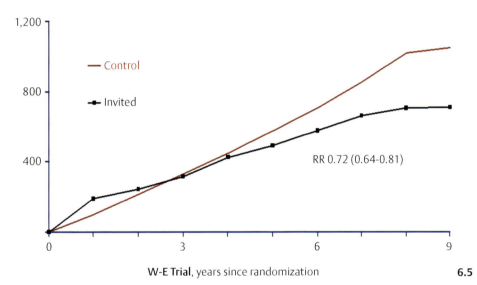

W-E Trial, years since randomization   **6.5**

Fig. **6.5** Cumulative incidence of Stage II or more advanced breast cancers in women aged 40–74 at randomization. Data are from the Two-County (W-E) Swedish Trial. A significant decrease in the incidence rate of advanced breast cancers is a prerequisite for the subsequent decrease in mortality from breast cancer.

■ The Most Important Task Is to Prevent Breast Cancer from Developing to Large, Advanced Tumors

Due to the close correlation between the incidence rate of advanced breast cancer and the mortality from the disease in a population, the frequency of advanced breast cancer is a sensitive predictor of the forthcoming breast cancer mortality in that population. Until recently, the major emphasis in combating the disease has been upon the development of combinations of therapeutic methods effective at all stages of the disease, particularly advanced, metastatic cancer. The results of the mammography screening trials demonstrated that breast cancer is not a systemic disease from its inception; it is rather a progressive disease, whose progression can be arrested by early detection in the preclinical detectable phase.[33, 39]

The recognition that early detection could more effectively lead to the desired goal, i.e., decreasing the rate of advanced tumors and the subsequent mortality from breast cancer, can be considered a paradigm shift in the approach to controlling breast cancer. This new paradigm focuses upon preventing breast cancer from growing to the metastatic stage. The best method to date is to offer high-quality mammography screening to asymptomatic women at regular intervals.

Paradigm shift for controlling breast cancer

Traditional emphasis	Modern emphasis
Applies various therapeutic combinations to all stages, including advanced disease	Employs early detection to arrest disease progression to advanced stage

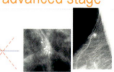

Fig. **6.6**   The shift to the new paradigm.

A new paradigm

A window of opportunity during the preclinical detectable phase

The tumor has not yet spread viable metastases, therefore curable by local treatment alone

Fig. **6.7**   The new paradigm.

Two Alternative Approaches

1 Development of therapeutic regimens effective at all stages, particularly against advanced cancer

Fig. **6.8**-1 Advanced breast cancer.

Fig. **6.8**-2 Bone metastasis from advanced breast cancer.

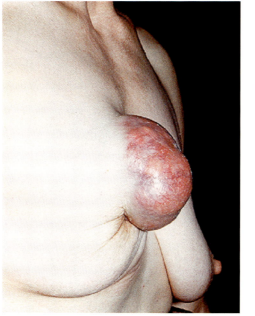
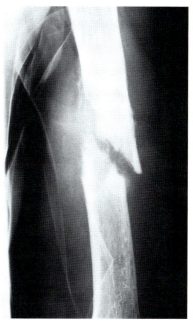

6.8-1
6.8-2

2 Prevention of the disease from progressing to advanced stages by early detection and surgical removal

Fig. **6.9**-1 to 4 Screen-detected 7 mm × 7 mm unifocal mucinous carcinoma.

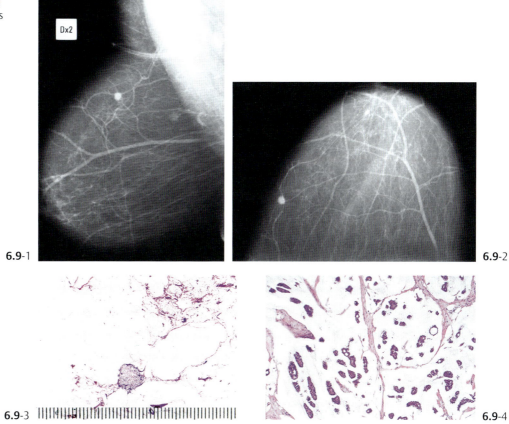

6.9-1
6.9-2
6.9-3
6.9-4

■ Nonpalpable, Screen-Detected Breast Cancer

Example 6.1

A 70-year-old asymptomatic woman, screening case. Physical examination shows no abnormality.

Ex. **6.1**-1 to 4   Left breast, MLO (**6.1**-1) and CC (**6.1**-2) projections. There are two small circular lesions on the mammogram, each measuring < 10 mm. The higher-density lesion (box) is ill-defined on microfocus magnification images taken at call-back (**6.1**-3, **6.1**-4). This is a mammographically malignant tumor. The low-density lesion (arrow, **6.1**-2) corresponds to a wart on the skin.

Ex. **6.1**-5   Ultrasound confirms the mammographic diagnosis.

Ex. **6.1**-6 to 8   Cytology from stereotactic FNAB shows malignant cells.

Ex. **6.1**-9   Specimen radiograph following preoperative localization using the bracketing technique. The tumor has been removed with wide margins.

Ex. **6.1**-10   Large-section histology demonstrates a 5 mm solitary tumor surrounded by adipose tissue.

Ex. **6.1**-11   Magnification radiography of the thinly sliced specimen.

Ex. **6.1**-12 & 13   Low- and high-power histological images demonstrate the structures of this 5 mm × 5 mm well-differentiated invasive ductal carcinoma.

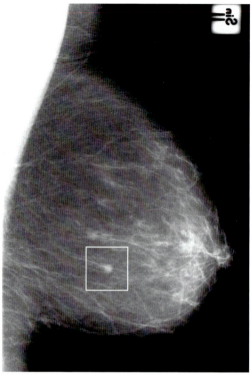

Ex. **6.1**-1

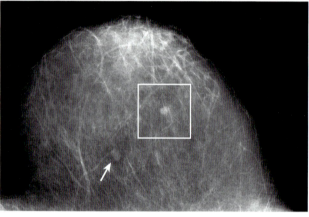

Ex. **6.1**-2

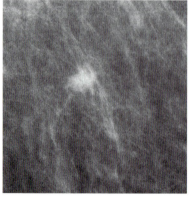

Ex. **6.1**-3

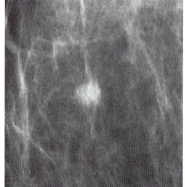

Ex.

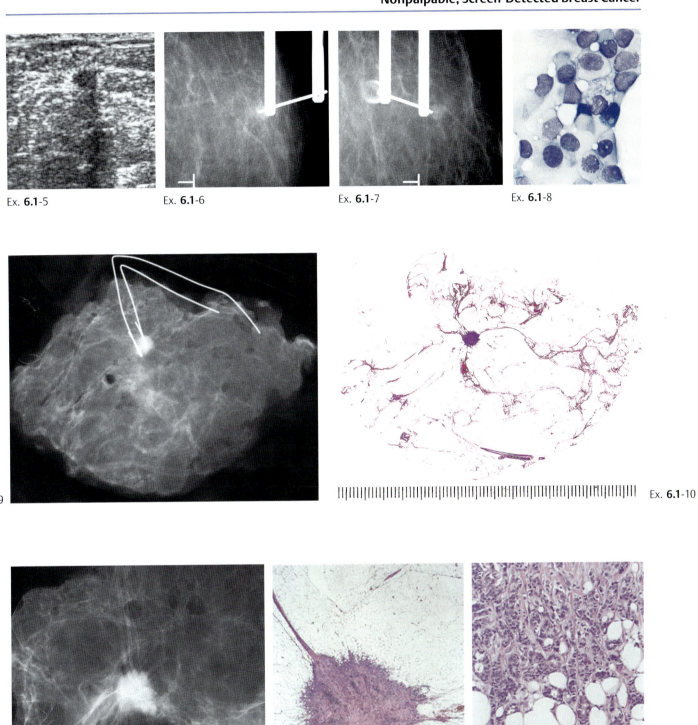

Ex. **6.1**-5

Ex. **6.1**-6

Ex. **6.1**-7

Ex. **6.1**-8

1-9

Ex. **6.1**-10

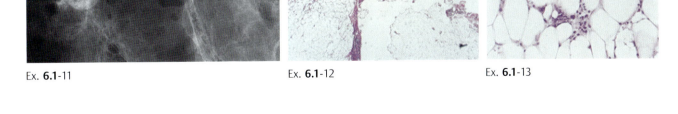

Ex. **6.1**-11

Ex. **6.1**-12

Ex. **6.1**-13

■ Mechanism for the Impact of Screening

The effect of screening will be primarily mediated through its impact upon the first-generation prognostic factors:
- **Tumor size**
- **Node status**
- **Histological malignancy grade**

Tumor Size

Regular mammography screening makes possible the detection of many (although not all) breast cancers early in their preclinical phase. Figure **6.10** graphically demonstrates the effect of tumor size upon long-term outcome. Treating breast cancer at its earliest phases leads to a profoundly better long-term outcome than can be accomplished by the use of any combination of therapeutic methods against large breast cancers.

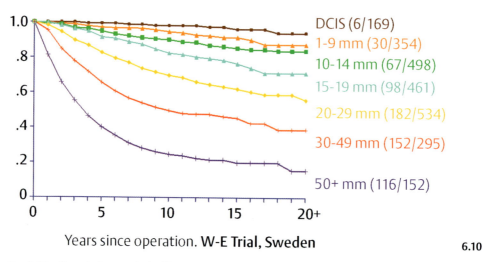

Fig. **6.10** Cumulative survival of breast cancer patients aged 40–74 as a function of tumor size.

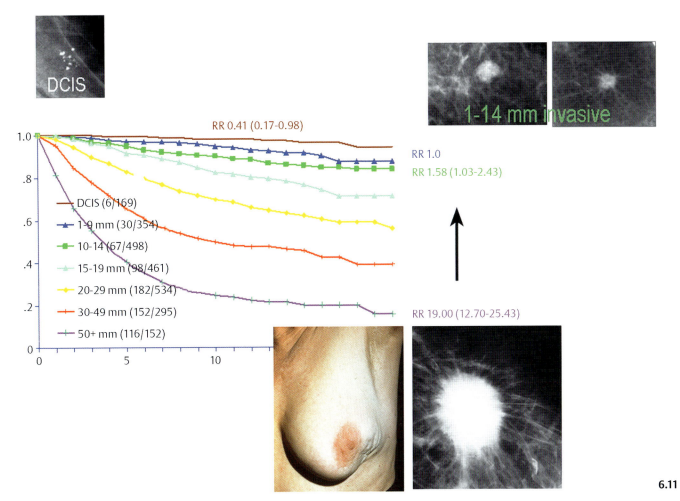

Fig. **6.11** Detecting breast cancer in 1–14 mm size ranges results in a 19-fold improvement in outcome. An equivalent improvement cannot be accomplished by any specific therapy or combination of therapeutic methods.

Node Status

With decreasing tumor size, the risk of node positivity decreases substantially. Data from the Swedish Two-County Trial (Table **6.1**) show that well over 90% of 1–9 mm breast cancers have no axillary lymph node metastases, regardless of histological malignancy grade.[35] Silverstein and colleagues confirm these findings and suggest using clinical and pathological features of the primary lesion to estimate the risk of axillary lymph node metastases.[29]

Kaufman and colleagues developed a treatment scale for the axillary management of breast cancer patients.[19] This scale is based on the preoperative values of tumor size, histological malignancy grade, and patient age to assist the clinician in relegating the patient to one of three axillary management groups: no axillary surgery, sentinel node mapping, or axillary dissection.

Table 6.**1** Axillary node positivity according to tumor size and malignancy grade for 526 invasive ductal cancers of 1–19 mm size

Size (mm)	Grade 1	Grade 2	Grade 3
1–9	2.2%	6.5%	4.9%
10–14	11.0%	18.1%	30.8%
15–19	11.2%	35.6%	32.5%

Histological Malignancy Grade

Microscopic examination of breast cancers often reveals multiple histological types and grades within the same tumor (intratumoral heterogeneity). The various tumor clones may grow at different rates. The more aggressive component(s) will grow more rapidly and may eventually dominate the histological image by the time a tumor becomes palpable. This phenomenon is interpreted as "worsening of malignancy potential," "dedifferentiation" associated with increasing tumor size. In other words, the larger the tumor, the more likely its malignancy grade has worsened (Table **6.2**).[3, 6, 11, 26, 48, 49]

Statistical evidence from the randomized controlled trials has shown that screening with mammography accomplishes a significant shift toward smaller tumor size in the population offered screening (Table **6.3**).[11] **The benefit of screening is brought about by finding the breast cancers at smaller size, with fewer lymph node metastases, and also by arresting tumor progression to higher malignancy grade** in those cases that have the propensity to dedifferentiate. Worsening of tumor malignancy potential is relatively more frequent in the age group 40–49 (81%) than in the age group 50–69 (50%).[35, 37] In women younger than 50 with palpable tumors, there is a significantly higher proportion of Grade 3 breast cancers than in older women. This may lead to the unsupported conclusion that younger women have a different spectrum of breast cancers. Alternatively, the malignancy grade of breast cancer worsens earlier and more frequently in younger women, as is supported by the data in Tables **6.4** to **6.7**. A study of the distribution of histological malignancy grade with tumor growth will help resolve this issue.

An important starting point is that **the vast majority (>80%) of breast cancers are Grade 1 or 2 in all age groups when the tumor size is 1–9 mm** (Table **6.4**).[35]

Table 6.**2** The probability of Grade 3 invasive breast cancers within a given size range (logistic regression). The larger the cancer, the higher the probability that it will be Grade 3

Size (mm)	Odds ratio
1–9	1.00
10–14	1.83
15–19	3.76
20–29	5.83
30–49	9.56
50+	9.33

Table 6.**3** Comparison of breast cancer size distribution in the control population and in the population invited to screening. There is a shift toward smaller tumor size in women invited to screening. The tumors detected at prevalence (first) screening have been deleted to avoid length bias

Size (mm)	Control (%)	Prevalence free (%)
1–9	6.7	18.7
10–14	15.4	23.3
15–19	20.5	20.8
20–29	29.7	24.0
30–49	19.9	9.2
50+	7.7	4.0

Table 6.**4** For tumors smaller than 10 mm, the proportion that are Grade 3 is similar in the three age groups shown

Tumor size (mm)	Age (years)	Grade 3 (%)
1–9	40–49	19.1
1–9	50–59	14.9
1–9	60–69	11.9

With increasing tumor size, the proportion of Grade 3 tumors increases at the expense of Grade 1 and 2 tumors in all age subgroups (Tables **6.5** to **6.7**), but this increase is considerably more rapid in younger women. By the time the tumors have reached the size of 15–19 mm, a significantly higher proportion of tumors are Grade 3 in younger women (54%) than in women aged >50 years (30.6% and 38.0%, respectively).

These data demonstrate that dedifferentiation of breast cancer in younger women occurs earlier in the preclinical detectable phase, takes place more rapidly, and occurs in a higher proportion of cases. This means that **younger women have more to gain from early detection**, provided that screening is performed at intervals sufficiently frequent to detect the more rapidly growing tumors before they have the opportunity to dedifferentiate. This is because early detection of potentially rapidly growing tumors can provide the greatest benefit.

Claims have often been made that detection of Grade 1, slowly-growing tumors by mammographic screening will have little long-term mortality benefit, since these tumors would allegedly never have caused the patient harm.[18, 22, 23] This contention ignores the fact that **breast cancer is a progressive disease** that not only grows in size but can and often does worsen in malignancy grade while it grows, as the above data clearly demonstrate.

Once a small tumor is found in a screening program, one cannot precisely predict what would have happened had the tumor not been detected and removed. It is, however, essential to detect and remove those cancers that, if not treated in their preclinical phase, would have ultimately progressed to fatal stage disease. The histological prognostic factors are used to predict patient outcome. Since the mammogram is a reflection of histology, correlation of histological and mammographic findings with long-term outcome will enable the radiologist to focus attention on the early mammographic signs of potentially fatal breast cancers.

Distribution of Histological Malignancy Grade by Tumor Size and Patient Age

Table 6.**5** Age group 40–49

Size (mm)	Grades 1 & 2 (%)	Grade 3 (%)
1–9	38 (80.9)	9 (19.1)
10–14	56 (70.0)	24 (30.0)
15–19	30 (46.2)	35 (53.8)
20–29	33 (45.2)	40 (54.8)
30+	16 (32.7)	33 (67.3)

Table 6.**6** Age group 50–59

Size (mm)	Grades 1 & 2 (%)	Grade 3 (%)
1–9	74 (85.1)	13 (14.9)
10–14	102 (73.9)	36 (26.1)
15–19	86 (69.4)	38 (30.6)
20–29	69 (47.9)	75 (52.1)
30+	22 (37.9)	36 (62.1)

Table 6.**7** Age group 60–69

Size (mm)	Grades 1 & 2 (%)	Grade 3 (%)
1–9	126 (88.1)	17 (11.9)
10–14	138 (75.8)	44 (24.2)
15–19	103 (62.0)	63 (38.0)
20–29	94 (51.1)	90 (48.9)
30+	40 (37.0)	68 (63.0)

■ The Relative Benefits of Downward Stage Shifting

Most breast cancers are **invasive** at the time of diagnosis, even those found at screening. On the mammogram, the vast majority of histologically proven breast cancers (64%) are noncalcified stellate or circular lesions, while calcifications comprise only a fraction of the findings (Fig. **6.12**). The mortality benefit from early detection results primarily from detecting invasive tumors at a smaller size than would have occurred without screening. Downward stage shifting from invasive breast cancer Stage II or worse to invasive Stage I tumors accounts for most of the mortality benefit. (Fig. **6.12**-1 to 6).[12, 50] Although there is a possibility that mammographic screening might lead to the detection of an excess number of breast cancer cases that would not otherwise have been diagnosed in the woman's lifetime (so-called "overdiagnosis"), careful analysis of the data showed no significant evidence of overdiagnosis of invasive cancers. Some DCIS cases detected at screening can be considered to belong to the "overdiagnosis" category, but on an individual basis it is not possible to predict which case would not have progressed to invasive cancer. In practical terms, **emphasis should be placed upon finding subtle spiculated and/or circular tumor masses that represent invasive carcinoma.** This is the most effective means we have for decreasing the rate of advanced breast cancer and mortality from the disease.

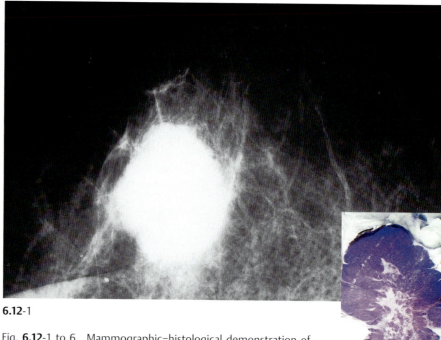

6.12-1

Fig. **6.12**-1 to 6   Mammographic–histological demonstration of downward stage shifting from a palpable, advanced cancer to a nonpalpable invasive carcinoma and to DCIS.

6.1.

95% of the mortality benefit originates from downward stage shifting of invasive breast cancers; 65% from Stage II–IV to Stage I; an additional 30% of the benefit originates from downward shifting within these stages.

Downward stage shifting

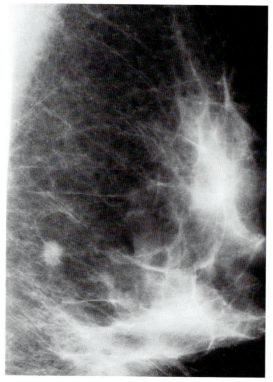

6.12-3

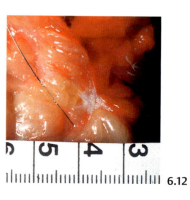

6.12

While removal of **in-situ carcinoma** may be important, the benefit in terms of mortality reduction is considerably less and tends to occur much later relative to the benefits of downward stage shifting from advanced invasive carcinoma to early invasive tumors. In practical terms, **the detection of calcifications on the mammogram is less important than the detection of small, invasive tumors.**

5% of the mortality benefit originates from downward stage shifting of small invasive breast cancers to DCIS.

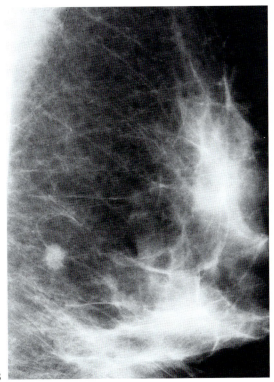

6.12-3

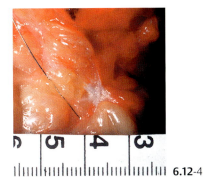

6.12-4

Downward stage shifting

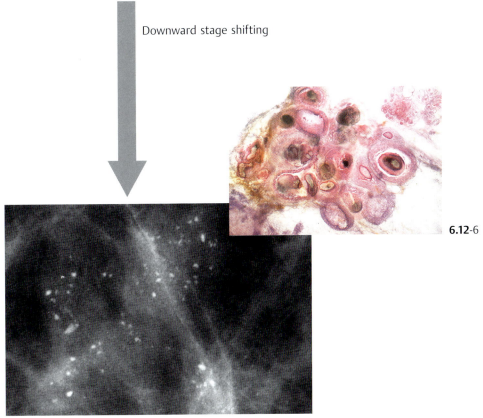

6.12-6

6.12-5

■ Mechanism for the Effect of Early Detection of Breast Cancer: Comments and Conclusions[41]

- The data indicate that the beneficial effect of screening is mediated mainly through its effect on tumor size, node status, and histological grade. **Mammographic screening can detect breast cancers in their preclinical, nonpalpable phase**, when they have, on average, a smaller size, less frequent lymph node metastases, and a more favorable histological grade in comparison to breast cancers detected by palpation.
- Tumor size of an invasive carcinoma will increase over time. The node status is also a time-related tumor characteristic. Tumor size and node status can therefore be used to quantify whether or not the time of diagnosis has been moved to an earlier point in time in comparison with detection by palpation. For screening to be effective, breast cancer should be detected as early in its natural history as possible, particularly the high-risk cases. **One important aim of mammographic screening is to detect invasive breast cancers when they are still in the size range of 1–14 mm and are node-negative.**[40]
- **The prognostic value of histological grade decreases with decreasing tumor size**. When the cancer is less than 10 mm in size, the histological grade no longer has useful prognostic significance partly because all these small tumors have an excellent prognosis, regardless of their histological grade, partly because women with Grade 2 invasive cancer have a slightly poorer outcome than women with Grade 3, 1–9 mm invasive cancer (Fig. **6.13**).
- While the **histological prognostic factors** have little predictive value for 1–9 mm invasive tumors, the "**mammographic prognostic features**" can successfully discriminate between (1) the vast majority of tumors with an extremely good long-term outcome (98% 15-year survival with surgical treatment alone) and (2) a small group of 1–9 mm cancers with high fatality (55% 15-year survival despite high rate of mastectomy).[32] The group with excellent prognosis comprising 86% of the 1–9 mm invasive breast cancers had a stellate or circular mammographic appearance with or without associated noncasting calcifications. The cases in the smaller group with high fatality had casting-type calcifications as a dominant feature on the mammogram. Tumors of this group behave as tumors do in the size-range 20–50 mm and should be reclassified accordingly. The very characteristic mammographic appearance of these cases (presence of casting-type calcifications) makes their identification easy. The present T1 a–c classification of breast cancers should be reevaluated to include the discriminatory mammographic features, since this classification is presently incapable of reliably discriminating between patients with exceptionally good (98%) and poor (55%) long-term prognosis (Fig. **6.14**).

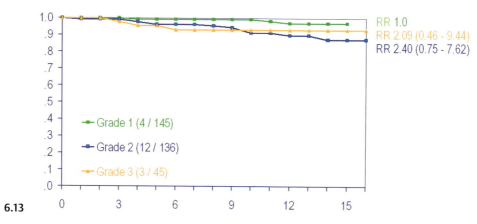

6.13

Fig. **6.13** Cumulative survival of women aged 40–74 with 1–9 mm invasive breast cancer by histological grade. Breast cancer deaths/number of breast cancer cases are shown according to years since operation. The relative risk estimates (RR) for long-term outcome are also shown (RR = 1.0 for Grade 1 invasive cancers; RR = 2.09 for Grade 3 invasive cancers; RR = 2.40 for Grade 2 invasive cancers).

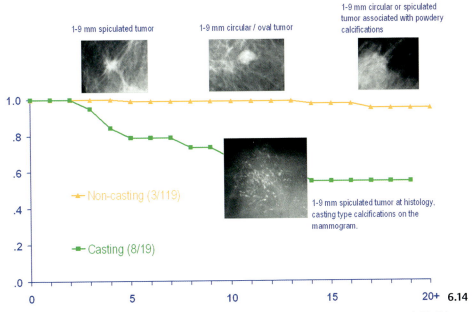

Fig. **6.14** Cumulative survival by mammographic prognostic features. Women aged 40–74 with 1–9 mm invasive breast cancer. The use of these mammographic prognostic features has a powerful discriminating effect in predicting the long-term outcome of women with 1–9 mm invasive cancers.

- It is more difficult to detect breast cancers while they are still node-negative, 1–14 mm size, and of lower histological grade in the age group 40–49. When tumors with these characteristics are detected, their outcome is not age dependent. Figure **6.15** demonstrates the excellent and essentially identical long-term survival of 40–49-year-old and 50–74-year-old women. Figures **6.16–6.18** demonstrate the long-term outcome of breast cancer cases as a function of tumor size, node status,

and malignancy grade in three different age groups. The data show no difference in long-term survival related to age. Therefore, early detection can reduce mortality from breast cancer throughout the age range 40–70 provided that the tumors are diagnosed and removed at similar size, node status, and histological grade. This will require a shorter interscreening interval in women aged 40–49 due to, on average, a shorter preclinical detectable period.[30, 46]

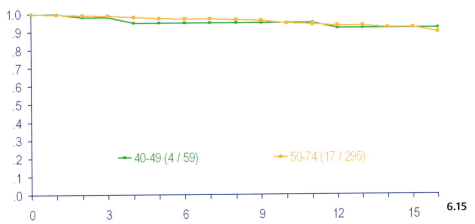

Fig. **6.15** Cumulative survival of women with 1–9 mm invasive breast cancer according to age . The long-term survival is equivalent in both 40–49 and 50–74 year age groups. Data from the W-E trial; horizontal axis is years since operation.

Cumulative Survival by Tumor Size and Age in the Two-County Swedish Screening Trial

Fig. **6.16**-1 to 3 Demonstration of long-term survival of breast cancer cases as a function of tumor size in three different age groups. The data show similar long-term outcomes in the three age groups. The risk of dying from a >2.0 cm breast cancer is 3.52, 3.82, and 5.89, respectively, for the age groups compared to the risk of dying from a breast cancer <2.0 cm.

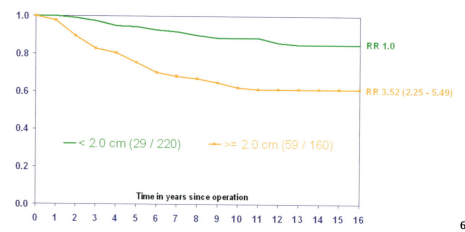

Fig. **6.16**-1   Age group 40–49.

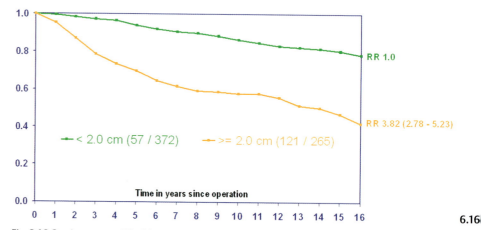

Fig.**6.16**-2   Age group 50–59.

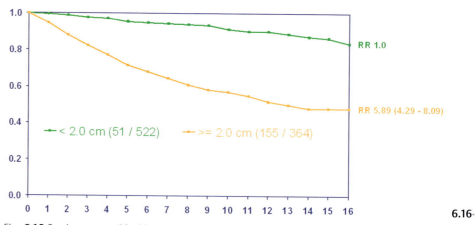

Fig. **6.16**-3   Age group 60–69.

Cumulative Survival by Node Status and Age in the Two-County Swedish Screening Trial

Fig. **6.17**-1 to 3   Demonstration of long-term survival of breast cancer cases as a function of node status in three different age groups. The data show similar long-term outcomes in the three age groups. The risk of dying from a node-positive breast cancer is 3.26, 4.17, and 5.08, respectively, for these age groups compared to the risk of dying from a node-negative breast cancer.

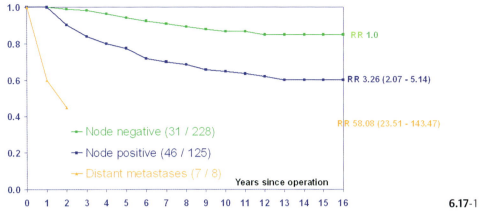

Fig. **6.17**-1   Age group 40–49.

6.17-1

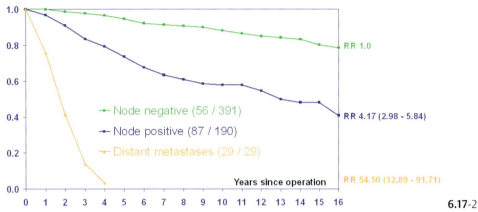

Fig. **6.17**-2   Age group 50–59.

6.17-2

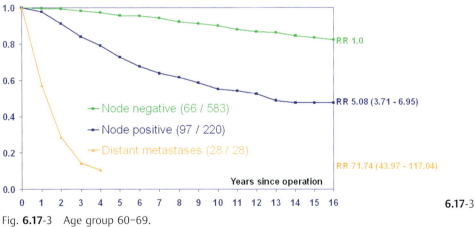

Fig. **6.17**-3   Age group 60–69.

6.17-3

Cumulative Survival by Histological Grade and Age in the Two-County Swedish Trial

Fig. **6.18**-1 to 3 Demonstration of long-term survival of breast cancer cases as a function of histological grade in three different age groups. The data show similar long-term outcomes in the three age groups. The risk of dying from a Grade 2 breast cancer is 2.80, 2.33, and 3.51, respectively, for the age groups compared to the risk of dying from a Grade 1 breast cancer. The corresponding relative risk values for Grade 3 invasive carcinoma are 7.11, 4.44, and 8.08.

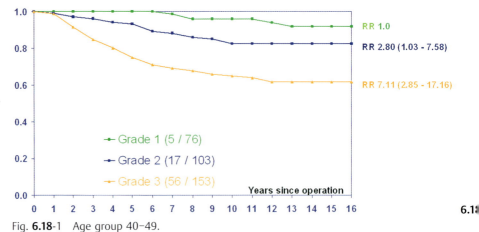

Fig. **6.18**-1 Age group 40–49.

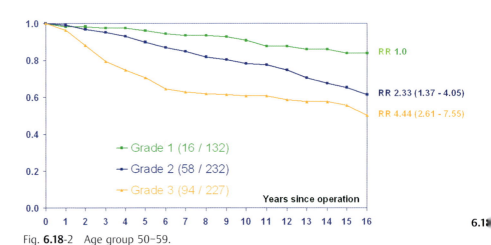

Fig. **6.18**-2 Age group 50–59.

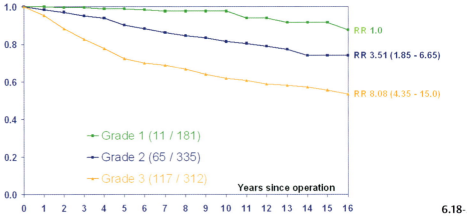

Fig. **6.18**-3 Age group 60–69.

184

■ Summary

- Correlating the tumor characteristics with the outcome of each individual case in the Two-County Trial has provided measures that can predict the effectiveness of other screening trials.[40] These measures include:
  - The vast majority of tumors found at screening should be invasive cancers. Finding DCIS cases will have only a small and delayed effect upon the mortality from breast cancer.[50]
  - 50–60% of all invasive tumors should be < 15 mm in diameter.
  - At least 30% of the poorly differentiated invasive cancers should be < 15 mm in diameter.
  - Analysis of histological grade and type of the breast cancer cases found at screening will further help predict whether a mortality decrease will follow and, if so, when.[50]
- Translating these measures into guidelines, the radiologist's goal is to find as many breast cancers as possible when the tumors are:
  - < 15 mm, preferably < 10 mm in diameter. This is particularly important for Grade 3 tumors.
  - Node-negative.
  - Still of histological malignancy Grade 1–2 (before the malignancy grade "worsens" to Grade 3).
- The biological parameters affecting and limiting the ability of mammography to detect breast cancer at its earlier phases make this a difficult enough task. We should therefore **strive to optimize all factors within our control** in order to maximize the benefits of early breast cancer detection.
- The results of the randomized controlled trials have demonstrated that **breast cancer is a progressive disease**, which does not behave as a systemic disease from its inception. Arresting disease progression in the preclinical detectable phase has a significant impact on the outcome. The point at which this progression is arrested (i.e., the time of diagnosis during the natural history of each individual case) is crucial in determining the outcome.

- The proposal that breast cancer is a **"systemic disease from its inception"**[14] is either mistaken or is not relevant to the treatment of tumors diagnosed while node-negative and less than 15 mm in diameter, as data from the W-E Trial clearly demonstrate.[39]
- Breast cancer **should be treated in its preclinical phase** if we are to save lives of women with the disease.[8]
- There is little evidence on a population basis for a significant mortality benefit from newer therapeutic methods in women who did not attend screening. When breast cancer mortality in women aged 20–39 at diagnosis (never screened) is compared over two consecutive 20-year periods, there is no statistically significant improvement in breast cancer mortality on a population level (RR = 0.73, 95% CI 0.50 to 1.06), despite the fact that 61% of the patients received modern chemotherapy. After adjustment for age, self-selection bias, and changes in incidence in the 40–49 age group, mortality from breast cancer was highly significantly reduced in women who attended screening (RR = 0.52, 95% CI 0.40 to 0.67), but not in women who declined to attend screening (RR = 0.81, 95% CI 0.60 to 1.09).[25, 31, 45]
- The United Kingdom used to have the highest breast cancer mortality rate in the world; ten years after the introduction of nationwide mammography screening, there was a sharp decline in breast cancer mortality rates. **Denmark, where screening is being slowly introduced** amid strenuous opposition, **currently has the highest breast cancer death rate in Europe.** There is no evidence that treatment of breast cancer is any different in Denmark from what it is in Sweden or the United Kingdom, but screening reaches only a minority of Danish women.[13]
- "Based on evidence accrued over decades of scientific research and countless, independent expert peer-reviews of the study design, data and conclusions of the trials, **the scientific foundation for the value of early detection with mammography is sound.**"[9]

The Impact of Early Detection on Breast Cancer Death

■ Mammography Screening and Treatment in Early Stage Can Dramatically Reduce Mortality from Breast Cancer in a Population

The new paradigm for breast cancer control emphasizes preventing breast cancer from developing to metastatic disease. The **randomized control trials** conducted over four decades demonstrated that invitation to regular mammographic screening can significantly reduce the rate of advanced breast cancer and subsequently also reduce mortality from the disease[1, 24, 27, 36, 42] As a result, **service screening programs** have been introduced in many countries. Evaluation of such programs has already confirmed that organized mammographic screening can also substantially reduce breast cancer mortality in a population. When evaluating service screening programs, there is an opportunity not only to compare breast cancer death in a population before and after the introduction of mammographic screening, but also to compare breast cancer death in contemporaneous women who actually attended versus those who declined participation in screening. When evaluating the results, one has, however, to take into account other, potentially influential factors such as an increased public awareness of the disease, the improved availability of diagnostic and treatment facilities, improvements in therapy and patient management, etc.[10, 17, 20, 25, 44, 45, 47]

The results of a comprehensive service screening program, covering one-third of the Swedish population, demon-strated a 40–45 % mortality reduction among women who actually attended mammographic screening. The vast majority of this benefit could be attributed to the earlier detection of breast carcinoma.[10]

Another study, spanning a 40-year period, compared death from breast cancers diagnosed in 40- to 69-year-old women during the 20-year period before the introduction of screening with death from breast cancers diagnosed during the 20-year period after the introduction of screening. After adjustment for age, self-selection bias, and changes in incidence, there was a highly significant 44 % reduction in breast cancer mortality in those women who regularly attended screening. The corresponding reduction was 16 % for women who did not attend screening, conclusively demonstrating that a considerable improvement of patient outcome requires treatment of the disease following detection in the preclinical phase.[45]

Figure **6.19** demonstrates the changes in cumulative survival of breast cancer patients over a 40-year period in Dalarna and Ostergotland counties of Sweden. During the 20 years before the introduction of screening, fewer than half of the breast cancer cases survived the disease (long-term survival curves from 1958 to 1967 and from 1968 to 1977). Following the introduction of mammographic screening, there was a dramatic improvement in the 20-year survival among the women who actually attended screening (RR = 0.29, 95 % CI 0.25 to 0.33). However, those women who declined screening during the period 1988–1998 had relatively little improvement in survival compared to the outcome of all women with breast cancer before screening was introduced, despite the use of modern therapeutic regimens (RR = 0.80, 95 % CI 0.64 to 1.01).

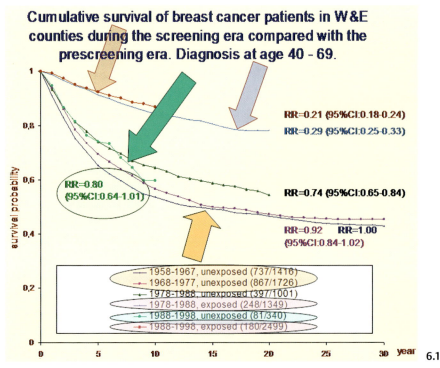

Fig. **6.19** Cumulative survival of breast cancer patients in the Swedish Dalarna and Ostergotland counties during the first 20 years following the introduction of screening compared with survival of breast cancer patients diagnosed during a 20-year period in the prescreening era. Diagnosis at age 40–69. Screen-detected and interval cancers in combination form the "exposed" group. Cases diagnosed outside of screening during the screening period and prior to the introduction of screening form the "unexposed" groups.[45]

■ Conclusion

The massive amount of data collected in the randomized controlled trials over the past four decades, combined with the supporting data from the ongoing service screening programs, confirms that **the most effective way to control breast cancer is to prevent it from growing to advanced stages by arresting its progression with early detection.** In their Editorial,[4] Cady and Michelson summarize: "[The] report from Sweden results from a nearly 30-year diligent and meticulous study of mammographic screening and sets the direction for our future efforts. The overall population impact is so impressive that technical concerns about false-positive and false-negative mammographic findings, while important and requiring improvement, can be put in perspective and should be secondary to this major public health achievement. This is especially important considering the difficulty, expense, and morbidity of our current focus on efforts to control poor prognosis and larger palpable breast carcinoma by systemic drugs and radical regional treatments."

The ultimate purpose of this book is to help physicians learn how to find as many breast cancers as possible in the preclinical stage.

Factors Influencing Early Detection

■ Multiple Factors That Determine How Early in the Preclinical Detectable Phase Individual Malignant Tumors Can Be Detected

Human, technical, and biological factors may all influence the time point at which a tumor is detected. The *human* and *technical* factors can and must be optimized to enable the earliest possible detection of breast cancer. The *human* factors can be most effectively improved through special training, preferably by subspecialization of radiology technologists and radiologists in breast imaging. The radiologist's skill in the perception and analysis of breast diseases and the technologist's skills in patient positioning are of vital importance (Chapters 7 and 9). *Technical* factors affecting image quality need to be optimized. The *biological* factors affecting breast cancer detection are largely beyond our control. The three major biological factors are:

- The nature of the surrounding breast tissue
- Heterogeneity of breast cancer at histology

- The progressive nature of breast cancer, including the variability in the rate of disease progression as a function of histological type and patient age.

The Nature of the Surrounding Breast Tissue

The diagnostic threshold may be considerably influenced by interference from the overlying normal breast tissue, which can be classified into five mammographic parenchymal patterns (Chapters 1 to 5).[16] Dense surrounding tissue (Patterns I, IV, and V) may seriously affect the detection of noncalcified small circular and stellate invasive cancers. When abnormal lesions develop within a breast that contains primarily adipose tissue, these lesions can be detected at the size of a few millimeters. The surrounding tissue has less of an influence on the detection of calcifications. To help overcome the limitations of detecting small invasive tumors in dense breasts, one must also rely upon indirect signs, such as parenchymal contour changes (Figs. **6.20** to **6.22**) and subtle architectural distortion (Figs. **6.23** and **6.24**).

Fig. **6.20**   Schematic image of parenchymal contour retraction of the posterior contour (tent-sign).

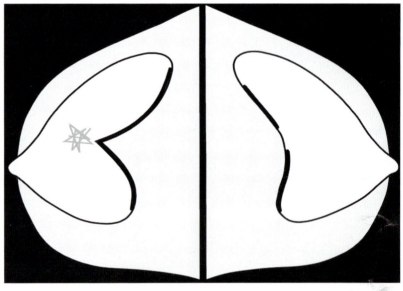

6.2

Fig. **6.21**-1 & 2   Parenchymal contour change is a useful indirect sign and may be the only sign leading to the detection of small invasive tumors without calcifications.

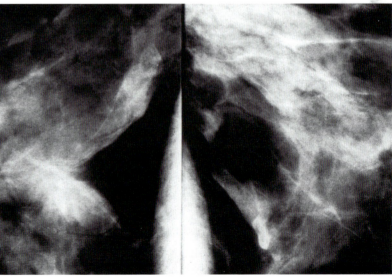

6.21-1

6.2

Ancillary imaging methods, including breast ultrasonography and occasionally breast magnetic resonance imaging, can provide additional information in selected cases. Unfortunately, a few cancers will escape detection by all imaging modalities in the preclinical phase and will eventually be detected by palpation. This is to be expected since breast cancer is a disease with many subtypes of widely differing histological and mammographic appearance; in addition, the mammographic parenchymal patterns of normal breasts vary considerably, and some of them may seriously interfere with the detection of small tumors.

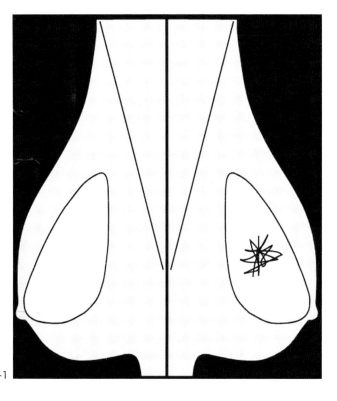

6.22-1

Fig. **6.22**-1 & 2   Schematic images of architectural distortion.

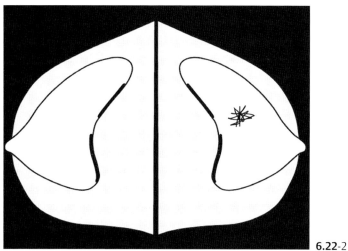

6.22-2

6.22-4

Fig. **6.22**-3 & 4   Detail of the left MLO and CC projections with architectural distortion.

2-3

Morphological Heterogeneity of Breast Cancer at Histology

The Disease We Call Breast Cancer Is, at Histology, a Heterogeneous Group of Numerous Disease Subtypes

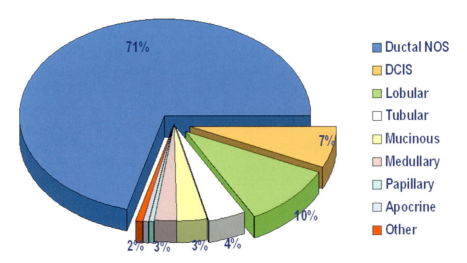

Fig. **6.23** Distribution of breast cancer subtypes.

The most frequently occurring invasive breast cancer is termed invasive ductal carcinoma NOS (not otherwise specified), in all age subgroups and irrespective of detection mode (clinical examination, mammographic screening, breast ultrasound, etc.). One-third of all invasive ductal carcinomas are associated with some of the special forms of breast cancers such as tubular cancer, invasive lobular carcinoma, colloid cancer, etc. The special forms of invasive breast cancers account for about 20–25 % of all invasive malignancies in the breast. Figures **6.24**-1 to 10 demonstrate the histological heterogeneity of different breast cancer subtypes using low-power large-section histological images.

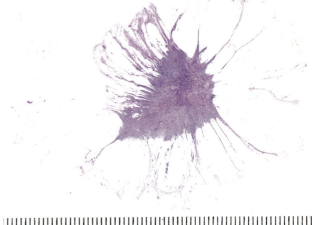

Fig. **6.24**-1 Low-power large-section histological image of a moderately differentiated invasive ductal carcinoma.

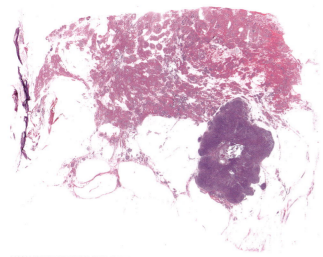

Fig. **6.24**-2 Medullary cancer.

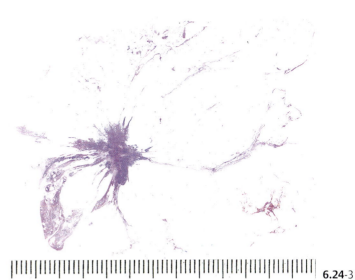

Fig. **6.24**-3 Well-differentiated invasive ductal carcinoma.

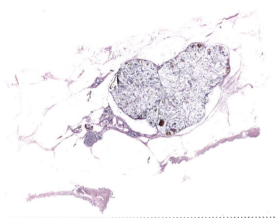

Fig. **6.24**-4 Colloid cancer.

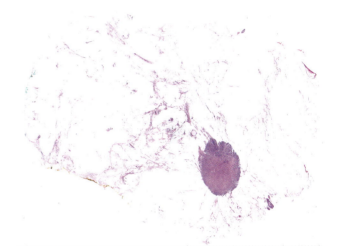

Fig. **6.24**-5 Well-differentiated invasive ductal carcinoma.

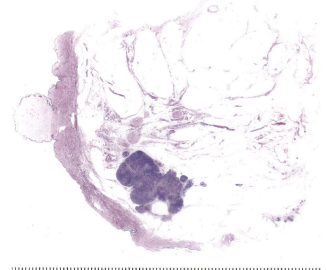

Fig. **6.24**-6 Invasive papillary carcinoma.

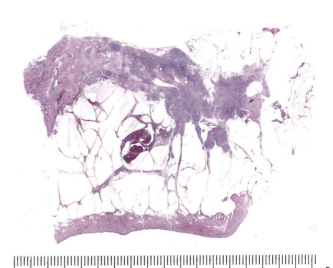

Fig. **6.24**-7 Invasive lobular carcinoma, classic type.

Morphological Heterogeneity of Breast Cancer at Histology

Fig. **6.24**-8   Intracystic papillary carcinoma.

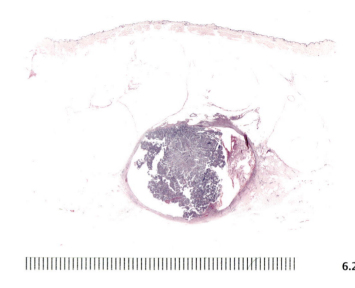

6.2

Fig. **6.24**-9   Multifocal invasive ductal carcinomas.

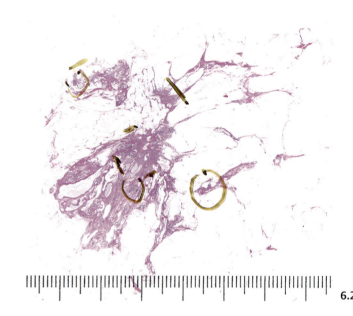

6.2

Fig. **6.24**-10   Extensive in-situ carcinoma.

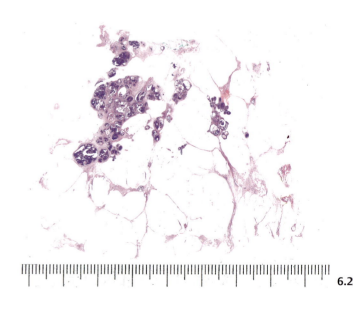

6.2

Intratumor Heterogeneity

Microscopic examination may often reveal one or more histological subtypes within the same tumor. This intratumor heterogeneity can be seen on the mammogram as, for example, a collection of microcalcifications within a spiculated/circular tumor mass, where the calcifications represent the in-situ component of the invasive tumor. Another example is a tumor mass that has a partially spiculated and partially lobulated contour (Fig. **6.25**-1 to 3).[2, 28]

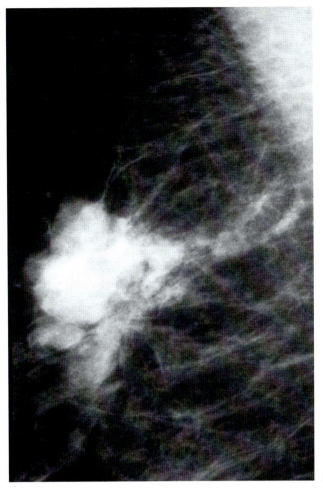

Fig. **6.25**-1   Right breast, detail of the MLO projection. There is a lobulated, oval tumor mass superimposed upon a stellate tumor.

6.25-1

Fig. **6.25**-2   Subgross, thick-section histological image of the stellate lesion (invasive ductal carcinoma) adjacent to a mucinous carcinoma, which corresponds to the lobulated tumor mass on Fig. **6.25**-1.

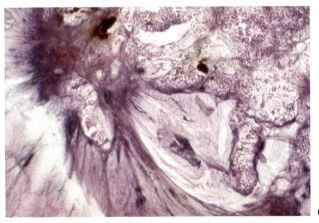

6.25-2

Fig. **6.25**-3   Low-power, conventional histological image of the ductal and mucinous carcinomas.

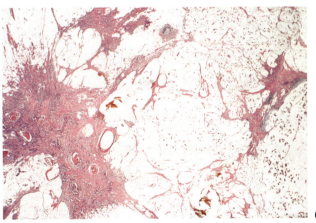

6.25-3

193

Morphological Heterogeneity of Breast Cancer at Mammography

Mammography is a simplified reflection of histology. Although there are a number of specific mammographic im-
ages corresponding to specific breast cancer subtypes (Fig. **6.26**-1 to 8), in general there is less variation in the mammographic image than there is in histology, since several different tumor types may have a common mammographic appearance (Figs. **6.29**, **6.38**, **6.41**).

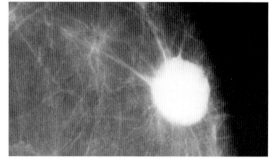

6.26-1

Fig. **6.26**-1   Circular invasive ductal carcinoma NOS.

6.26-2

Fig. **6.26**-2   Architectural distortion: atypical form of DCIS.

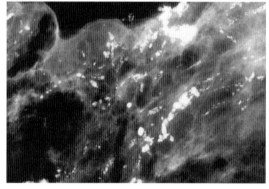

6.26-3

Fig. **6.26**-3   Casting-type calcifications in Grade 3 DCIS.

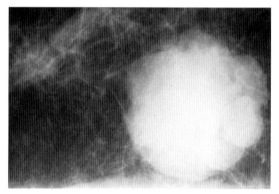

6.26-4

Fig. **6.26**-4   Lobulated, ill-defined mucinous carcinoma.

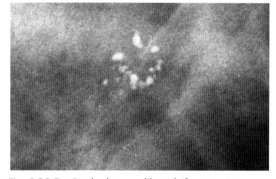

6.26-5

Fig. **6.26**-5   Crushed stone–like calcifications in Grade 2 DCIS.

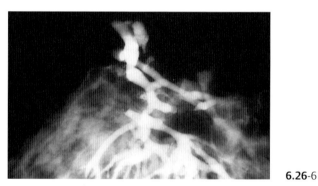

6.26-6

Fig. **6.26**-6   Galactogram showing multiple foci of DCIS.

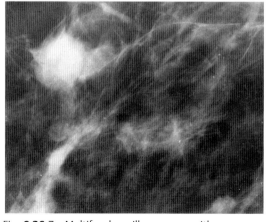

6.26-7

Fig. **6.26**-7   Multifocal papillary cancer with interconnecting bridges.

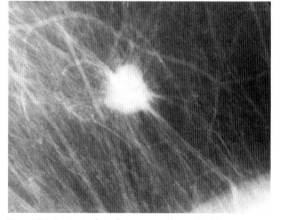

6.26-8

Fig. **6.26**-8   Spiculated tumor with central tumor mass surrounded by spicules.

Mammographic Appearance of Histologically Malignant Lesions

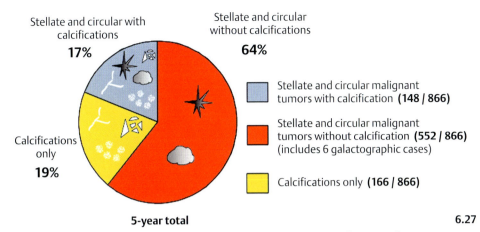

Stellate and circular with calcifications
17%

Stellate and circular without calcifications
64%

Calcifications only
19%

Stellate and circular malignant tumors with calcification **(148 / 866)**

Stellate and circular malignant tumors without calcification **(552 / 866)** (includes 6 galactographic cases)

Calcifications only **(166 / 866)**

5-year total

6.27

Fig. **6.27** Distribution of mammographic findings in 866 histologically proven breast cancers.

The series of 1168 open surgical biopsies from the Department of Mammography, Falun, Sweden included 866 histologically proven malignancies. The mammographic findings are distributed as shown in Fig. **6.27**:

- **Stellate or circular tumor mass** with no associated calcifications in 64% of the cases (552/866).
- **Calcifications and an associated tumor mass** in 17% of the cases (148/866).
- **Calcifications with no associated tumor mass** accounted for 19% of all malignancies detectable on the mammogram (166/866).

Consequently, the most common manifestation of breast cancer on the mammogram is a tumor mass without calcifications. Among the tumor masses with no associated calcifications, **it is the stellate/spiculated tumor that accounts for two-thirds of all breast cancers** (Fig. **6.28**). These data emphasize the priorities in searching for breast malignancies. Since most of the tumor masses will represent invasive tumors, special emphasis should be placed on detecting subtle stellate and circular tumors on the mammogram.

Ratio of Stellate/Circular Malignant Tumors

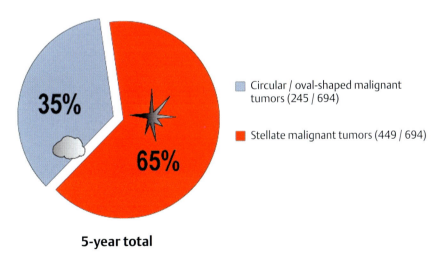

35%

65%

Circular / oval-shaped malignant tumors (245 / 694)

Stellate malignant tumors (449 / 694)

5-year total

6.28

Fig. **6.28** Distribution of spiculated/stellate and circular/oval tumor masses with no associated calcifications in 694 histologically proven breast cancers; the spiculated/stellate tumors are twice as common as circular/oval tumors among breast cancers with no associated calcifications.

Morphological Heterogeneity of Breast Cancer at Mammography

Stellate/Spiculated Tumors

The characteristic mammographic appearance of stellate/spiculated malignant breast tumors is a solid, central tumor mass surrounded by straight, radiating spiculations. More than 90% of the stellate lesions seen on the mammo-gram will be malignant at histology (Fig. **6.24**). A stellate/spiculated mammographic image may be the representation of invasive ductal carcinoma, tubular carcinoma, or certain types of invasive lobular carcinoma.

Figures **6.24**-1 to 7 demonstrate the similar stellate mammographic appearance of tubular cancer, invasive ductal carcinoma, and certain subtypes of invasive lobular carcinoma.

Fig. **6.29**-1 & 2   Tubular cancer.

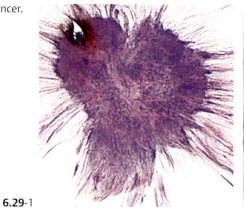

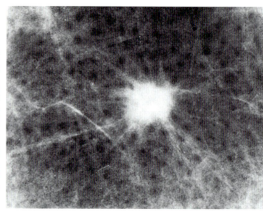

6.29-1

6.2!

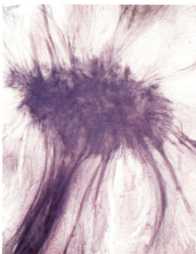

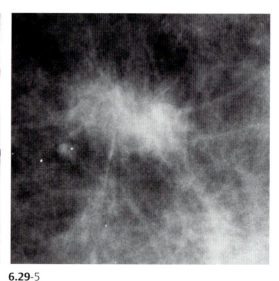

6.29-3

6.29-4

6.29-5

Fig. **6.29**-3 to 5   Invasive ductal carcinoma.

Fig. **6.29**-6 & 7   Invasive lobular carcinoma.

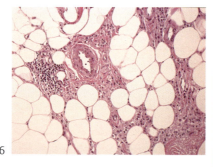

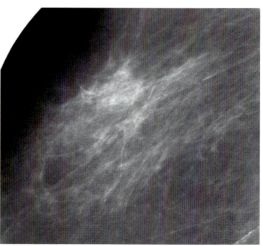

6.29-6

6.29

Malignancy Ratio of Stellate Lesions

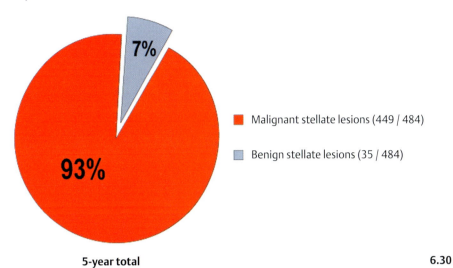

■ Malignant stellate lesions (449 / 484)

■ Benign stellate lesions (35 / 484)

5-year total

6.30

Fig. **6.30**   Spiculated/stellate lesions on the mammogram represent a malignant breast tumor in 93% of cases.

Histology of Malignant Stellate Lesions

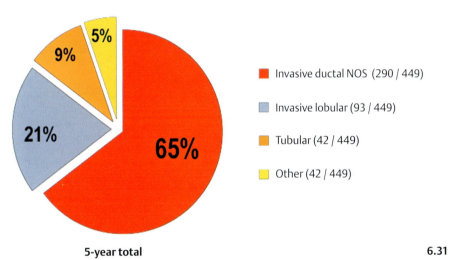

■ Invasive ductal NOS (290 / 449)

■ Invasive lobular (93 / 449)

■ Tubular (42 / 449)

■ Other (42 / 449)

5-year total

6.31

Fig. **6.31**   Based on 449 malignant breast tumors all having a stellate or spiculated mammographic appearance, the histological diagnosis was, in order of decreasing frequency:
(a) invasive ductal carcinoma;
(b) certain types of invasive lobular carcinoma;
(c) tubular carcinoma.

*Clinical Image and Mammographic Demonstration
of Advanced Ductal Carcinoma*

Fig. **6.32**   Extensive skin retraction is
typically seen over an advanced carcinoma.

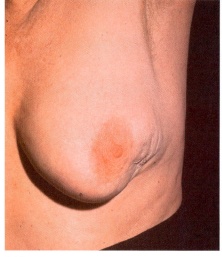 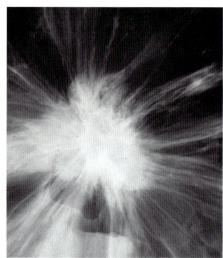

Fig. **6.33**   Classic stellate mammographic image of an invasive ductal
carcinoma with a well-developed central tumor mass surrounded by individual, straight spiculations.

6.32   **6.33**

Figs. **6.34** and **6.35**   In its early
phase of development, the spiculated
mass will often have a fairly nonspecific appearance. At this stage an
asymmetric density may be the only
abnormality seen on the mammogram and a more specific stellate
image will evolve as the tumor grows.
The time difference was 25 months
between the two examinations in this
case.

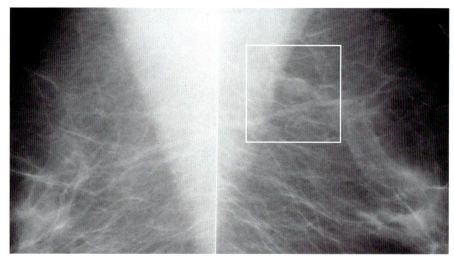

6.34-1   **6.34**-2

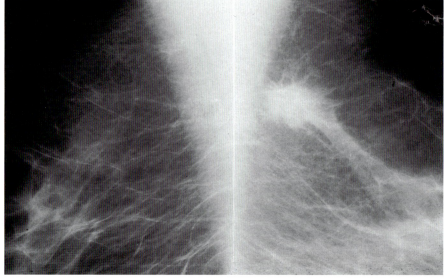

6.35-1   **6.35**-2

Histology of Benign Stellate Lesions

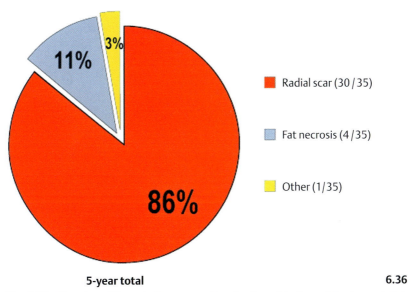

Radial scar (30 / 35)

Fat necrosis (4 / 35)

Other (1/35)

5-year total

6.36

Fig. **6.36**   Based on 35 surgically removed benign breast lesions all having a stellate or radiating mammographic appearance, the histological diagnosis was, in order of decreasing frequency:
(a) radial scar (most often);
(b) traumatic fat necrosis (often postsurgical);
(c) granular cell tumor (an infrequent finding).

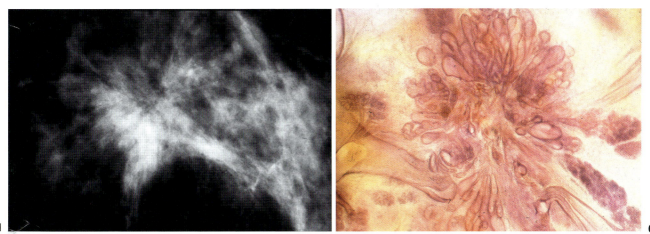

6.37-1

6.37-2

Fig. **6.37**-1 & 2   Mammographic and thick-section histological images of a radial scar.

Morphological Heterogeneity of Breast Cancer at Mammography

Circular/Oval-shaped Tumors

Since the contour of normal fibroglandular tissue bordering adipose tissue is concave, the presence of lesion(s) with a convex contour should alert the reader. Cancers with widely varying histological features may have a similar circular/oval-shaped mammographic appearance: medullary carcinoma, colloid cancer, moderately and poorly differentiated invasive ductal carcinoma, intracystic papillary carcinoma in situ, invasive papillary carcinoma, etc.

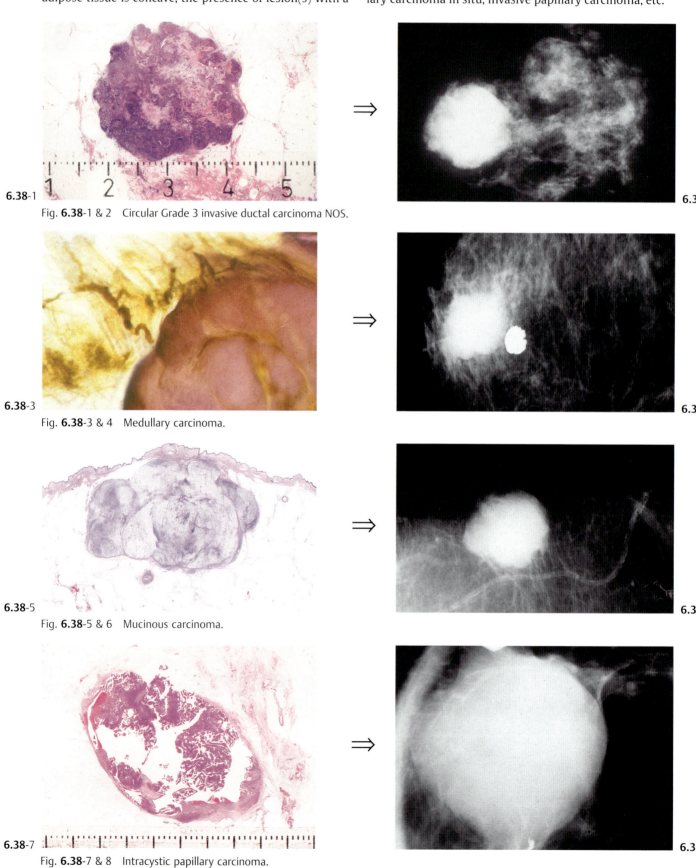

6.38-1

Fig. **6.38**-1 & 2   Circular Grade 3 invasive ductal carcinoma NOS.

6.38-3

Fig. **6.38**-3 & 4   Medullary carcinoma.

6.38-5

Fig. **6.38**-5 & 6   Mucinous carcinoma.

6.38-7

Fig. **6.38**-7 & 8   Intracystic papillary carcinoma.

Most of the circular lesions seen on the mammogram will be benign, being caused by cysts or fibroadenomas. One-third of all invasive breast cancers will have a circular/oval shape on the mammogram. Circular/oval malignant tumor masses tend to maintain their shape throughout their pre-clinical detectable phase. Their mammographic appearance changes only in size and density.

Histology of Malignant Circular/Oval-shaped Lesions

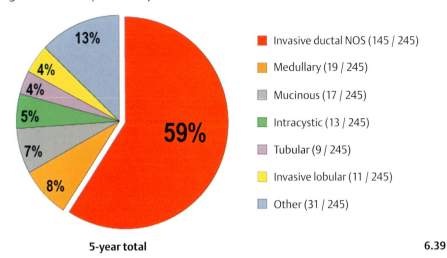

Invasive ductal NOS (145 / 245)

Medullary (19 / 245)

Mucinous (17 / 245)

Intracystic (13 / 245)

Tubular (9 / 245)

Invasive lobular (11 / 245)

Other (31 / 245)

5-year total

6.39

Fig. **6.39** Distribution of histological subtypes of 245 **malignant** breast tumors with a circular/oval-shaped mammographic appearance.

Histology of Benign Circular/Oval-shaped Lesions

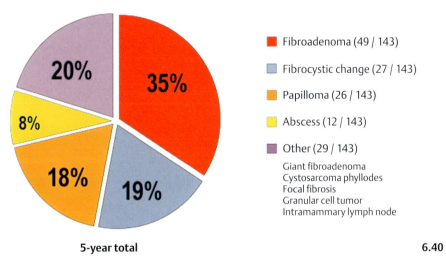

Fibroadenoma (49 / 143)

Fibrocystic change (27 / 143)

Papilloma (26 / 143)

Abscess (12 / 143)

Other (29 / 143)

Giant fibroadenoma
Cystosarcoma phyllodes
Focal fibrosis
Granular cell tumor
Intramammary lymph node

5-year total

6.40

Fig. **6.40** Distribution of histological subtypes of 143 surgically removed **benign** breast lesions with a circular/oval-shaped mammographic appearance.

Morphological Heterogeneity of Breast Cancer at Mammography

Calcifications on the Mammogram

The purpose of searching for microcalcifications on the mammogram is to detect those subtypes of ductal carcinoma in situ (DCIS) that are associated with calcifications visible on the mammogram. There is a much better correlation between the histological and mammographic features of DCIS subtypes than that observed with invasive carcinomas. For example, a change in the cellular architecture of Grade 3 DCIS (from solid to micropapillary cell proliferation) results in an altered mammographic image (Fig. **6.41**-1 to 8). The positive correlation between the histological and mammographic presentation of the different subtypes of DCIS makes it possible to identify the individual DCIS subtypes from the mammogram.

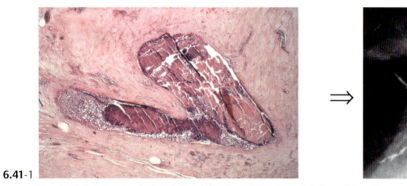
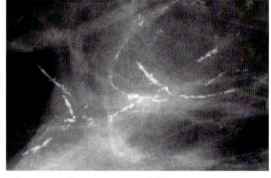

6.41-1
6.41-2

Fig. **6.41**-1 & 2   Grade 3 DCIS, solid cell proliferation with branching, fragmented casting-type calcifications.

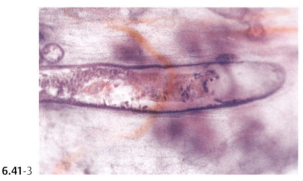
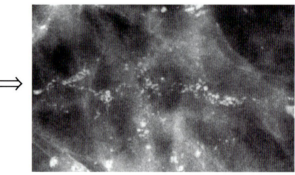

6.41-3
6.41-4

Fig. **6.41**-3 & 4   Grade 3 DCIS, micropapillary cell proliferation with dotted casting-type calcifications.

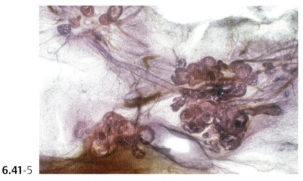
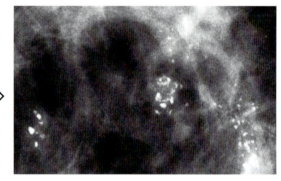

6.41-5
6.41-6

Fig. **6.41**-5 & 6   Grade 2 DCIS with crushed stone–like calcifications.

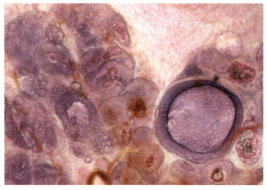
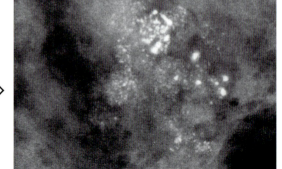

6.41-7
6.41-8

Fig. **6.41**-6 & 7   Grade 1 DCIS with powdery calcifications.

Calcifications on the Mammogram

Mammographic–histological correlation of 1168 surgical breast biopsies over a five-year period during the 1990s at the Department of Mammography, Falun Central Hospital, Falun, Sweden, included 264 cases (23 %) in which calcifications on the mammogram were the only preoperative finding. Of these cases 166 proved to be malignant at histology (63 %) with a varying malignancy ratio depending upon the type of calcification. Detailed results of this correlation appear in Figure **6.42**-1.

Mammographic Appearance of All Calcifications Sent to Open Breast Surgery

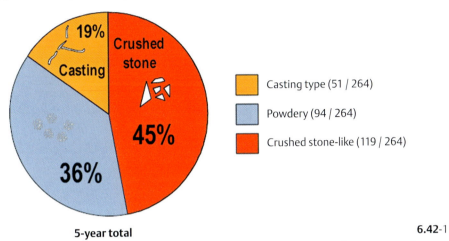

Casting type (51 / 264)

Powdery (94 / 264)

Crushed stone-like (119 / 264)

5-year total

6.42-1

Fig. **6.42**-1   Distribution of calcification subtypes referred to surgery for suspicion of malignancy.

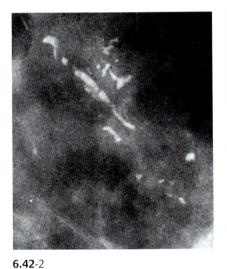

6.42-2

Fig. **6.42**-2   Casting-type calcifications (BIRADS: linear, branching).

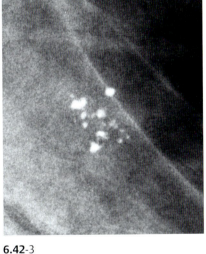

6.42-3

Fig. **6.42**-3   Crushed stone–like calcifications (BIRADS: pleomorphic).

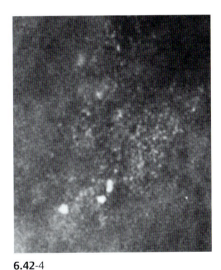

6.42-4

Fig. **6.42**-4   Powdery calcifications (BIRADS: indistinct, amorphous).

Malignancy Ratio of Casting-Type Calcifications

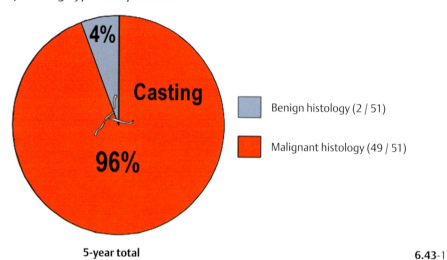

Benign histology (2 / 51)

Malignant histology (49 / 51)

5-year total

6.43-1

Fig. **6.43**-1   Distribution of **malignant** and **benign** histology of 51 casting-type (BIRADS: linear, branching) calcification cases undergoing breast surgery.

Fig. **6.43**-2   Right breast MLO projection with casting-type calcifications.

Fig. **6.43**-3   MLO microfocus magnification image.

Fig. **6.43**-4   Right CC projection, microfocus magnification.

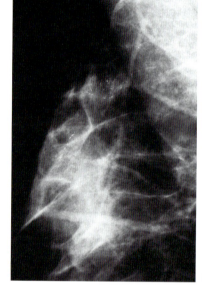

6.43-2

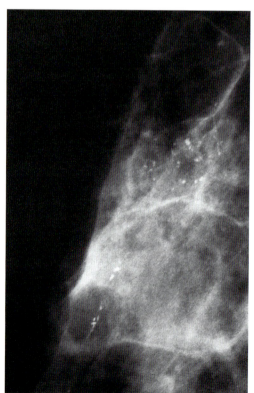

6.43-3

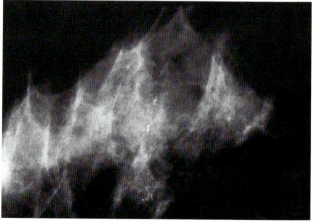

6.43-

Calcifications on the Mammogram

Fig. **6.43**-5   Specimen radiograph.

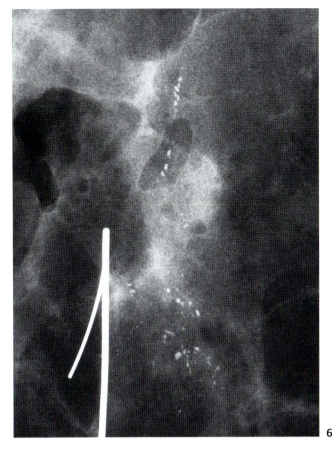

6.43-5

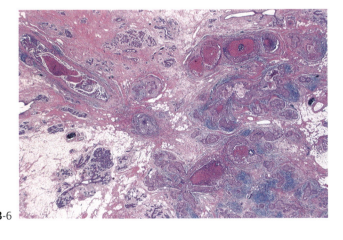

43-6

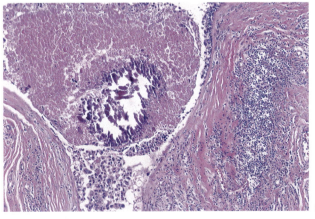

6.43-7

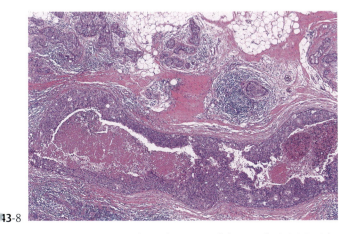

43-8

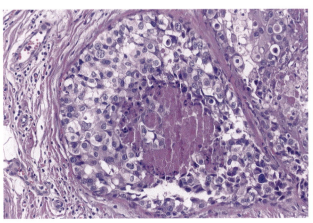

6.43-9

Fig. **6.43**-6 to 9   Histological images of this Grade 3 DCIS with central necrosis and calcifications.

Malignancy Ratio of Crushed Stone-like Calcifications

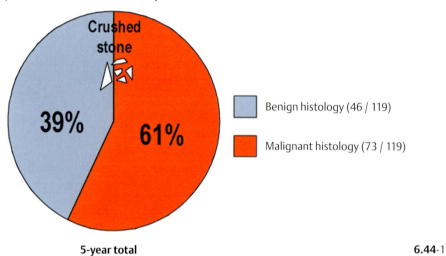

Benign histology (46 / 119)

Malignant histology (73 / 119)

5-year total

6.44-1

Fig. **6.44**-1   Distribution of **malignant** and **benign** histology of 119 crushed stone–like (BIRADS; pleomorphic) calcification cases undergoing breast surgery.

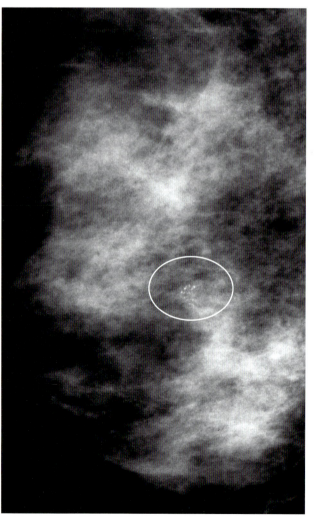

6.44-2

Fig. **6.44**-3   Microfocus magnification shows the varying size, density and shape of the calcifications.

Fig. **6.44**-2   Right breast, MLO projection. There is a cluster of centrally located, crushed stone–like calcifications with no associated tumor mass.

Calcifications on the Mammogram

Fig. **6.44**-4   Operative specimen radiograph.

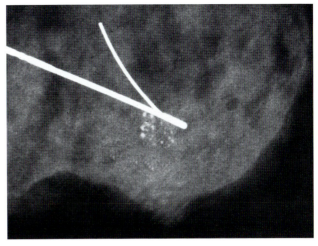

6.44-4

Fig. **6.44**-5   Radiograph of the paraffin block.

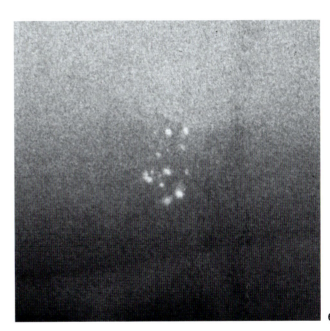

6.44-5

Fig. **6.44**-6 & 7   Histology images, H&E staining. Grade 2 DCIS with central necrosis and amorphous calcifications.

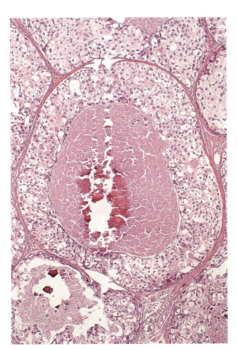

6.44-6

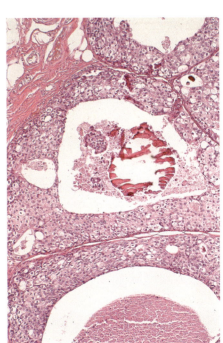

6.44-7

Crushed Stone–like Calcification Cases—Benign

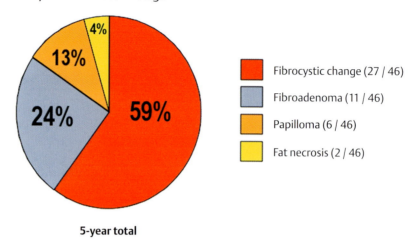

5-year total

6.45-1

Fig. **6.45**-1 Distribution of **benign** histological subtypes of 46 crushed stone–like (BIRADS: pleomorphic) calcification cases undergoing breast surgery.

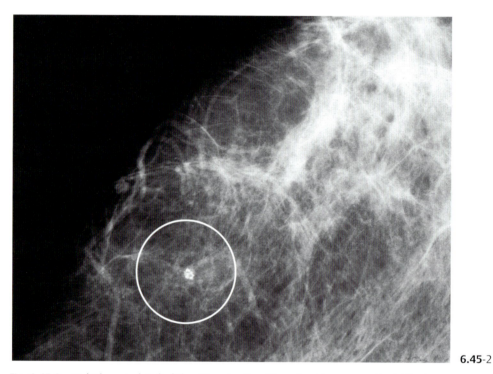

6.45-2

Fig. **6.45**-2 Right breast, detail of the CC projection. There is a tiny group of calcifications without associated tumor mass in the lateral portion of the breast.

Calcifications on the Mammogram

Fig. **6.45**-3   Microfocus magnification with spot compression demonstrates the cluster, crushed stone–like calcifications that vary in size, shape, and density. The final diagnosis can only be made by histological examination.

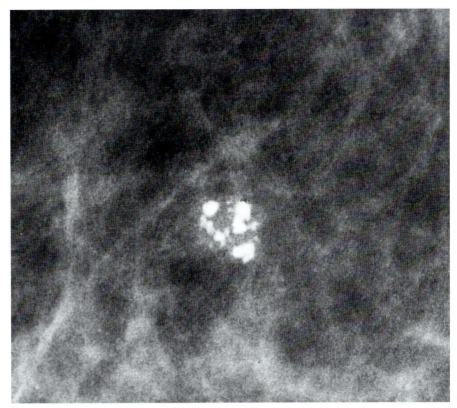

6.45-3

Fig. **6.45**-4   Subgross, thick-section histology shows the cystically dilated acini of a TDLU. The calcifications shown in **6.45**-2 and **6.45**-3 are localized in the accumulated cyst-fluid. **Diagnosis:** fibrocystic change without epithelial cell proliferation.

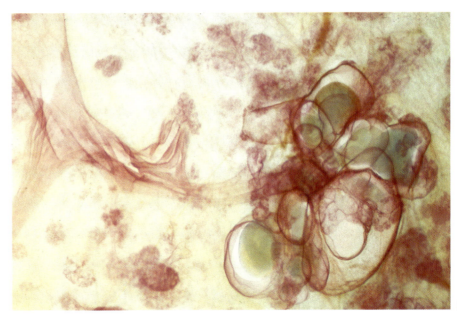

6.45-4

Malignancy Ratio of Powdery Calcification Cases

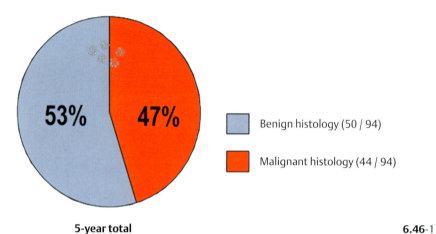

Benign histology (50 / 94)

Malignant histology (44 / 94)

5-year total   **6.46**-1

Fig. **6.46**-1   Distribution of **malignant** and **benign** histology of 94 powdery (BIRADS: indistinct, amorphous) calcification cases undergoing breast surgery.

Fig. **6.46**-2 & 3   Right breast, detail of the MLO microfocus magnification view. There are "tea cup–like" and powdery calcifications surrounded by dense fibrosis. **Histology:** Grade 1 DCIS associated with psammoma body–like calcifications. These correspond to the powdery calcifications on the mammogram.

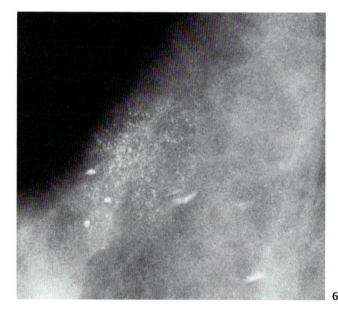

6.4

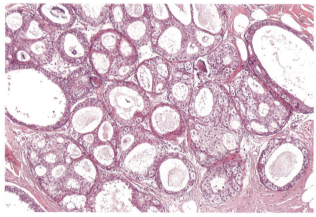

6.4

Malignant Histology of Powdery Calcification Cases

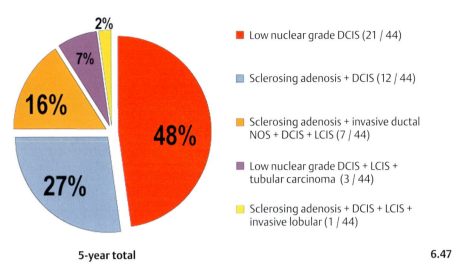

5-year total

6.47

Fig. **6.47**   Distribution of **malignant** histological subtypes of 94 powdery (BIRADS: indistinct, amorphous) calcification cases undergoing breast surgery.

Benign Histology of Powdery Calcification Cases

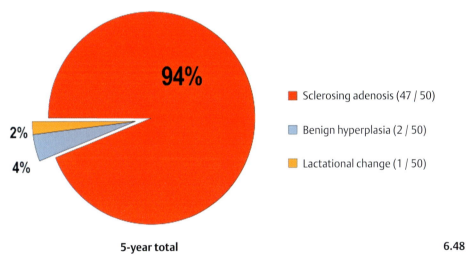

5-year total

6.48

Fig. **6.48**   Distribution of **benign** histological subtypes of 46 powdery (BIRADS: indistinct, amorphous) calcification cases undergoing breast surgery.

Microcalcifications with or without an associated tumor mass are usually **easily detectable**, although their **differential diagnosis may be difficult.** Calcifications with no associated tumor mass will most often represent a benign process.

Histology: 30 mm × 200 mm micropapillary ductal carcinoma in situ with multiple foci of microinvasion. Micrometastases were found in one of the 11 surgically removed axillary nodes.

Treatment: Segmentectomy, postoperative irradiation and chemotherapy.

Outcome: No evidence of recurrence was found during 11 years of follow-up.

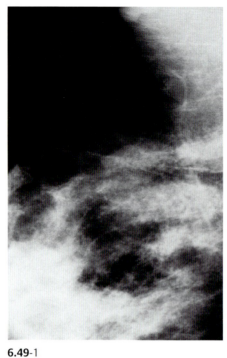 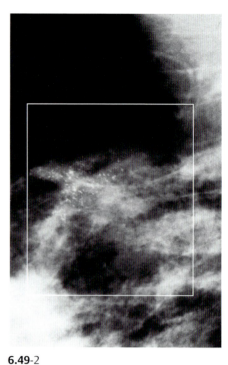

6.49-1

6.49-2

Fig. **6.49**-1   44-year-old woman, right breast, detail of the MLO projection. Normal screening examination.

Fig. **6.49**-2   At next screening a large number of newly developed calcifications were detected. They are mammographically malignant, crushed stone–like and casting-type calcifications with no associated tumor mass.

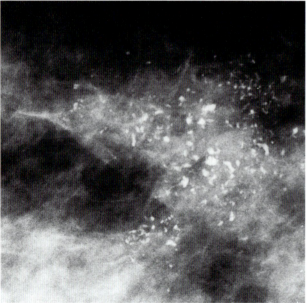 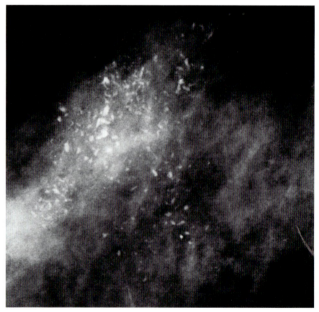

6.49-3

6.4

Fig. **6.49**-3 & 4   Spot compression with microfocus magnification in the MLO and CC projections.

Calcifications on the Mammogram

When calcifications on the mammogram represent one of the subtypes of DCIS, the **number, appearance and extent of these calcifications may change during the preclinical detectable phase;** they may increase in number, or they may decrease in number, and they can also occasionally disappear entirely.

In this case of increasing calcifications in a 70-year-old woman, a tiny group of nonspecific calcifications was missed at screening. Two years later, still asymptomatic, a group of coarse, crushed stone–like calcifications have developed.

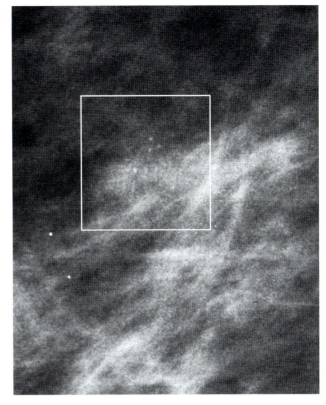

6.50-1

Fig. **6.50**-1   Left breast, detail of the MLO projection. The area with the faint, nonspecific calcifications is outlined by the rectangle, not perceived at this examination.

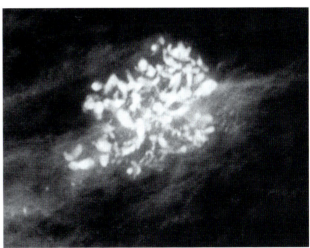

6.50-2

Fig. **6.50**-2   The calcifications have increased considerably in number and appearance during the interscreening interval of 25 months, but have remained restricted to a single, large cluster.

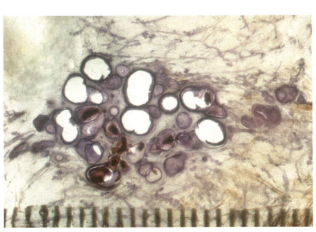

0-3

Fig. **6.50**-3   Subgross, thick-section histology: Grade 2 DCIS. The TDLU has been greatly distended and measures 22 mm in diameter (about 25× the original size).

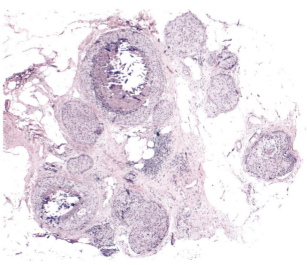

6.50-4

Fig. **6.50**-4   Low-power histological image shows Grade 2 DCIS with extensive intraluminal necrosis and amorphous calcifications.

Morphological Heterogeneity of Breast Cancer at Mammography—Calcifications on the Mammogram

When the missed or underdiagnosed malignant-type calcifications begin to decrease in number and sometimes disappear, it is likely that tumor invasion has already begun (Figs. **6.51**-1 to 8 and **6.52**-1 to 5).

Fig. **6.51**-1 to 5 Five consecutive screening examinations performed at two-year intervals on a woman who was 61 years old at first screening. Details of the right MLO projection. The series of mammograms demonstrate the gradual decrease in the number of calcifications associated with the development of an invasive tumor.

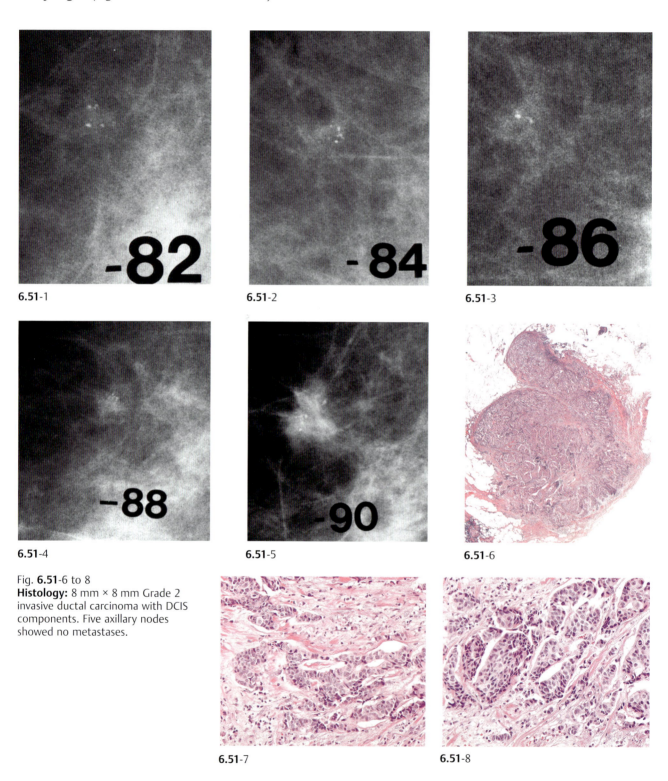

6.51-1

6.51-2

6.51-3

6.51-4

6.51-5

6.51-6

Fig. **6.51**-6 to 8
Histology: 8 mm × 8 mm Grade 2 invasive ductal carcinoma with DCIS components. Five axillary nodes showed no metastases.

6.51-7

6.51-8

Treatment: Segmentectomy. **Outcome**: A 6 mm × 6 mm local recurrence was detected at the fifth yearly mammographic follow-up examination. Reexcision was followed by postoperative irradiation. **Follow-up:** The patient was recurrence-free at the most recent follow-up, 13 years after the initial treatment.

Calcifications on the Mammogram

Another Example of Calcifications Disappearing Concurrently with the Development of an Invasive Tumor

Fig. **6.52**-1 to 5   Five consecutive screening examinations starting at age 57 show little, if any, change in the first four examinations until the development of a small (8 mm) invasive ductal carcinoma. The calcifications have been completely dissolved by the enzyme stromelysin-3.

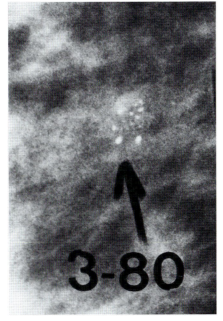

6.52-1

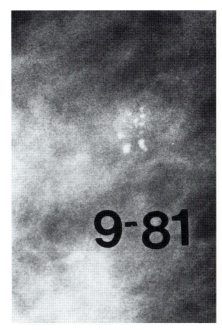

6.52-2

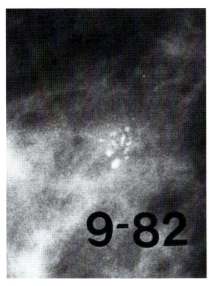

6.52-3

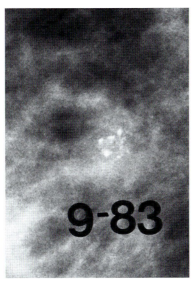

6.52-4

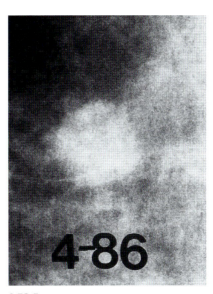

6.52-5

Important note: As long as the *malignant type*, crushed stone–like calcifications on the mammogram are unchanged or even increase in number, it is likely that the proliferating cells are still confined within the basement membrane. As soon as the calcifications start to decrease in number, invasion has most likely begun.

The Progressive Nature of Breast Cancer and the Variability in the Rate of Disease Progression according to Histological Type and Patient Age

Sojourn Time

Another factor affecting the tumor size at detection is the **duration of the preclinical detectable phase** (sojourn time, an expression of tumor growth rate). Accomplishment of the goal of early detection is seriously complicated by the rate of tumor growth, which varies greatly according to histological type and patient's age.[6, 37] At one extreme, the rapidly growing, high-risk tumors have a short mean sojourn time. When the interscreening interval is longer than the sojourn time, fewer of these tumors will be imaged during their preclinical phase. At the other extreme, slowly growing tumors, which will benefit less from early detection, are more likely to be imaged during their sojourn time (Fig. **6.53**). As we learn more about the growth rates of the breast cancer subtypes, we can partially counteract the detrimental effect of high growth rates by adjusting the length of the interscreening interval. The relationship of the tumor growth rates to the length of the time interval between two consecutive screening examinations will greatly influence the success of early detection. The length of the preclinical detectable phase, also called the mean sojourn time, varies by tumor type and patient age, and is longer and more variable in older women (Table **6.8** and Fig. **6.54**-1 to 4).

In premenopausal women, the mean sojourn time is about 1¹/₂ years and varies little by tumor type. (Table **6.9** and Fig. **6.55**-1 & 2). To maximize the effect of screening, the length of the interscreening interval should preferably not exceed 12 months in premenopausal women. Unfortunately for premenopausal women, biological factors make early detection more difficult. Although dense breasts are somewhat more common in the age group 40–49, more importantly, the cancers that arise have a more rapid rate of progression. These factors in combination make control of breast cancer a more elusive goal in younger women, but when we succeed in detecting breast cancer at a size of < 10–15 mm, the long-term outcome is equally good in pre- and postmenopausal women.[7, 30, 35, 37] (Figs. **6.15** to **6.18**).

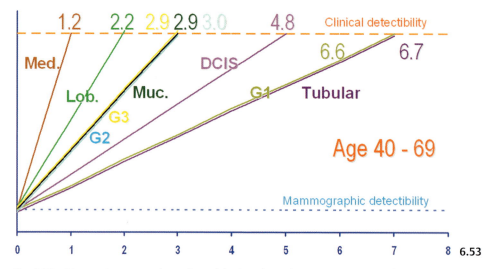

Fig. **6.53**   Mean sojourn time (growth rate) by histological type in women aged 40–69.

Sojourn Time

Estimated Growth Rates by Histological Tumor Type in Women Aged 50–69

Tumor type	MST (years)
Medullary cancer	1.2
Invasive lobular	2.3
Mucinous cancer	2.9
Grade 2 ductal	3.0
Grade 3 ductal	3.1
DCIS	5.1
Tubular cancer	7.1
Grade 1 ductal	7.7

Table 6.**8** In postmenopausal women the estimated mean sojourn time (MST) is longer than in younger women and it varies considerably according to histological tumor type

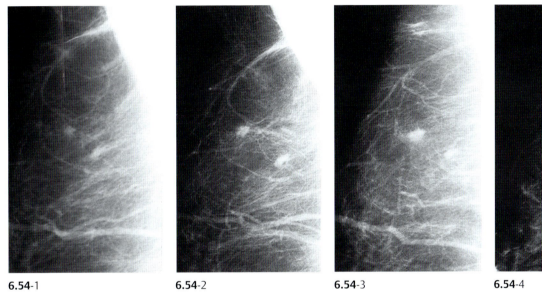

6.54-1   **6.54**-2   **6.54**-3   **6.54**-4

Fig. **6.54**-1 to 4   Example of a slowly growing tumor (40-month interval between first and fourth mammograms) in a 65-year-old woman, demonstrating a slow growth rate/long sojourn time. **Histology:** moderately differentiated 11 mm invasive ductal carcinoma without metastases in four surgically removed axillary lymph nodes. **Treatment:** mastectomy. The patient died of a cerebrovascular lesion six years and two months after treatment.

Estimated Tumor Growth Rates by Histological Type in Women Aged 40–49

Tumor type	MST (years)
Medullary cancer	1.2
Grade 2 ductal	1.7
Grade 3 ductal	1.7
Mucinous cancer	1.9
Grade 1 ductal	2.0
Invasive lobular	2.2
Tubular cancer	3.2
DCIS	3.2

Table 6.**9** The estimated mean sojourn time (MST) is considerably shorter in women aged 40–49 and varies much less with tumor type in this age range. The practical implication is that the interscreening interval must not exceed 12 months in premenopausal women

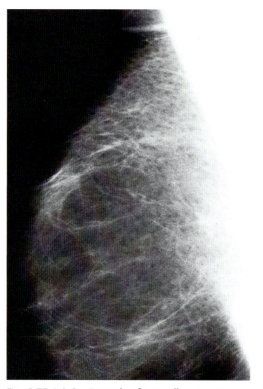
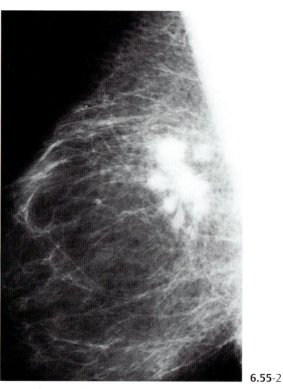

6.55-1   6.55-2

Fig. **6.55**-1 & 2   Example of a rapidly growing tumor (22-month interval) in a 42-year-old woman, demonstrating a fast growth rate/short sojourn time.

Sojourn Time

Demonstration of the Influence of Age upon Mean Sojourn Time in Different Tumor Types

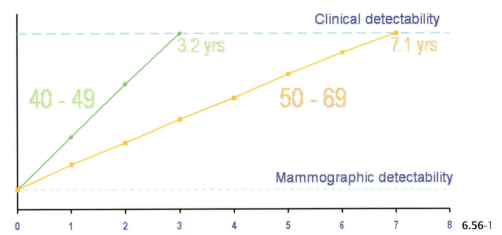

Fig. **6.56**-1   Estimated mean sojourn time in tubular cancer by age range. The mammographically detectable tubular carcinoma becomes a palpable tumor during a mean interval of 3.2 years in women aged 40–49, while the corresponding period is 7.1 years in women aged 50–69.

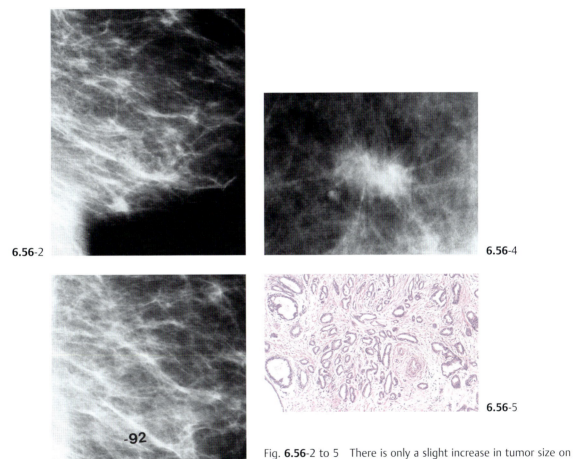

6.56-2

6.56-3

6.56-4

6.56-5

Fig. **6.56**-2 to 5   There is only a slight increase in tumor size on the mammograms of this 67-year-old woman after a two-year interscreening interval. **Histology:** 10 mm, Grade 1, invasive ductal carcinoma with tubular features without metastases in the nine surgically removed axillary nodes (pN0/9). **Treatment:** Segmentectomy and postoperative irradiation.

Demonstration of the Influence of Age upon Mean Sojourn Time in Different Tumor Types

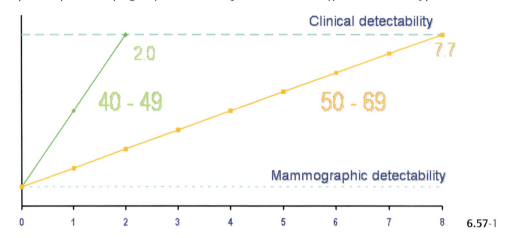

Fig. **6.57**-1   Estimated mean sojourn time in Grade 1, well-differentiated invasive ductal carcinoma by age range. The mammographically detectable well-differentiated invasive ductal carcinoma becomes a palpable tumor during a mean interval of 2.0 years in women aged 40–49, while the corresponding period is 7.7 years in women aged 50–69.

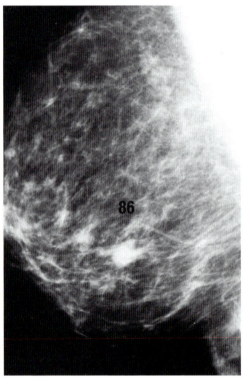

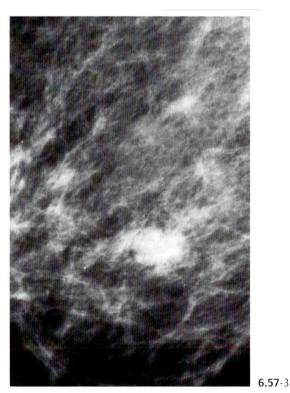

Fig. **6.57**-2   A 7 mm × 7 mm solitary tumor mass is seen on the MLO projection of this asymptomatic, 71-year-old woman.

Fig. **6.57**-3   Microfocus magnification view. The lesion was considered benign at mammographic work-up. However, a considerable change occurred during the next seven years (see Fig. **6.57**-4 to 7).

Sojourn Time

Fig. **6.57**-4   Right breast, CC projection. The patient is now 78 years old. A high-density, hour glass–shaped lesion consists of a sharply outlined anterior portion and a spiculated posterior component, suggesting a compound tumor.

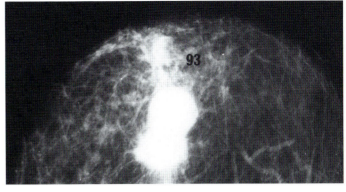

6.57-4

Fig. **6.57**-5   Microfocus magnification image of the compound tumor.

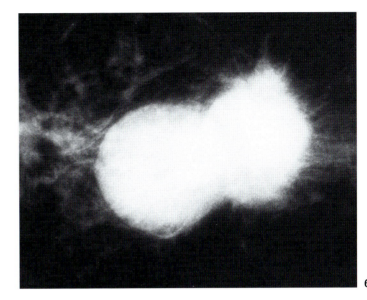

6.57-5

Fig. **6.57**-6   The heterogeneous nature of the lesion is well-demonstrated at ultrasound. There is a cystic cavity containing an intracystic tumor. Immediately adjacent to this, there is a lesion with acoustic shadowing which corresponds to the spiculated tumor on the mammogram.

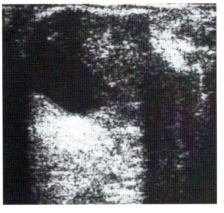

6.57-6

Fig. **6.57**-7   Large-section histology shows an intracystic papillary carcinoma adjacent to the 15 mm invasive ductal carcinoma.

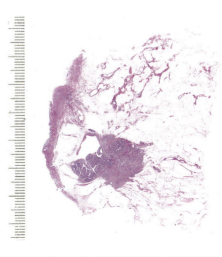

6.57-7

Fig. **6.57**-8   The stellate lesion on the mammogram corresponds to a well-differentiated invasive ductal carcinoma at histology.

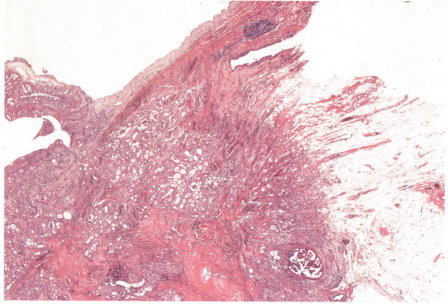

6.5

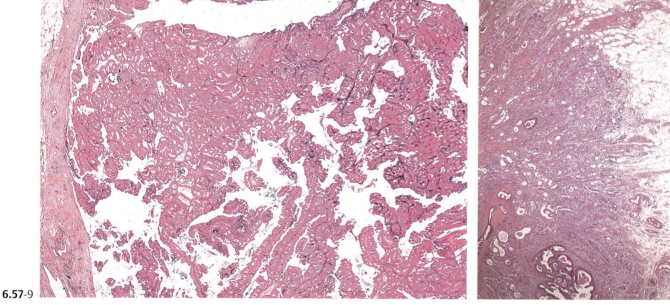

6.57-9

6.57

Fig. **6.57**-9 & 10   The circular lesion on the mammogram corresponds to an intracystic papillary carcinoma (**6.57**-9) on histology. Adjacent to it (**6.57**-10) a portion of the stellate, invasive ductal carcinoma is seen.

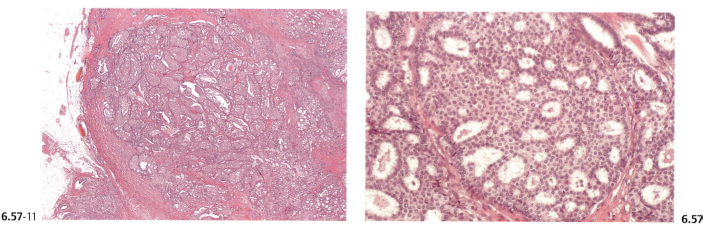

6.57-11

6.57

Fig. **6.57**-11 & 12   Higher-power magnification of the intracystic carcinoma (**6.57**-11). Histological examination also reveals Grade 1 DCIS foci in the surrounding tissue (**6.57**-12).

Sojourn Time

Demonstration of the Influence of Age upon Mean Sojourn Time in Different Tumor Types

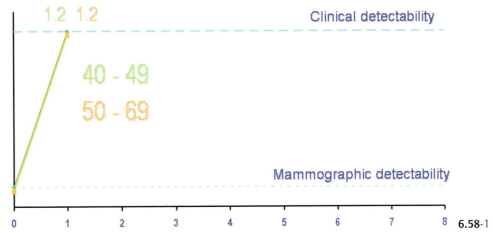

Fig. **6.58**-1   Estimated mean sojourn time in medullary carcinoma by age range. The growth rate is rapid, and the mean sojourn time is correspondingly short in all age subgroups. Thus, medullary carcinoma is seldom discernible on the previous mammogram and seldom detected at screening.

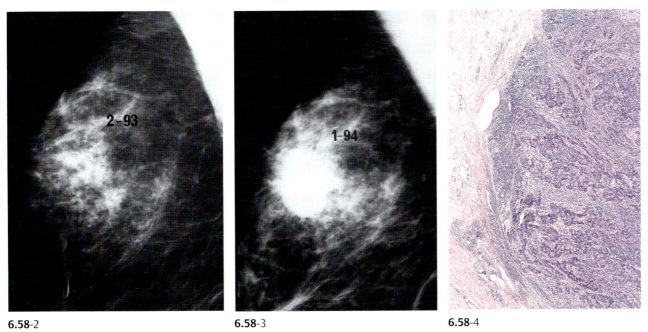

6.58-2

6.58-3

6.58-4

Fig. **6.58**-2 to 4   Comparative right MLO projections of a 52-year-old woman with 11 months interval. This 30 mm × 20 mm medullary carcinoma has developed over an interval of 11 months. There were no axillary lymph node metastases and the patient has had no recurrence following mastectomy during nine years of follow-up.

Demonstration of the Influence of Age upon Mean Sojourn Time in Different Tumor Types

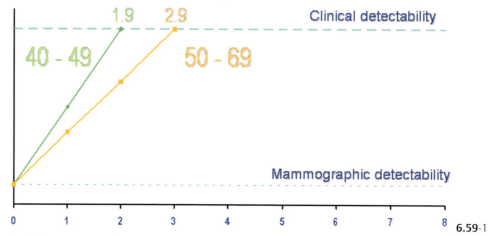

Fig. **6.59**-1   Estimated mean sojourn time in years in mucinous (colloid) carcinoma by age range. The mammographically detectable mucinous carcinoma becomes a palpable tumor during a mean interval of 1.9 years in women aged 40–49, while the corresponding period is 2.9 years in women aged 50–69.

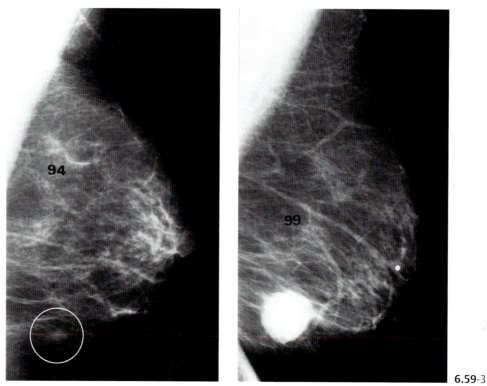

Fig. **6.59**-2 & 3   A 75-year-old woman. Left breast, MLO-projections five years apart. The final screening mammogram at age 70 (**6.59**-2) shows a tiny nonspecific density in the lower-inner quadrant of the left breast. The patient presented with a palpable tumor five years later (**6.59**-3). This case demonstrates the time difference between mammographic and clinical detectability, which is called the sojourn time or the preclinical detectable phase. **Follow-up:** Four years following treatment the patient was recurrence-free.

Sojourn Time

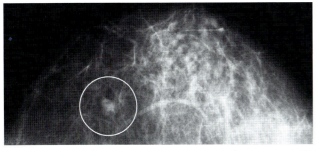
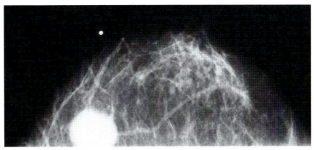

9-4   6.59-5

Fig. **6.59**-4 & 5   The CC projections corresponding to Fig. **6.59**-2 & 3

Fig. **6.59**-6   Typical ultrasound appearance of mucinous carcinoma.

Fig. **6.59**-7   Low-power histological image demonstrates a pure mucinous carcinoma (22 mm, pN0/6).

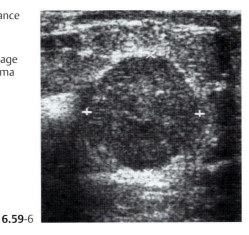
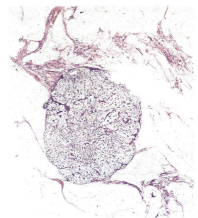

6.59-6   6.59-7

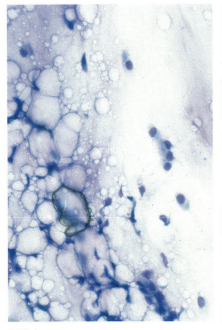
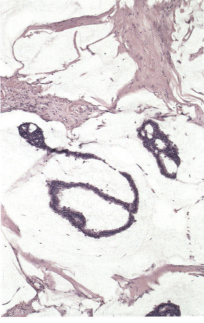
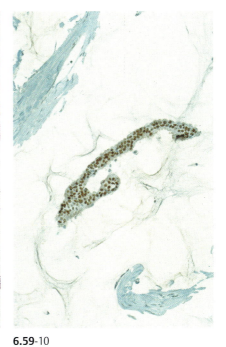

6.59-8   6.59-9   6.59-10

Fig. **6.59**-8   Preoperative cytology: malignant cells.

Fig. **6.59**-9   Medium-power histological image, H&E stain. Clusters of well-differentiated cancer cells are surrounded by the mucin they produce.

Fig. **6.59**-10   Immunohistological staining highlights the estrogen receptor-positive cluster of cells.

Demonstration of the Influence of Age upon Mean Sojourn Time in Different Tumor Types

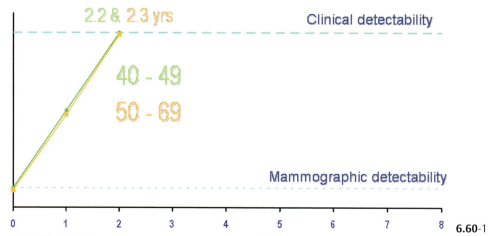

Fig. **6.60**-1   Estimated mean sojourn time in invasive lobular carcinoma by age. According to our estimates, there is no difference in length of sojourn time by age range in invasive lobular carcinoma (2.2 vs. 2.3 years).

Fig. **6.60**-2 to 5   Details of right and left MLO views demonstrate the development of invasive lobular carcinoma (rectangle) over an interval of two years.

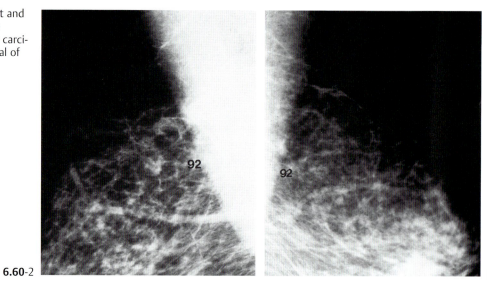

6.60-2

6.60

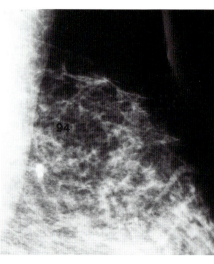

6.60-4

6.60

Sojourn Time

Fig. **6.60**-6 Low-power, large-section histological image of the 4 cm × 3 cm invasive lobular carcinoma, corresponding to the mammographic image in Fig. **6.60**-4.

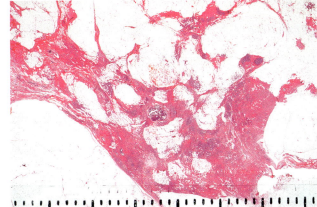

6.60-6

Fig. **6.60**-7 & 8 Subgross, thick-section histology images of this invasive lobular carcinoma.

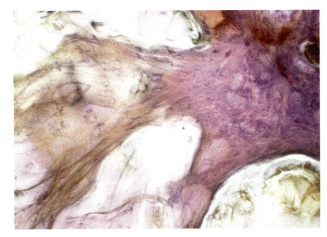

6.60-7

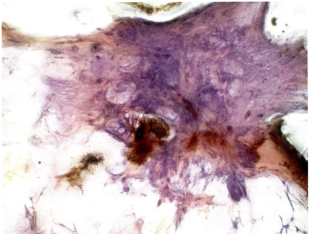

6.60-8

Fig. **6.60**-9 High-power H&E histological image of the classic invasive lobular carcinoma, which invades the adipose tissue.

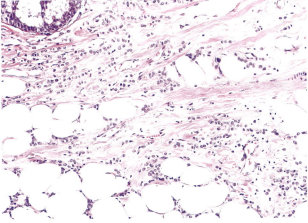

Lymph node status: One of the 17 surgically removed axillary nodes had metastases at histological examination.
Treatment: Segmentectomy and postoperative irradiation.
Outcome: No recurrence has been detected during the first 10 years after treatment.

6.60-9

Heterogeneity over Time

The malignancy grade of some breast cancers may worsen over time as they dedifferentiate from Grade 1 or 2 to Grade 3 (see page 176). This phenomenon is termed tumor progression or heterogeneity over time.

The combination of the various types of heterogeneity discussed in this chapter makes detection, diagnosis, differential diagnosis, and treatment of breast cancer an extremely complex issue.

The following series of mammograms (Fig. **6.61**-1 to 6) chronicles the progression of a malignant tumor over a period of seven years.

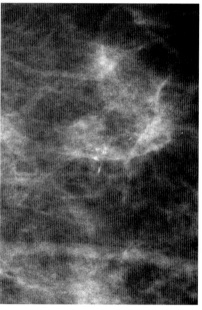 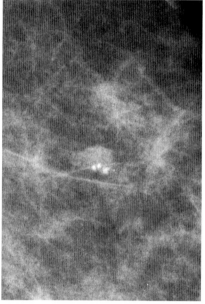 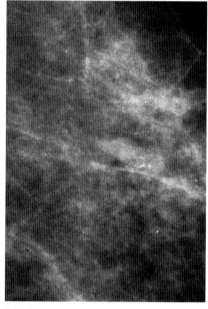

6.61-1

Fig. **6.61**-1   In this first image, at age 50, there is a cluster of irregular, mammographically malignant type calcifications, which were underdiagnosed.

6.61-2

Fig. **6.61**-2   Twenty-four months later: the calcifications are easy to perceive but have changed their appearance due to extensive necrosis and now appear to represent a benign process.

6.61-3

Fig. **6.61**-3   An additional 23 months later: the calcifications are now faint and seem to be disappearing.

Heterogeneity over Time

Histology: 13 mm moderately differentiated invasive ductal carcinoma associated with 25 mm high-grade DCIS. One of the 11 removed axillary nodes contained metastases.

Treatment: Mastectomy. Postoperative irradiation. Tamoxifen.

Outcome: No signs of recurrence 12 years following treatment.

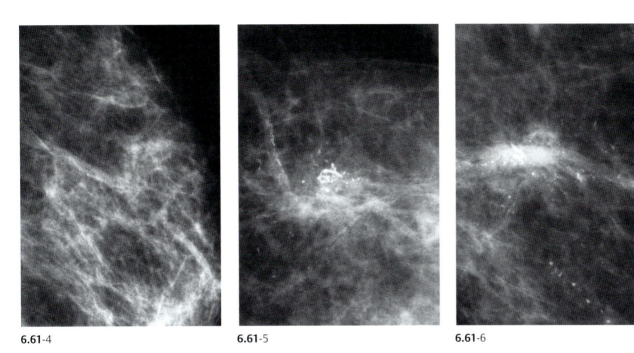

6.61-4

6.61-5

6.61-6

Fig. **6.61**-4   Nineteen months after the previous examination (Fig. **6.61**-3): the calcifications are no longer detectable.

Fig.**6.61**-5 & 6   Reappearance of malignant type calcifications after another 19 months. The presence of casting-type calcifications and the architectural distortion suggest dedifferentiation of the tumor to a higher malignancy grade.

Heterogeneity in Outcome

Breast cancer is also a heterogeneous disease in terms of outcome. The general belief—based on experience gained with palpable tumors—is that breast cancer cases can be classified by histological type into groups having good, intermediate, and poor outcome (Fig. **6.62**). According to this, Grade 3 invasive ductal carcinomas will inevitably belong to the group with a poor outcome. However, long-term follow-up of the different types of breast cancers detected and treated in their earliest detectable stage clearly shows that any subtype can have a very good outcome (Fig. **6.63**). The prerequisite for this good outcome is early detection and removal in the 1–9 mm tumor size range.

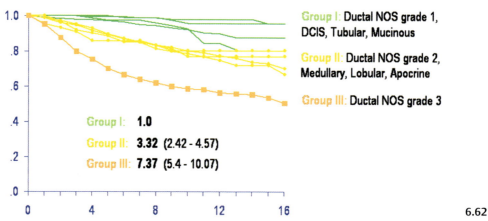

Fig. **6.62** Grouping of histological subtypes by survival. W-E Trial, Sweden. (NOS = not otherwise specified, i.e., invasive ductal cancer without any associated special forms of invasive carcinoma).

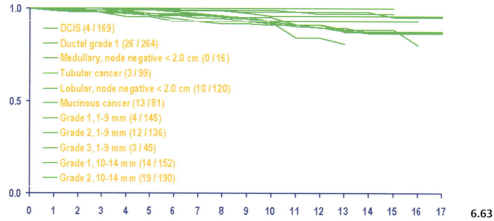

Fig. **6.63** The long-term outcome of many different tumor types can be uniformly good provided they are treated early in the preclinical detectable phase.

Heterogeneity in Outcome

Figures **6.64** and **6.65** demonstrate the extent to which we lose control as tumor size increases and lymph node metastases appear.

Detecting and treating breast cancer early enough in its natural history will result in very good long-term outcome irrespective of the histological subtype.

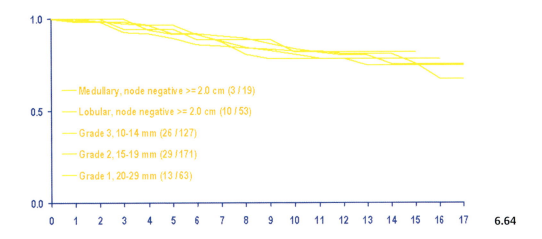

6.64

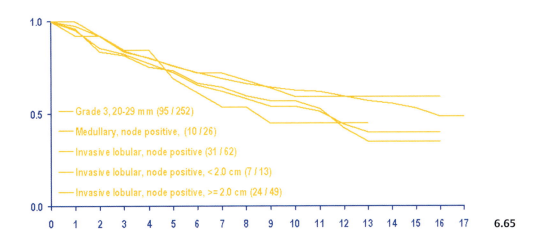

6.65

Example 6.2

Demonstration of how the outcome of medullary carcinoma depends upon early detection (Ex. **6.2**-1 to 7)

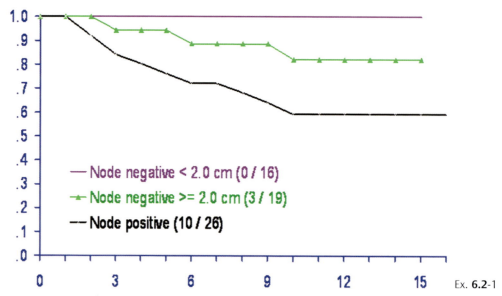

Ex. **6.2**-1   Cumulative survival of women aged 40–74 years with medullary cancer according to tumor size and node status. Data from the Swedish W-E Trial. Women with node-negative, <20 mm medullary carcinoma have a truly excellent long-term survival. Also, women with >20 mm, node-negative medullary carcinoma have fairly good survival. However, node-positive cases, irrespective of tumor size, have poor survival.

Illustrative Case

A 56-year-old asymptomatic woman, first screening study. Called back for evaluation of a tiny, oval-shaped tumor mass located in the medial portion of her left breast.

Ex. **6.2**-2   Detail of the left MLO projection shows a tiny oval-shaped, lobulated lesion (rectangle).

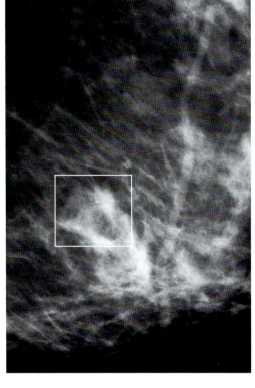

Ex. **6.2**-2

Ex. **6.2**-3   Left breast, CC projection. The finding is situated in the medial portion of the breast.

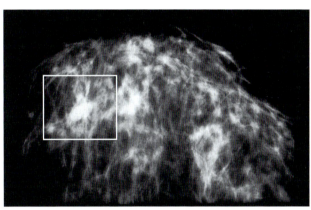

Ex. **6.2**-3

Ex. **6.2**-4   Microfocus magnification, MLO projection.

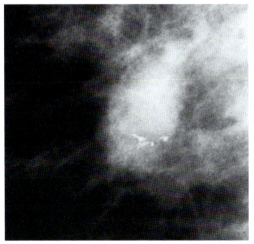

Ex. **6.2**-4

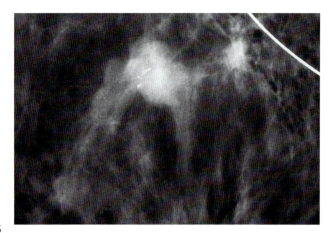

Ex. **6.2**-5 Microfocus magnification radiograph of the operative specimen. The tumor mass appears as two adjacent oval-shaped, ill-defined lesions, associated with malignant type calcifications.

Ex. **6.2**-5

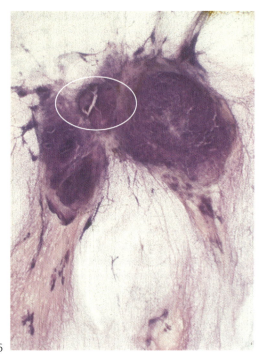

Ex. **6.2**-6 Subgross, thick-section histological image of the tumors. The in-situ component, containing calcifications, is encircled, and magnified in **6.2**-7.

Ex. **6.2**-6

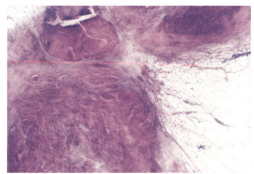

Ex. **6.2**-7

Histology: 10 × 10 mm medullary carcinoma.
Lymph node status: No metastases were found at histological examination in six surgically removed axillary nodes.
Treatment: Segmentectomy and postoperative irradiation.
Outcome: Yearly follow-up examinations for 10 years after treatment showed no signs of recurrence.

Guidelines for Optimization of Screening Efficacy

- The interscreening interval should be optimized according to the estimated mean sojourn time in the age groups screened.
- Properly positioned, high-quality mammographic images facilitate lesion detection.
- Special training of the radiologist in reading a large volume of screening mammograms should be a prerequisite for this task.
- Regular audit of performance is an essential aspect of continuing medical education.
- Double reading of all screening mammograms with consultation between the radiologists for all call-back cases is essential to maintain high sensitivity and specificity. The benefits of double reading are self-evident to those radiologists who practice it. In addition to the available evidence, it can be aptly defended with the old adage, "Two heads are better than one."
- It is highly desirable that the radiologist who calls women back from screening also performs the workup of the suspected findings and conveys the results to each patient. This feedback is an essential part of the continuous education of the radiologist, resulting in improved specificity.

Conclusions

In summary, multiple factors determine how early in the preclinical detectable phase we will indeed be able to detect the individual malignant tumors. The following three factors are predetermined:

- Mammographic parenchymal pattern
- Histological tumor type
- Rate of tumor growth (influenced by both tumor type and patient's age)

These factors, particularly in combination, make the task of early detection difficult enough. The following factors must be optimized if we are to achieve the aim of early detection:

- Length of interscreening interval
- Image quality
- Patient positioning
- Radiologist's skill

There is no room for compromise in breast positioning, in image quality, or in the training of the radiologist in the perception and analysis of breast diseases. Early detection can be best achieved through special training and by subspecialization of radiology technologists and radiologists in breast imaging.

Chapter 7: Finding Breast Cancer When It Is Still Small: Use of Systematic Viewing Methods

A Systematic Method for Viewing Mammograms

■ Basic Philosophy

The essence of screening is to confidently reassure women that their normal mammograms are indeed normal, while at the same time to find the occasional abnormality with great reliability. The vast majority of mammograms will reflect variations in normal anatomy. Familiarity with the basic mammographic patterns down to the finest details of the four structural components enables the reader to differentiate with confidence between the normal and the abnormal tissue by accounting for the radiopaque structural components that are seen against the radiolucent background. Using this approach, the challenging decision of whether or not the mammogram is normal will not become an insurmountable problem.

■ Prerequisites

For effective reading and interpretation of mammograms, a number of prerequisites should be met.

Superb Mammographic Technique Is Essential

- Properly positioned images with adequate breast compression will spread out the breast parenchyma for better evaluation.
- Images with consistently high contrast and high resolution will demonstrate the finer details of normal anatomy and small pathological lesions.

Viewing Conditions during Image Reading Will Have a Decisive Impact upon the Diagnostic Outcome

- Distractions can only impair a radiologist's reading ability.
- Making notes or reports during screening is a function that should be delegated to the clerical staff.
- Investment in good viewing facilities is as important as investment in imaging equipment.
- The reading of large numbers of mammograms requires motorized multiviewers.
- The films of the current and the second most recent examinations should be pre-hung by the clerical staff in a standard format to facilitate perception of any changes.

Perception of Subtle Radiographic Abnormalities Can Be Enhanced by the Use of a Hand-held Mammography Viewer

The limited field of view provided by the viewer (Fig. **7.1**-1) has the following advantages:
- Extraneous light is eliminated.
- Attention can be better focused as peripheral distractions are decreased.
- Magnification of the mammographic image by the low-power lenses in the viewer further improves the perception of small details.
- The combination of these factors makes the use of the viewer superior to the use of an ordinary magnifying glass.
- Improvements in perception are helpful in any radiological study, but are particularly important in mammography.

■ A Systematic Approach Is Essential for Viewing Any Diagnostic Image

Practicing systematic, **side-by-side, step-by-step viewing** (Fig. **7.1**-2 to 4) ensures that all regions of the mammogram will be viewed in detail. At the same time, a comparison should be made with each corresponding region in the contralateral breast.

Special attention is given to asymmetric densities in regions with a high frequency of malignant lesions.

When reading screening mammograms, there should be **a constant search for the normal structural elements of the breast. The pathological lesions will stand out as aberrations of the normal structure.**

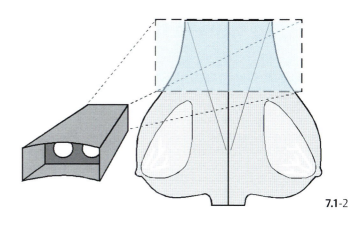

7.1-2

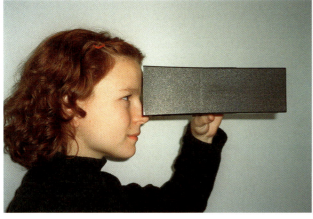

7.1-1

Fig. **7.1**-1   Use of the mammography viewer.

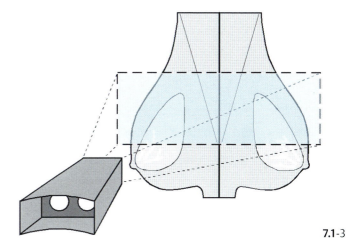

7.1-3

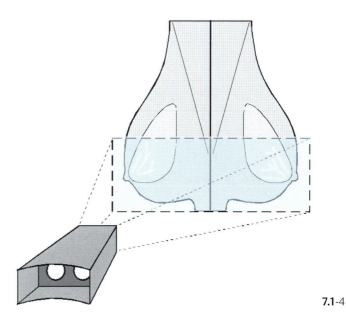

7.1-4

Systematic Approach to the Analysis of the Findings

The careful, systematic viewing of mammograms should be applied to all studies, both to screening and to clinically referred cases. In **screening**, the primary decision to be made is whether the examination is normal or whether there is an abnormality requiring further examination of the patient. Even if the findings at screening appear to be straightforward, the two-view screening mammograms should not be considered sufficient for definitive diagnosis or description of the extent of the disease. **Screening is not yet diagnosis**. A complete mammographic work-up using spot compression and/or microfocus magnification mammography and involving the use of adjunctive tools (ultrasound examination, percutaneous needle biopsies) is needed to reach the diagnosis necessary for the planning of further management. Microfocus magnification mammography, with its superior spatial and contrast resolution, will often reveal additional tumor foci or microcalcifications.

When managing **clinically referred cases and call-backs** from screening, the primary goal is to arrive at a diagnosis of the clinical findings and/or the suspicious lesions seen on the mammogram. Systematic viewing of the mammograms, which should be an integral part of every mammographic study, may reveal additional findings. These should also be further evaluated in order to reach a diagnosis.

The aim of perception is to find:

1 *Asymmetric densities*
   - Circular lesions
   - Stellate/spiculated lesions
   - Nonspecific asymmetric densities seen in "forbidden areas"
2 *Disruption of the harmonic structure*
   - Architectural distortion
   - Parenchymal contour change
3 *Microcalcifications with or without associated tumor mass*
4 *Abnormalities occurring in the nipple/retroareolar areas*

■ Asymmetric Densities on the Mammogram

The most frequently occurring finding at mammography is an asymmetric density, caused by:
- Normal fibroglandular tissue or focal fibrosis (pp. 243–249)
- Nonspecific asymmetric density (pp. 250–255)
- Definite pathological lesion (pp. 256–404)

Once an asymmetric density has been perceived, its nature should be unequivocally determined. Familiarity with and a constant search for the normal structural components of the fibroglandular tissue will enable the reader to conclude that the asymmetric density in question consists of **normal breast tissue**. Coned-down compression combined with microfocus magnification can be very helpful in reaching this conclusion. Double spot compression using Mammospot®, developed by Dr. G. L. Hixson, compresses the breast both from underneath and from above, spreading the tissue apart more effectively and resulting in a sharper image (Fig. **7.3**-1 & 2).

The pathological lesions will have to be worked up mammographically according to basic principles. This requires:
- Additional views
- Spot compression
- Microfocus magnification
- Combination(s) of the above

In addition, ancillary methods such as breast ultrasound (Fig. **7.3**-4) and interventional methods (fine-needle aspiration biopsy [FNAB], larger-core needle biopsy) (Fig. **7.3**-5) should be used to reach a diagnosis of either a benign or a malignant lesion.

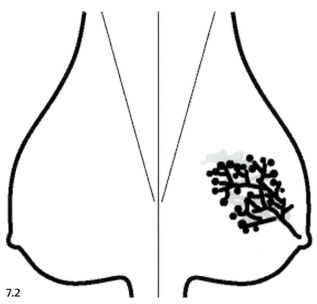

7.2

Fig. **7.2**   Schematic representation of an asymmetric density.

Fig. **7.3**-1   Double compression using Mammospot®.

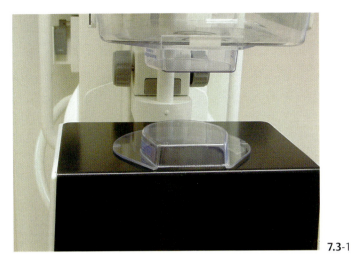

7.3-1

Fig. **7.3**-2   Double compression combined with microfocus magnification.

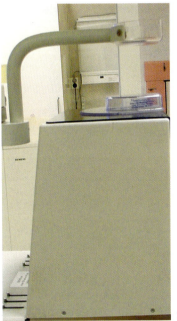

7.3-2

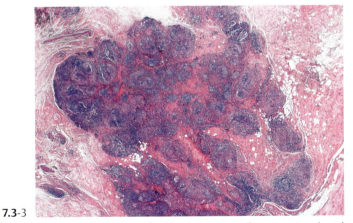

7.3-3

Fig. **7.3**-3   Low-power histological image of an invasive ductal carcinoma surrounded by extensive fibrosis, which makes detection by mammography difficult.

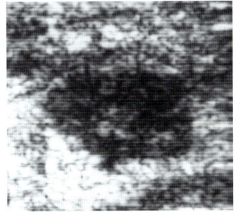

7.3-4

Fig. **7.3**-4   Breast ultrasound examination is a very useful ancillary method in the diagnostic work-up of breast lesions, especially in dense breasts.

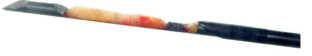

Fig. **7. 3**-5   Large core (14-gauge) needle biopsy enables us to arrive at the preoperative histological diagnosis.

7.3-5

Systematic Work-up of Asymmetric Densities on the Mammogram

The vast majority of asymmetric densities consist of normal breast tissue.

Normal fibroglandular tissue or focal fibrosis producing asymmetric densities on the mammogram include the following examples:

- **Accessory breast** (pp. 243–245)
- **Asymmetric involution** (pp. 246–248)
- **Hormonal effect** (p. 249)
  - Premenopausal
  - Exogenous hormones
- **Fibrosis/scar tissue** (p. 248)
  - Posttraumatic
  - Postinflammatory

The fibroglandular tissue and the supporting connective tissue will be visualized on the mammogram as:

- **Nodular densities**
  - Normal TDLUs: 1–2 mm circular/oval-shaped densities surrounded by radiolucent adipose tissue (Fig. **7.4**-1).

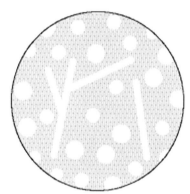

7.4-1

Fig. **7. 4** Schematic representation of the building blocks as they are seen on the mammogram. Fig. **7.4**-1 Normal sized TDLUs and ducts surrounded by adipose tissue. Fig. **7.4**-2 Enlarged TDLUs and prominent ducts surrounded by adipose tissue, as in adenosis. Fig. **7.4**-3 Both nodular and linear densities are hidden in the homogeneous, ground glass-like density corresponding to fibrosis.

  - Adenosis: 3–5 mm circular/oval-shaped densities surrounded by radiolucent adipose tissue (Fig. **7.4**-2).

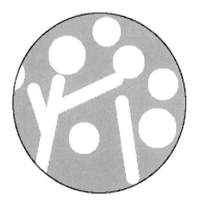

7.4-2

- **Fibrosis:** structureless, "ground glass–like" density with concave contours (Fig. **7.4**-3).

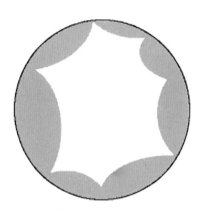

7.4-3

- **Linear densities and adipose tissue:** the ducts and their branches surrounded by adipose tissue.
- **Adipose tissue:** outlines the nodular and linear densities.

Normal Fibroglandular Tissue

Accessory Breast

Fig. **7.5**-1 & 2   Mediolateral oblique projection, right and left breasts. An asymmetric density is seen in the axillary tail of the left breast.

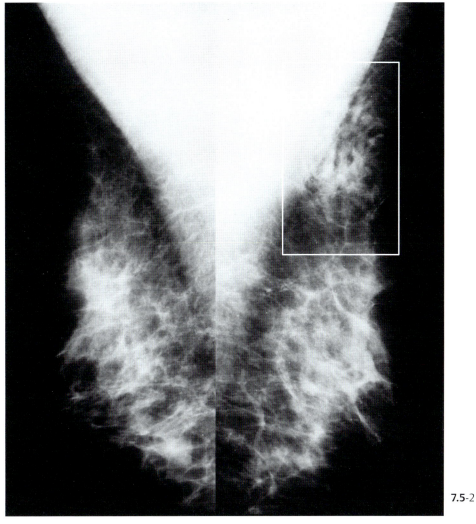

7.5-1

7.5-2

Fig. **7.5**-3   Microfocus magnification shows ducts (linear densities) and TDLUs (nodular densities) outlined by adipose tissue.

Fig. **7.5**-4   Thick-section histology of the accessory breast shows normal breast tissue, TDLUs, and ducts.

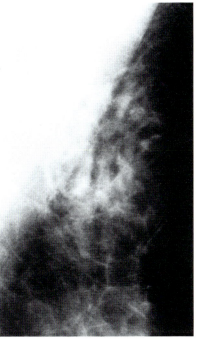

7.5-3

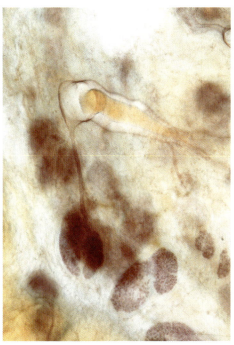

7.5-4

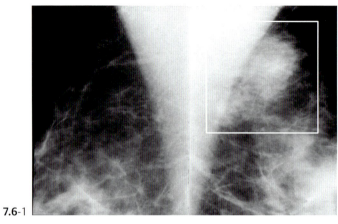

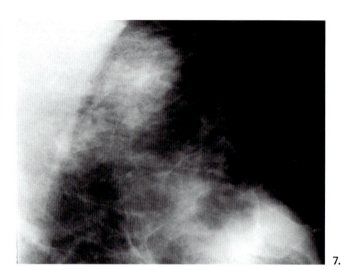

7.6-1

Fig. **7.6**-1 & 2   Accessory fibroglandular tissue in the axillary tail: the most frequent location of an accessory breast.

7.6

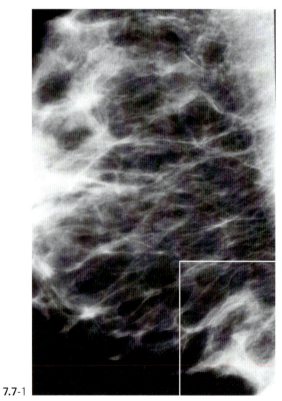

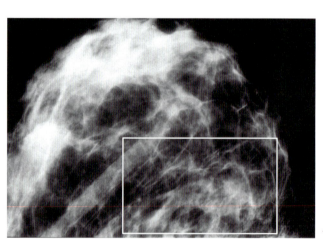

7.7-1

7.7

Fig. **7. 7**-1 & 2   Accessory fibroglandular tissue close to the abdomen: less frequent location of an accessory breast.

Fig. **7.8**-1 & 2   Fibroadenolipoma developing in an axillary accessory breast.

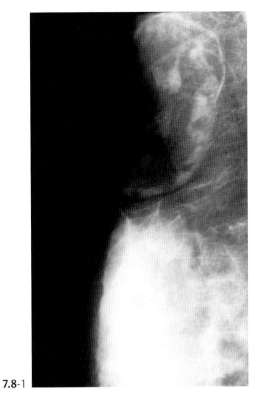
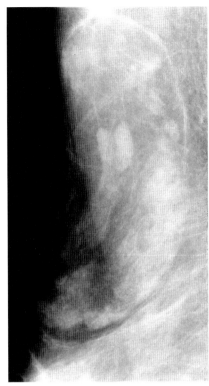

7.8-1

7.8-2

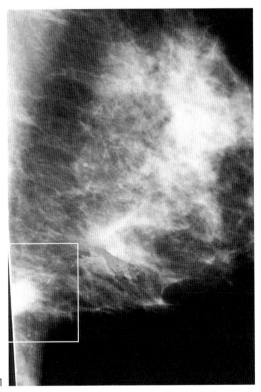

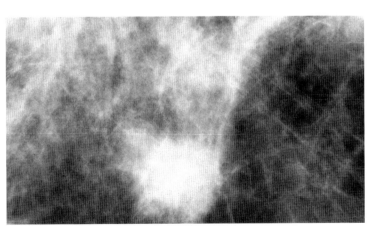

9-1

7.9-2

Fig. **7.9**-1 & 2   Invasive ductal carcinoma developing in the accessory breast located close to the abdomen.

Normal Fibroglandular Tissue

Asymmetric Involution without Architectural Distortion

Fig. **7.10**-1 & 2   Right and left MLO projections. The asymmetric density has scalloped contours, and consists of homogeneous, radiopaque fibrous, and radiolucent adipose tissue. There are no signs of malignancy.

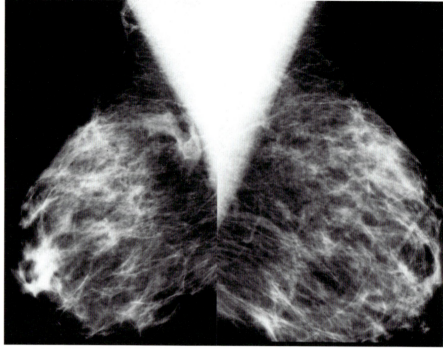

7.10-1   7.10

Fig. **7.10**-3 & 4   Right and left CC projections. The asymmetric density is localized to the retroglandular clear space of the right breast.

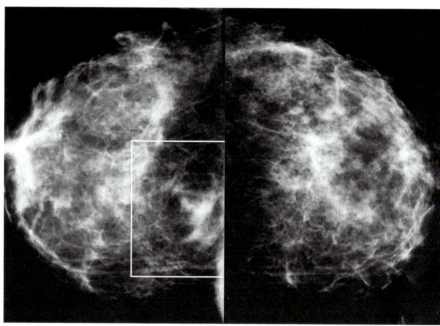

7.10-3   7.10

Fig. **7.10**-5 & 6   Microfocus magnification views, MLO and CC projections: the asymmetric fibroglandular tissue contains three of the four building blocks (TDLUs, fibrosis and adipose tissue), and it has scalloped contours. No architectural distortion is demonstrable. The density is projected over the retroglandular clear space on the CC projection.

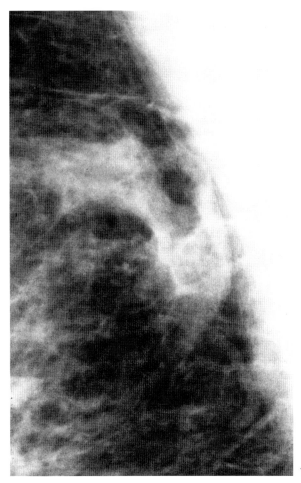

7.10-5

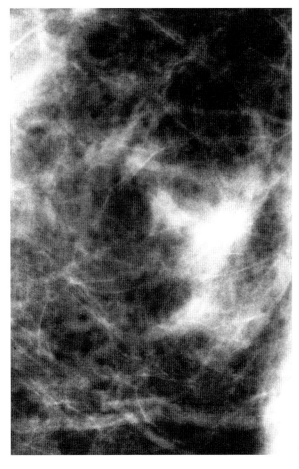

7.10-6

Asymmetric Fibroglandular Tissue without Architectural Distortion

● **Asymmetric gynecomastia**

Fig. **7.11**-1 & 2   Right and left male breasts, mediolateral oblique projections. The obvious asymmetric density in the central portion of the left breast corresponds to fibroglandular tissue (asymmetric gynecomastia).

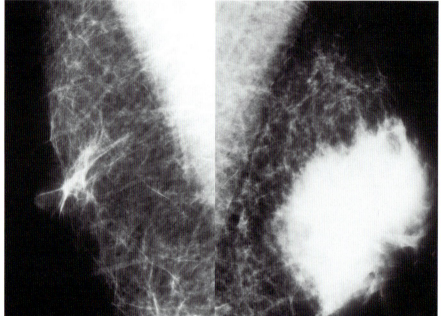

7.11-1

7.11

● **Asymmetric involution** is the most frequent reason for uncertainty in mammographic interpretation and unnecessary callbacks.

Fig. **7.12**-1 & 2   Asymmetric involution may result in islands of fibroglandular tissue. The presence of the building blocks (TDLUs, adipose and fibrous tissue) ensures the correct diagnosis. Asymmetric involution is the most frequent reason for uncertainty in mammographic interpretation and unnecessary call-backs.

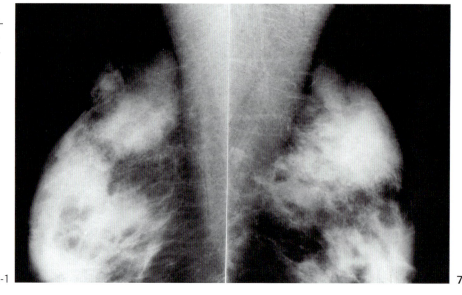

7.12-1

7.12

● **Focal fibrosis/scar tissue**. Surgery/trauma/inflammation causing fibrosis can result in an asymmetric density on the mammogram.

Fig. **7.13**-1 & 2   Focal fibrosis detected on the screening mammogram. The density has concave contours and consists of homogeneous, ground glass–like, structureless fibrosis (collagen). There is no demonstrable pathological lesion.

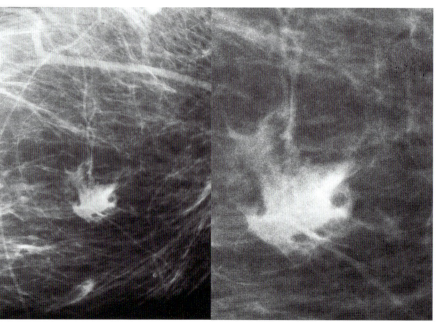

7.13-1

7.13

- **Exogenous hormone effect.** Hormone replacement therapy (HRT) can lead to the reappearance of the basic building blocks. This can impose some limitations on mammographic interpretation.

Fig. **7.14**-1 & 2   Before HRT (Pattern II).

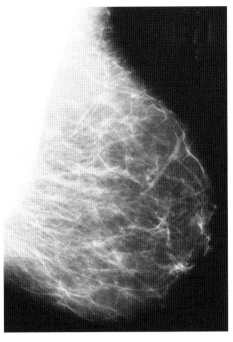
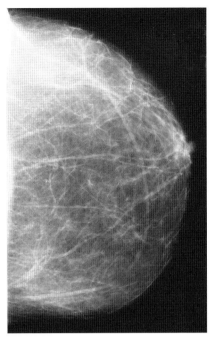

7.14-1

7.14-2

Fig. **7.14**-3 & 4   One year on HRT (Pattern II has been "reversed" to Pattern I).

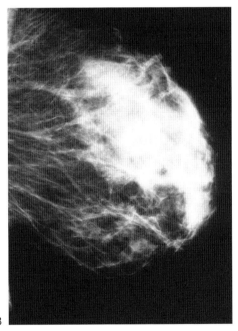
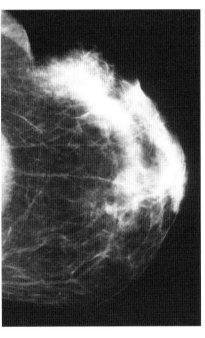

7.14-3

7.14-4

Nonspecific Asymmetric Density with Architectural Distortion on the Mammogram

When an asymmetric density does not display normal structural components, and especially when there is concurrent architectural distortion, the presence of a pathological lesion must be suspected. The distortion may be caused by a desmoplastic reaction associated with a mammographically occult carcinoma in situ or a radial scar.

Nonspecific asymmetric density
- Desmoplastic reaction/fibrosis with architectural distortion
- De-novo fibrosis without trauma or inflammation

Example 7.1

A 45-year-old asymptomatic woman.

Ex. **7.1**-1 & 2   Right and left breasts, details of the CC projections. Subtle architectural distortion is seen in the retroglandular clear space of the right breast.

Ex. **7.1**-3 & 4   The architectural distortion is more obvious on side-by-side comparison obtained through the mammographic viewer.

Ex. **7.1**-5 & 6   Highlighting the concave contours of the radiopaque fibroglandular tissue makes the architectural distortion in the right breast stand out as an abnormal, although nonspecific, density.

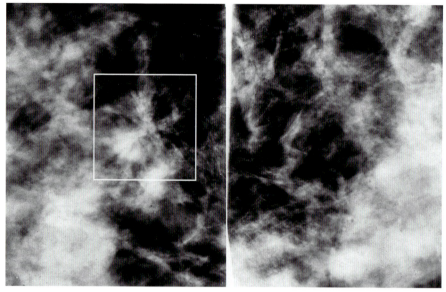

Ex. **7.1**-1   Ex. **7.1**-2

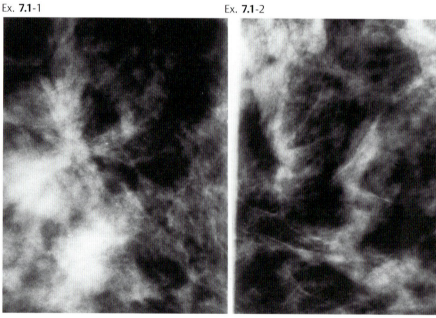

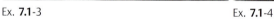

Ex. **7.1**-3   Ex. **7.1**-4

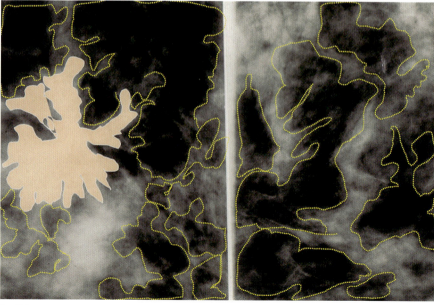

Ex. **7.1**-5   Ex. **7.1**-6

Example 7.1

Ex. **7.1**-7 Microfocus magnification image of the architectural distortion.

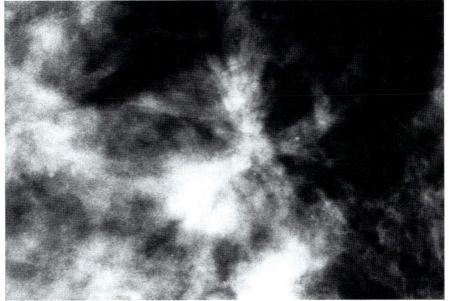

Ex. **7.1**-7

Ex. **7.1**-8 Low-power histological image of the 40 mm ductal carcinoma in situ corresponding to the architectural distortion seen on the mammogram.

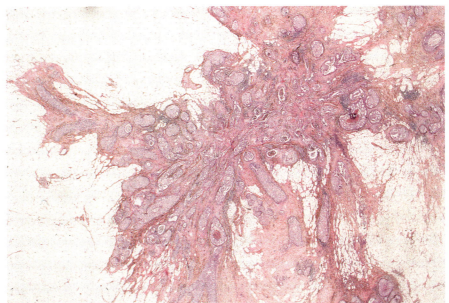

Ex. **7.1**-8

Ex. **7.1**-9 Higher-power histological image of this Grade 2 DCIS.

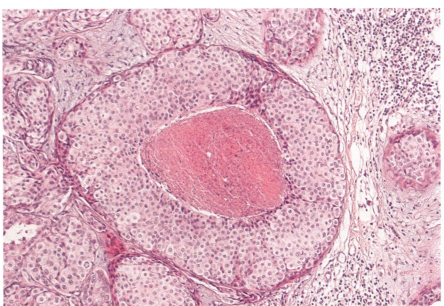

Treatment: Mastectomy.
Outcome: No recurrence found at the yearly follow-up examinations during the 12-year period following treatment.

Ex. **7.1**-9

Example 7.2

Ex. **7.2**-1   Right and left MLO projections: asymmetric density in the upper half of the left breast.

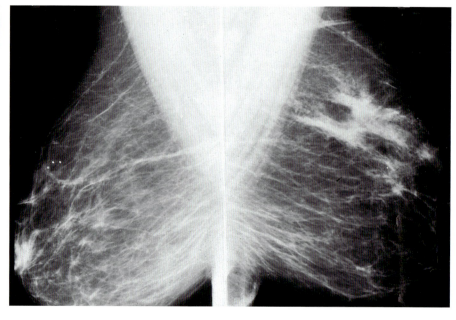

Ex.

Ex. **7.2**-2 & 3   MLO and CC microfocus magnification views show architectural distortion within the density.

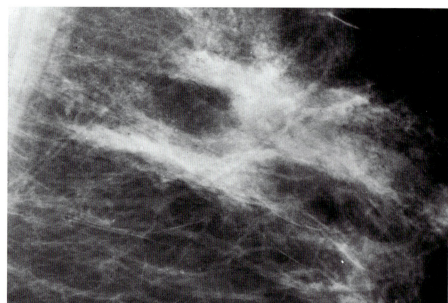

Ex.

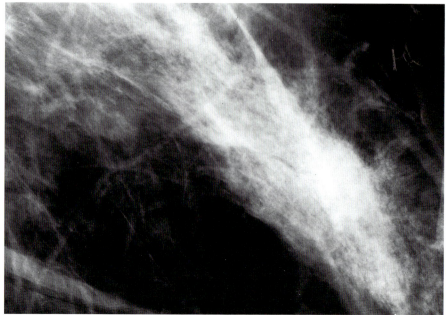

Ex.

Example 7.2

Ex. **7.2**-4   Specimen radiograph following preoperative localization using the "bracketing" technique.

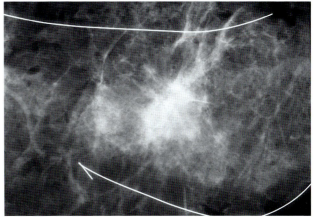

Ex. **7.2**-4

Ex. **7.2**-5 to 7   Histological examination shows ductal carcinoma in situ (**7.2**-5, **7.2**-6) and multiple papillomas (**7.2**-7).

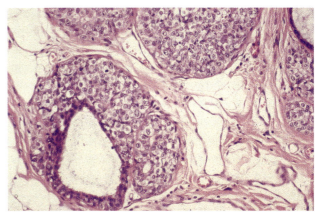

Ex. **7.2**-5

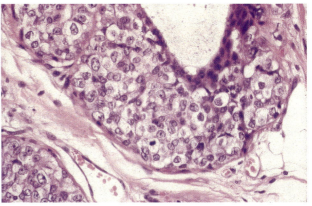

Ex. **7.2**-6

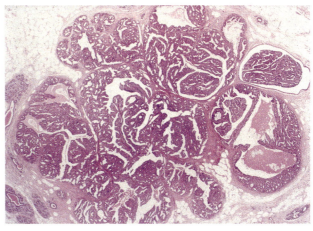

Ex. **7.2**-7

Nonspecific Asymmetric Density with Architectural Distortion on the Mammogram

Example 7.3

A 71-year-old asymptomatic woman, screening examination.

Ex. **7.3**-1 & 2   Right breast, MLO and CC projections. There is a large area with architectural distortion in the upper outer quadrant. There is no history of previous trauma or surgery.

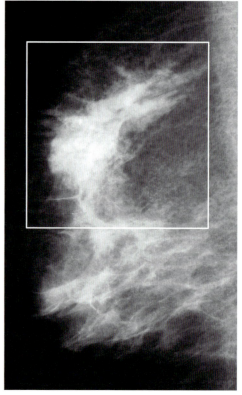

Ex. **7.3**-1

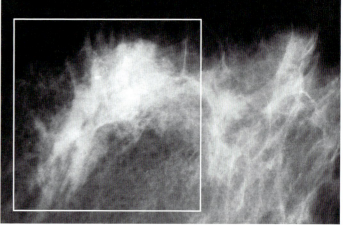

Ex.

Example 7.3

Ex. **7.3**-3 & 4 Microfocus magnification mammogram and the specimen radiograph show the nonspecific architectural distortion associated with nonspecific calcifications.

Ex. **7.3**-5 Radiograph of a specimen slice.

Ex. **7.3**-6 Large-section histology: 4 cm × 3 cm DCIS associated with desmoplastic reaction, accounting for the mammographic finding.

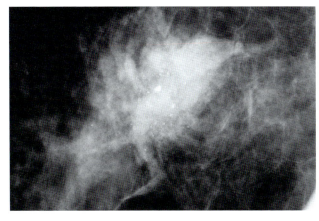

Ex. **7.3**-3

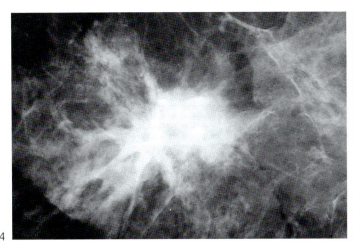

3-4

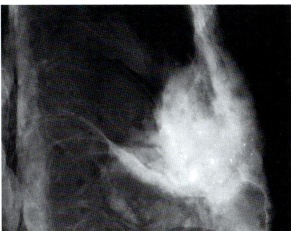

Ex. **7.3**-5

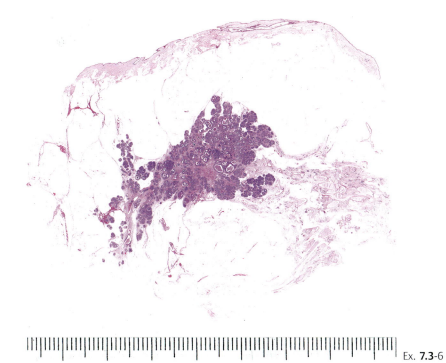

Ex. **7.3**-6

Lymph node status: No metastasis was found at histological examination of eight surgically removed axillary nodes. **Treatment**: Mastectomy.

Outcome: Sixteen years after treatment the patient is free of recurrence.

Definite Pathological Lesion Causing an Asymmetric Density on the Mammogram

The mammographic image is a reflection of the underlying histology, but it tends to simplify the histological heterogeneity into the following basic patterns:

> **Definite pathological lesions**
> - Stellate/spiculated tumor
> - Circular/oval tumor mass
> - Calcifications
> - Tumor mass with calcifications

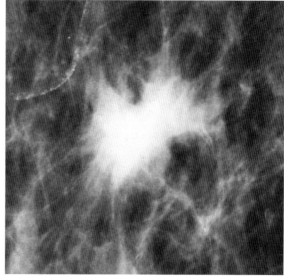

7.16

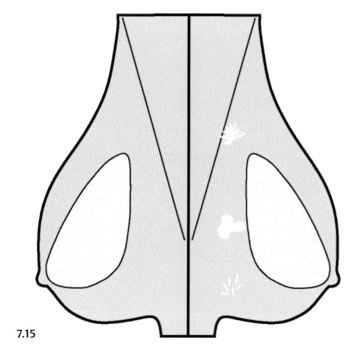

7.15

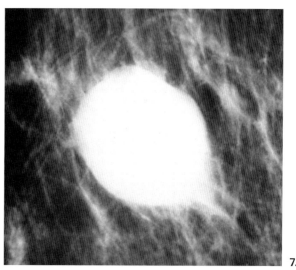

7.17

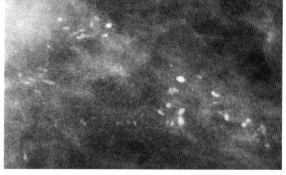

7.18

Fig. **7.16**   Spiculated lesion.

Fig. **7.17**   Circular/oval lesion.

Fig. **7.18**   Microcalcifications.

Fig. **7.19**   Stellate or oval tumor associated with calcifications.

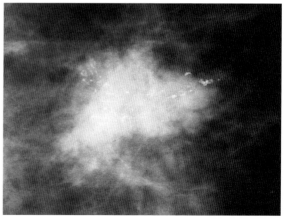

7.19

■ Distribution of Histological Diagnoses at Open Biopsy

Mammographic screening discloses a wide spectrum of benign and malignant breast abnormalities as well as numerous variations of the normal fibroglandular tissue, hyperplastic breast changes, etc. An adequate preoperative work-up using a systematic approach and a combination of the tools available to the radiologist will help in the differential diagnosis and management of each individual case. The diagnostic procedures have been developed to a high degree of accuracy, enabling us to provide detailed gross morphological and histological information about the nature of the underlying disease processes. Management can thus be far more precisely planned and unnecessary procedures can be minimized.

Summary of 1168 Cases Sent to Open Surgery

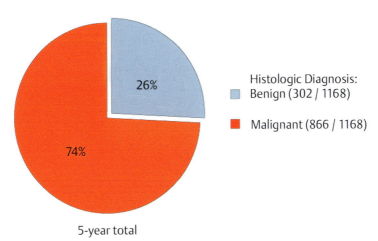

7.20   5-year total

Fig. **7.20**   Relative distribution of malignant and benign histological diagnoses in a series of 1168 cases referred to open surgery from the Department of Mammography, Falun Central Hospital. The indications for surgery included mammographic and ultrasound findings, preoperative needle biopsy, and patient concern. Various subsets of this patient material of 1168 cases are presented on the following pages in pie charts.

■ Algorithm for the Work-up and Management of an Asymmetric Density on the Mammogram

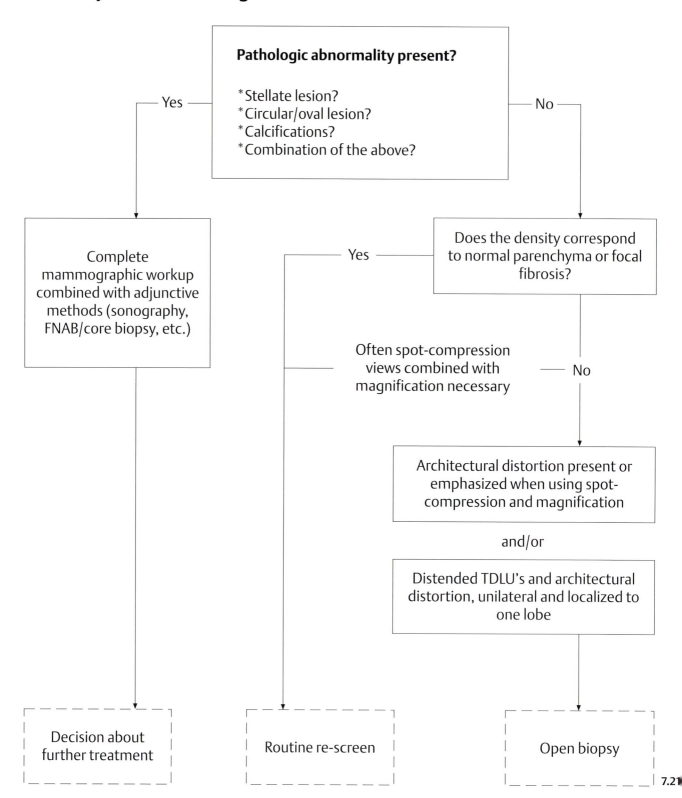

Pathologic abnormality present?

*Stellate lesion?
*Circular/oval lesion?
*Calcifications?
*Combination of the above?

Yes — No

Complete mammographic workup combined with adjunctive methods (sonography, FNAB/core biopsy, etc.)

Yes — Does the density correspond to normal parenchyma or focal fibrosis?

Often spot-compression views combined with magnification necessary — No

Architectural distortion present or emphasized when using spot-compression and magnification

and/or

Distended TDLU's and architectural distortion, unilateral and localized to one lobe

Decision about further treatment

Routine re-screen

Open biopsy

7.21

Practice in Perception and Work-up of Findings

■ Breast Regions with a Higher Frequency of Breast Cancer

Breast cancer occurs with a varying frequency in different quadrants of the breast. These figures appear to be related to the relative proportions of glandular tissue in these quadrants (Fig. **7.22**).

Knowing where the different regions of the breast are projected on the mammogram will help the radiologist search more effectively for breast cancer. The majority of breast cancers will be found in one of the following **four regions of the mammogram** (these so-called **"forbidden areas"** will contain nonspecific asymmetric densities representing early phases of malignant lesions, and require special attention):

1 The upper outer quadrant projected to the region parallel with the edge of the pectoralis major muscle on the MLO view ("milky way")
2 The medial half of the breast, best seen on the CC projection
3 The retroglandular, clear space on the CC projection
4 The retroareolar area

Lesions Localized in the Upper Outer Quadrant

Breast cancer is most frequently found in the **upper outer quadrant** of the breast. On the mammogram, most of the upper outer quadrant will be projected over an area **several centimeters in width and parallel to the pectoralis major muscle** on the mediolateral oblique view (see Fig. **7.23**). As this is the area with the highest frequency of breast cancer, any asymmetric density occurring here should be carefully evaluated. The highest yield from breast cancer screening will be obtained by searching for small stellate lesions; for their precursors, the nonspecific asymmetric densities; for the circular/oval lesions; and for calcifications in the shaded area of Figure **7.23**. The term "milky way" is used figuratively, since the region shown on Figure **7.23** is the most frequent site for breast cancer, and most breast cancers will appear as stellate (starlike) lesions.

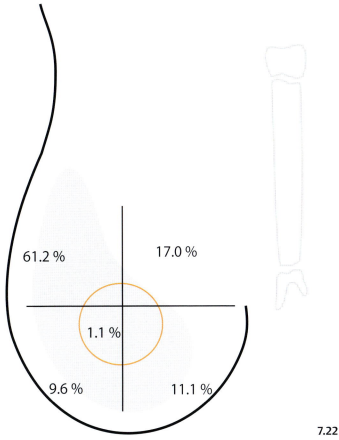

7.22

Fig. **7.22** Frequency of breast cancers by location in the breast from a series of 961 consecutive, histologically confirmed cases from the Falun Central Hospital.

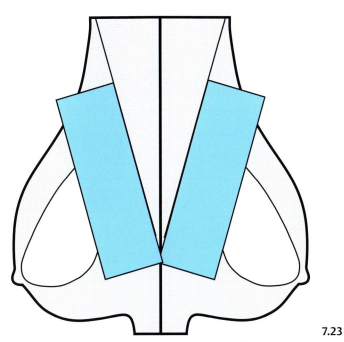

7.23

Fig. **7.23** The region on the mammogram where the upper outer quadrant is projected ("milky way").

Lesions localized in the upper outer or upper inner quadrant, closer to the chest wall, are projected over **an area several centimeters in width and parallel to the pectoralis major muscle** ("milky way").

Example 7.4

A 66-year-old asymptomatic woman, screening examination.

Ex. **7.4**-1 & 2   Right and left breasts, MLO projections.

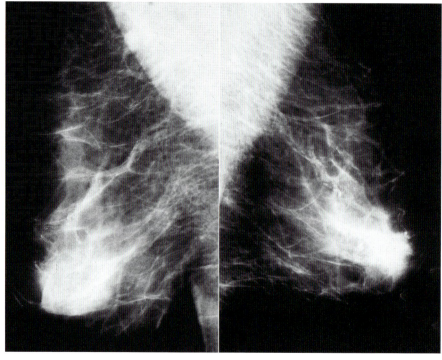

Ex. **7.4**-1

Ex.

Ex. **7.4**-3 & 4 and 6 & 7   Systematic application of the side-by-side, step-by-step viewing method can be of great help in detecting subtle lesions on the mammogram, as demonstrated in these images.

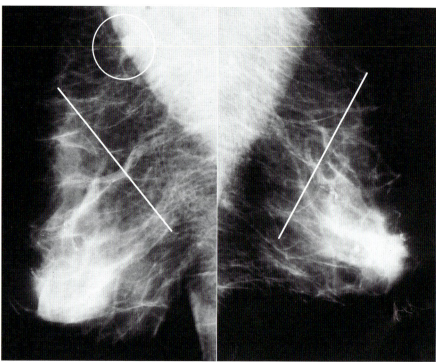

Ex. **7.4**-3

Ex.

Example 7.4

Ex. **7.4**-5 Schematic presentation of side-by-side viewing using the hand-held viewer.

Comment
- Pathological lesions projected over the pectoral muscle may be difficult to perceive. Side-by-side comparison aids in detection.
- A comet-tail associated with a lesion may often contain DCIS, and should be removed.

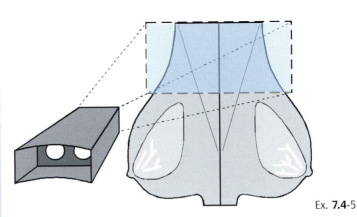

Ex. **7.4**-5

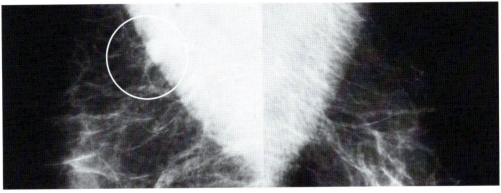

Ex. **7.4**-6

Ex. **7.4**-7

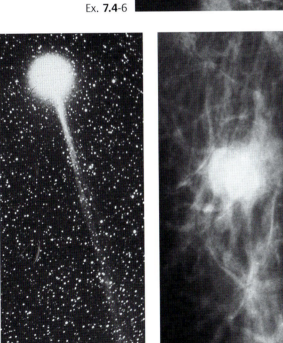
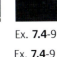

Ex. **7.4**-8

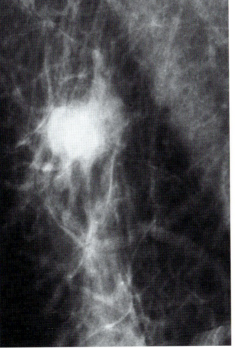
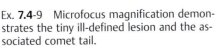

Ex. **7.4**-9

Ex. **7.4**-9 Microfocus magnification demonstrates the tiny ill-defined lesion and the associated comet tail.

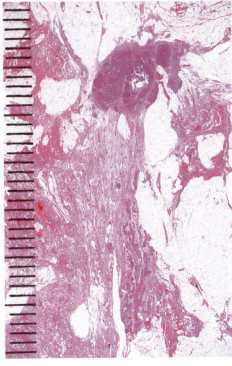

Ex. **7.4**-10

Ex. **7.4**-10 Large-section histology image of the 8 mm × 8 mm moderately differentiated invasive ductal carcinoma. The comet tail consists of >20 mm Grade 1 ductal carcinoma in situ.

Lymph node status: 2 of 12 axillary nodes showed metastases. **Treatment:** Mastectomy, postoperative irradiation and Tamoxifen. **Outcome:** The patient died 10 years after treatment; the cause of death was stroke.

Example 7.5

Ex. **7.5**-1 & 2   Right and left breasts, MLO projections. No abnormality was perceived at this screening examination.

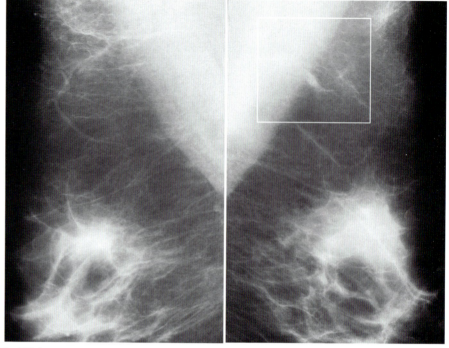

Ex. **7.5**-1   Ex. **7.5**-2

Ex. **7.5**-3 & 4   23 months later there was a palpable tumor in the axillary tail of the left breast. The mammograms also show pathological lymph nodes in the left axilla.

Comment
- Pathological lesions consist of an excess amount of tissue, causing the normally concave border of fibroglandular tissue to become convex.
- Pathological lesions, when small, are often nonspecific in appearance.
- When the nonspecific density is situated on one of the so-called "forbidden areas" on the mammogram (p. 259), a thorough work-up is recommended.

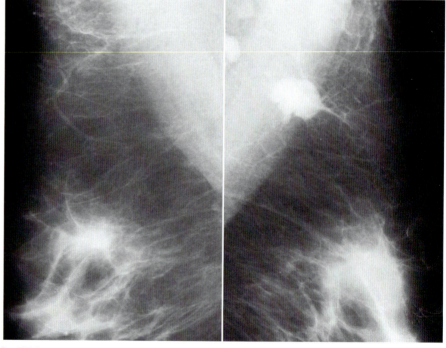

Ex. **7.5**-3   Ex. **7.5**-4

Example 7.5

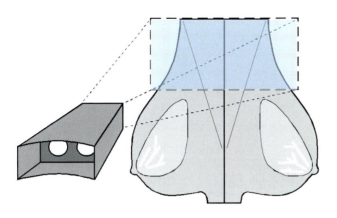

5-5

Ex. **7.5**-6 to 9   Simulating the images as seen through the viewer, a nonspecific density with convex contours can already be perceived on the left "milky way" at the first examination. Failure to detect this rapidly growing tumor allowed it to progress to metastatic disease.

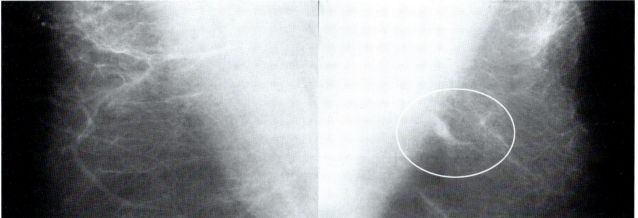

5-6   Ex. **7.5**-7

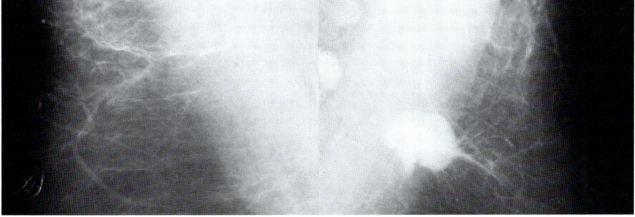

5-8   Ex. **7.5**-9

Ex. **7.5**-10   Specimen radiograph of the dissected tumor with the adjacent axillary nodes, some of which are pathological.

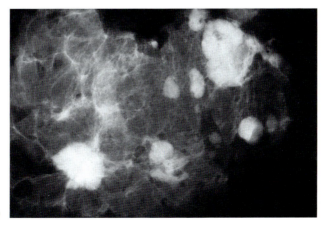

Ex. **7.5**-10

Example 7.6

A 44-year-old asymptomatic woman, screening examination.

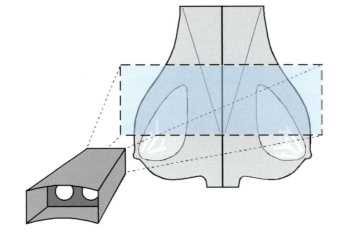

Ex. **7.6**-1 & 2   Detailed view of the right and left MLO projections.

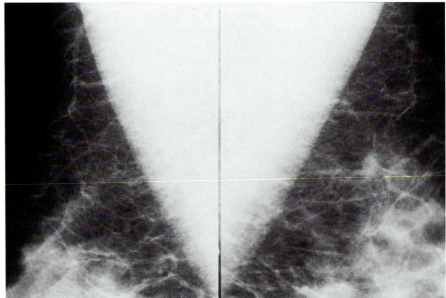

Ex. **7.6**-1   Ex.

Ex. **7.6**-3 & 4   Detection of the asymmetric density in the left breast is easy when the "milky way" is outlined. Attention is thus focused to the area on the mammogram with the highest frequency of breast cancer.

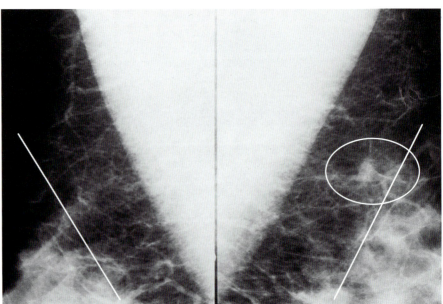

Ex. **7.6**-3   Ex.

Example 7.6

Ex. **7.6**-5 & 6   Alternatively, use of the viewer facilitates comparison with the corresponding area in the opposite breast.

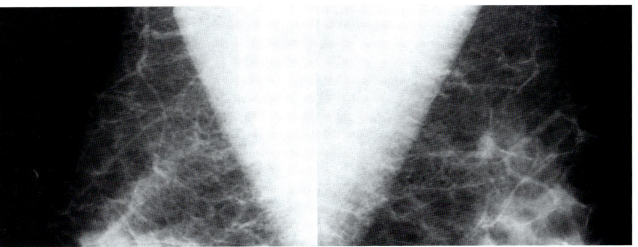

6-5

Ex. **7.6**-6

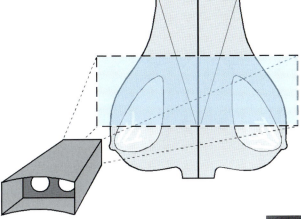

Ex. **7.6**-7

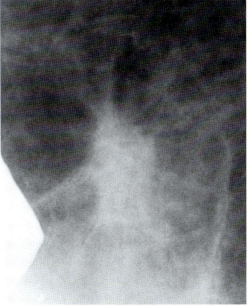

Ex. **7.6**-8

Ex. **7.6**-8   Microfocus magnification spot compression view demonstrates a spiculated, mammographically malignant lesion.

Comment
- After having found a lesion, continue to search for more.
- Multifocality is more common than unifocality.

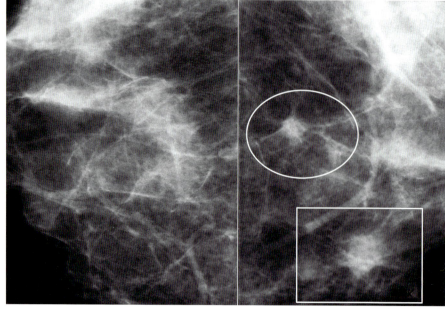

Ex. **7.6**-9 & 10   Details of the right and left CC projections show two spiculated lesions with no associated calcifications.

Ex. **7.6**-9   Ex.

Ex. **7.6**-11   Microfocus magnification view of the lesion within the oval on Fig. **7.6**-10. There is an additional, smaller, nonspecific density close to the stellate lesion.

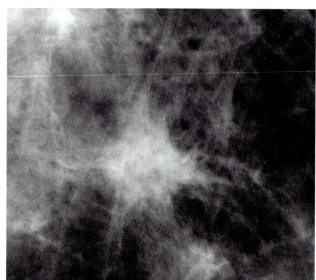

Ex.

Ex. **7.6**-12   Microfocus magnification of the larger lesion in the rectangle on Fig. **7.6**-10.

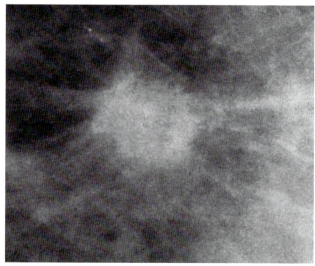

Ex.

Example 7.6

Ex. **7.6**-13   Specimen radiograph.

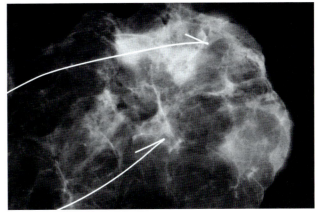

Ex. **7.6**-13

Ex. **7.6**-14   Large-section histology demonstrates two foci of invasive ductal carcinoma in different levels (6 mm × 5 mm and 4 mm × 4 mm). In addition, there are multiple foci of low-grade DCIS and LCIS on a large area in the breast.

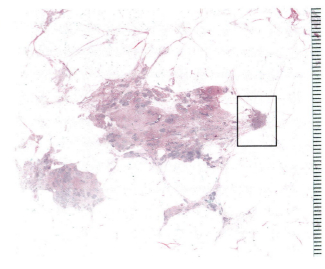

Ex. **7.6**-14

Ex. **7.6**-15   High-power histological image of the encircled well-differentiated invasive ductal carcinoma focus.

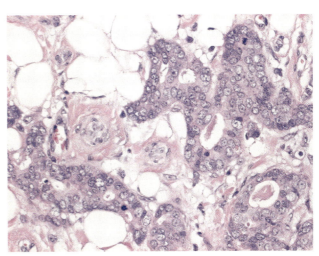

Ex. **7.6**-15

Lymph node status: No metastases were demonstrated at histological examination in five axillary lymph nodes.
Treatment: Mastectomy.
Outcome: A de-novo cluster of crushed stone–like calcifications were detected at the sixth yearly follow-up examination in the opposite breast. Histological examination showed Grade 2 in-situ carcinoma corresponding to the mammographic finding. In addition, a large area with a lobular carcinoma in situ (LCIS) and a 9 mm × 4 mm invasive lobular carcinoma was detected at histology.
Right mastectomy was performed due to asynchronous multifocal carcinoma.
Twelve years following mastectomy for multifocal breast cancer in the left breast and six years after mastectomy for multifocal breast cancer in the right breast, the patient is recurrence-free.

Lesions Localized in the Upper Outer Quadrant

Example 7.7

A 68-year-old asymptomatic woman, screening examination.

Ex. **7.7**-1 & 2   Right and left breasts, detailed view of the MLO projections.

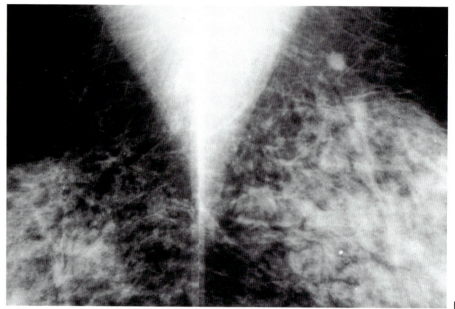

Ex. **7.7**-1

Ex.

Ex. **7.7**-3 & 4   Perception of a tiny, noncalcified invasive carcinoma may be difficult in a Pattern IV-type breast. However, outlining the "milky way" can aid in finding a small pathological lesion.

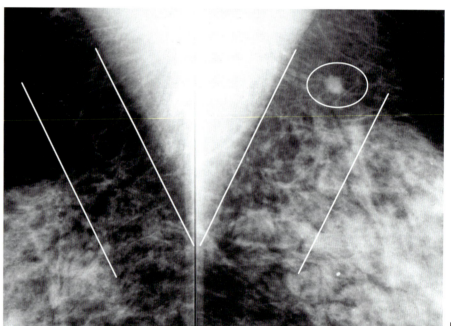

Ex. **7.7**-3

Ex.

Ex. **7.7**-5 & 6   Right and left breasts, detailed views of the right and left CC projections. The tumor mass is less convincingly demonstrated; thus the mammographic work-up should begin with the MLO view.

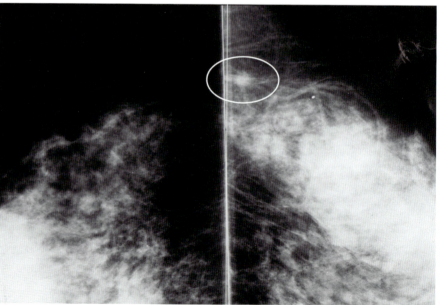

Ex. **7.7**-5

Ex.

Example 7.7

Comment
- When the pathological lesion is well seen on one projection but is difficult to discern on the other projection, work-up should begin with the projection on which the lesion is best seen.
- The radiologist's triple tasks are to perceive a lesion; to arrive at the diagnosis through work-up; and to attempt to determine whether it is unifocal or multifocal.

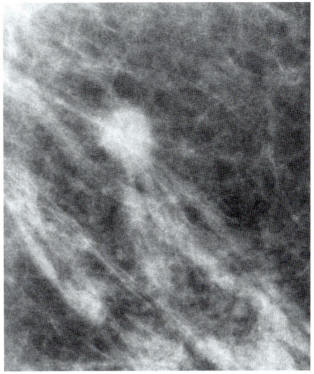

Ex. **7.7**-7

Ex. **7.7**-7 Microfocus spot magnification on the MLO projection demonstrates a solitary, ill-defined, mammographically malignant tumor.

Ex. **7.7**-8 Microfocus spot magnification view of the tumor on the exaggerated MLO projection.

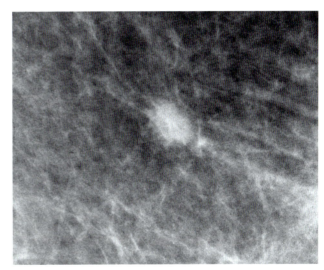

Ex. **7.7**-8

Ex. **7.7**-9 Subgross, thick-section histology of the excised malignant tumor.

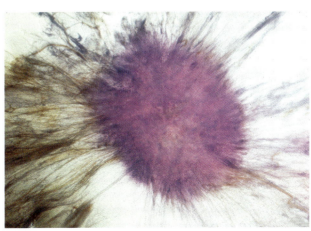

Ex. **7.7**-9

Lesions Localized in the Upper Outer Quadrant—Example 7.7

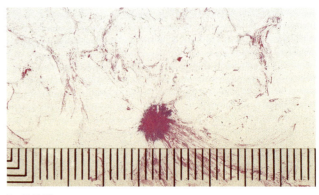

Ex. **7.7**-10

Ex. **7.7**-10   Large-section histology shows a solitary, 6 mm × 6 mm invasive carcinoma.

Ex. **7.7**-11   Low-power histological image of the tumor.

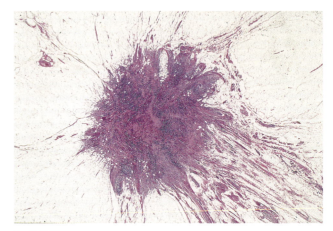

Ex. **7.7**-11

Ex. **7.7**-12 & 13   Medium-power histological image showing moderately differentiated invasive ductal carcinoma with lobular components.

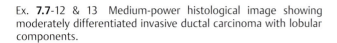

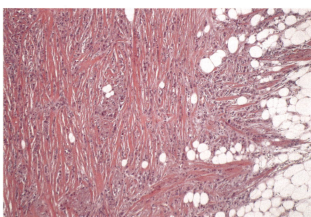

Ex. **7.7**-12

Lymph node status: No metastasis was found at histological examination of 10 surgically removed axillary nodes.
Treatment: Segmentectomy and postoperative irradiation.
Outcome: Yearly examination during the 11 years following treatment did not reveal signs of recurrence.

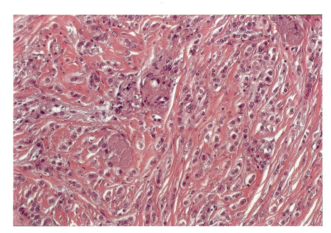

Ex. **7.7**-13

Example 7.8

Nonspecific appearance of early breast cancer. A 67-year-old woman, asymptomatic screening case.

Ex. **7.8**-1   The nonspecific tiny density (arrow) on the "milky way" did not trigger call-back for further evaluation in this case.

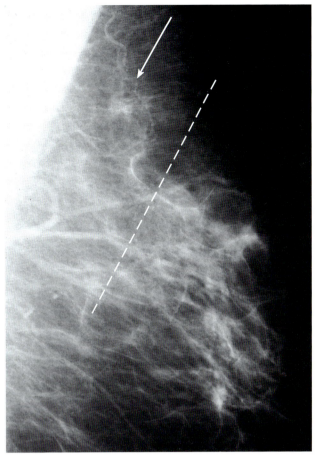

Ex. **7.8**-1

Ex. **7.8**-2   Same patient 25 months later, detail of the left MLO projection. During the intervening 25-month interval the tiny nonspecific density has developed into a mammographically malignant lesion.

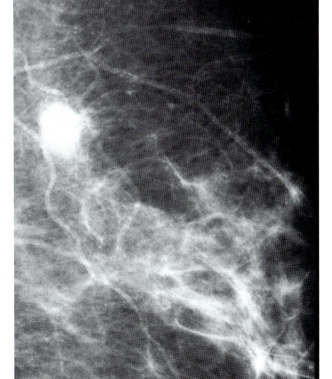

Ex. **7.8**-2

Comment
- Systematically viewing the four areas on the mammogram that are listed on page 259 will help the reader to react to subtle asymmetric densities, some of which may be the earliest signs of an invasive cancer.

Histology: 10 mm × 10 mm moderately differentiated invasive ductal carcinoma.
Lymph node status: No metastasis was found in the four removed axillary lymph nodes.
Treatment: Segmentectomy and postoperative irradiation.
Outcome: Yearly follow-up for 13 years did not show any sign of recurrence or de-novo tumor.

Example 7.9

A 66-year-old asymptomatic woman, screening examination.

Analysis of the findings: The calcifications may represent DCIS distributed over a large area, associated with two invasive foci, which should all be removed at surgery. Preoperative 14-gauge core needle biopsy of the small tumor masses indicated invasive ductal carcinoma.

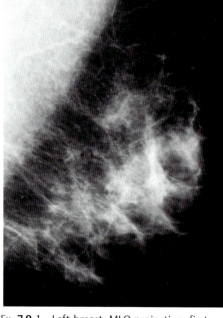

Ex.**7.9**-1

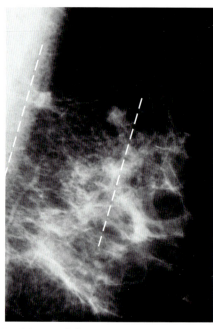

Ex.7

Ex. **7.9**-1   Left breast, MLO projection, first screening examination. No abnormality is seen.

Ex. **7.9**-2   Left breast, MLO projection, second screening examination 24 months later. Two tumor masses have developed during the interscreening interval, projected over the "milky way."

Ex. **7.9**-3   Left breast, detail of the CC projection. The two tumor masses are located in the medial half of the breast.

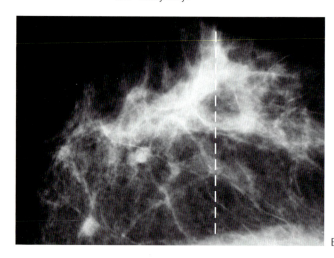

Ex.7

Ex. **7.9**-4   CC projection, microfocus magnification of the medial half of the left breast. The two *de novo* tumors are mammographically malignant. The increased resolution from magnification reveals microcalcifications over a large area.

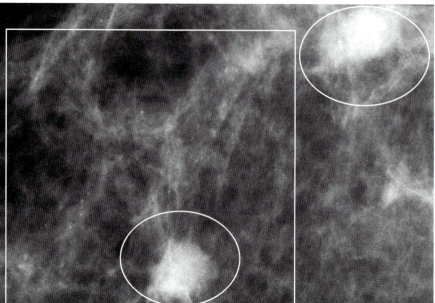

Ex.7

Example 7.9

Ex. **7.9**-5 The bracketing technique was used for preoperative localization. Specimen radiograph shows both the ill-defined tumors and a large area of adjacent fibroglandular tissue.

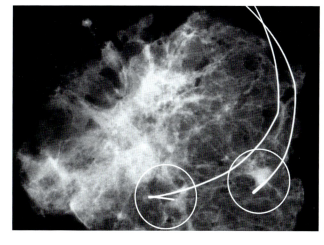

Ex.**7.9**-5

Ex. **7.9**-6 Large-section histology image of the excised specimen showing two invasive tumors (encircled), and the adjacent fibroglandular tissue.

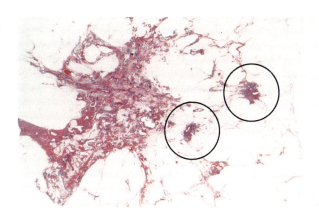

Ex.**7.9**-6

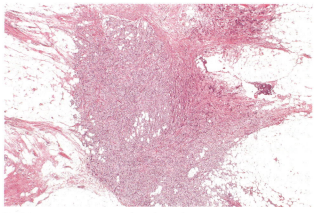

9-7

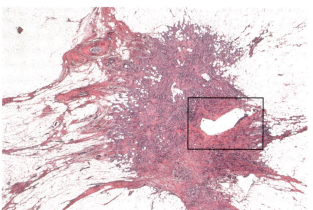

Ex.**7.9**-8

Ex. **7.9**-7 & 8 Low-power histological images of the two invasive tumors. Note the defect in **7.9**-8 caused by core biopsy.

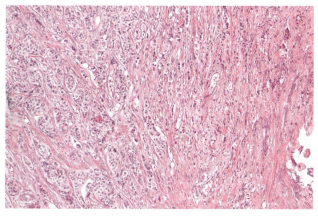

9-9

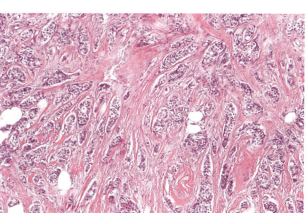

Ex.**7.9**-10

Ex. **7.9**-9 & 10 Higher-power histological images of the two invasive breast cancer foci.

273

Lesions Localized in the Upper Outer Quadrant—Example 7.9

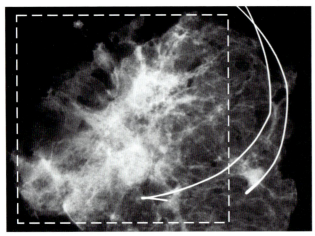

Ex.**7.9**-11

Ex. **7.9**-11   The fibroglandular tissue containing the calcifications and which is adjacent to the invasive tumors (rectangle) contains different manifestations of DCIS.

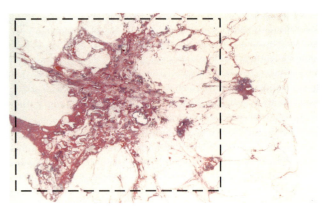

Ex.**7**

Ex. **7.9**-12   Large-section histological image (H&E stain) from the same tissue shown on **7.9**-11. Two invasive cancers measuring 6 mm × 5 mm and 6 mm × 6 mm are seen. Adjacent to them, there is an area measuring 60 mm × 40 mm with DCIS.

Ex. **7.9**-13   Large-section histology showing dilated ducts with micropapillary DCIS and intraluminal secretion.

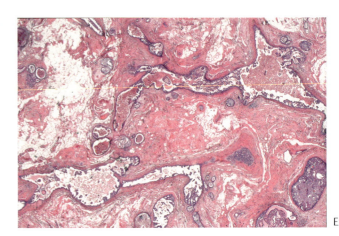

Ex.**7**

Ex. **7.9**-14   Magnification of the sub-gross image of micropapillary DCIS and the so-called roman arches consisting of proliferating malignant cells.

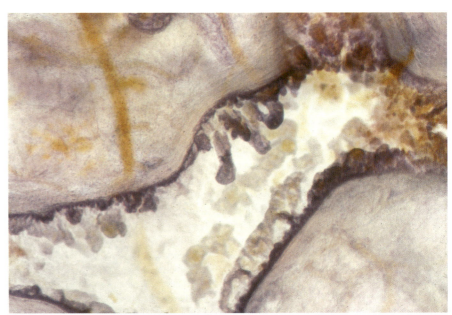

Ex.**7**

Example 7.9

Ex. **7.9**-15 to 18   Low-power histological images of the micropapillary DCIS (60 mm × 40 mm area).

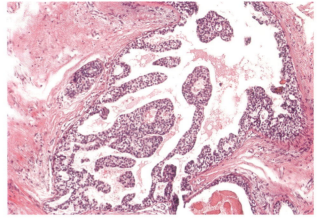

Ex.**7.9**-15

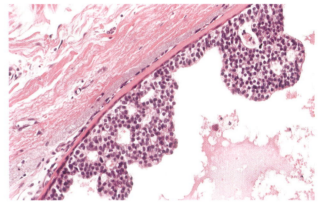

Ex.**7.9**-16

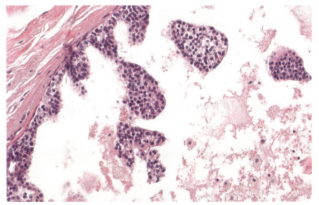

Ex.**7.9**-17

Ex. **7.9**-18   Subgross, thick-section histology of the micropapillary DCIS.

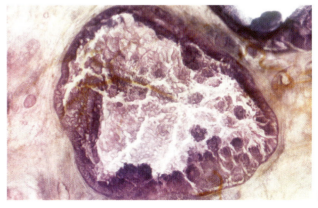

Ex.**7.9**-18

Ex. **7.9**-19 to 22   The resected tissue (outlined by a rectangle in Ex. **7.9**-11 & 12) contains all of the common growth patterns found in DCIS:
(1) Solid cell proliferation is shown in **7.9**-19 & 20.
(2) Micropapillary cell proliferation is shown in **7.9**-21.
(3) Cribriform cell proliferation in **7.9**-22.

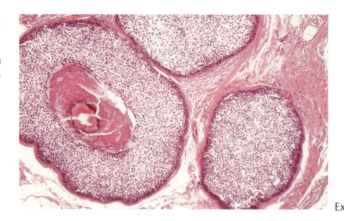

Ex.7

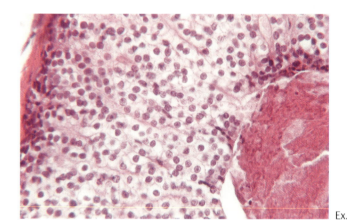

Ex.7

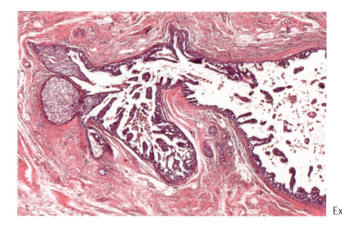

Ex.7

Comment
● Multifocality of breast cancer has many manifestations. Whenever two or more obviously invasive foci are detected on the mammogram, one should search for the presence of associated DCIS. Subtle asymmetric densities, non-specific calcifications, nipple discharge, etc. may lead to the detection of additional tumor foci.

Lymph node status: No metastasis shown at histological examination of 12 surgically removed lymph nodes.
Treatment: Mastectomy.
Outcome: Ten years following treatment the patient has no demonstrable recurrence.

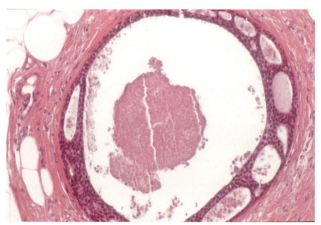

Ex.7

Example 7.10

A 63-year-old asymptomatic woman, screening examination.

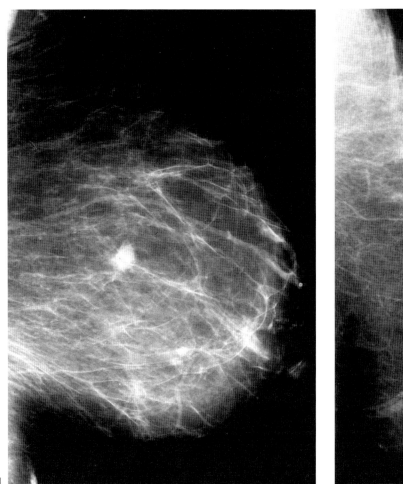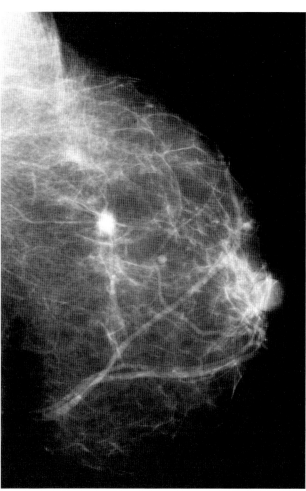

Ex. **7.10**-1 & 2   Left breast, MLO and CC projections. Pattern II-type breast, fatty involution. The surrounding adipose tissue makes detection of this small density easy.

Lesions Localized in the Upper Outer Quadrant—Example 7.10

Ex. **7.10**-3 & 4   Microfocus magnification images, MLO and CC projections. The solitary, high-density, ill-defined tumor mass is mammographically malignant.

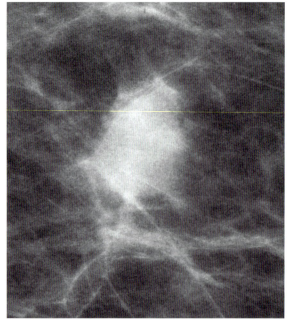

Ex. **7.10**-3

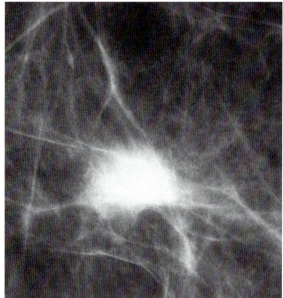

Ex. **7.10**-4

Ex. **7.10**-5 Ultrasound examination supports the mammographic diagnosis and facilitates percutaneous needle biopsy.

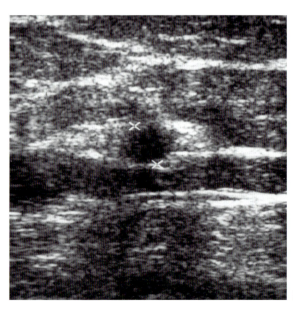

Ex. **7.10**-5

Example 7.10

Ex. **7.10**-6   Fine-needle aspiration biopsy shows malignant cells.

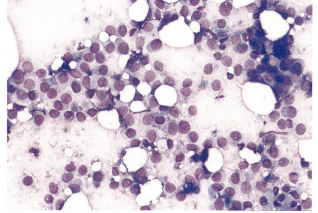

Ex. **7.10**-6

Ex. **7.10**-7   Large-section histology, H&E stain. The tumor is solitary and measures 9 mm × 7 mm.

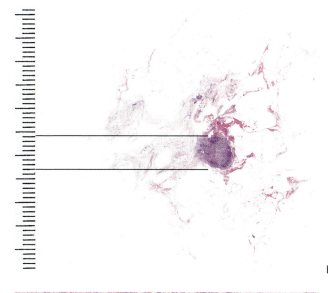

Ex. **7.10**-7

Ex. **7.10**-8 & 9   Low-power (**7.10**-8) and high-power (**7.10**-9) histological image of a well-differentiated invasive ductal carcinoma.

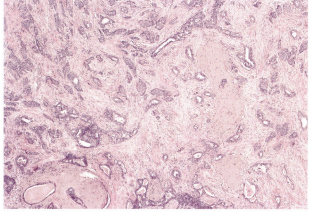

Ex. **7.10**-8

Comment
- In Pattern II-type breasts perception of small tumors is not difficult.
- Preoperative evaluation of unifocality or multifocality is also relatively easy, and assists in planning treatment.

Treatment: Segmentectomy and postoperative irradiation.

Outcome: Disease-free during the first 36 months following treatment.

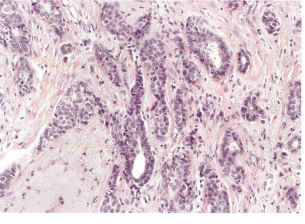

Ex. **7.10**-9

Lesions Localized in the Upper Outer Quadrant

Example 7.11

This 41-year-old woman, when attending her first screening examination, reported a palpable lesion in her left breast. Physical examination confirmed a "thickening" in the upper outer quadrant of the left breast.

Ex. **7.11**-1 & 2 and 3 & 4   Details of the right and left MLO and CC projections. The area with the palpable "thickening" is outlined.

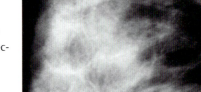
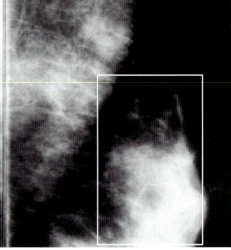

Ex. **7.11**-1

Ex.

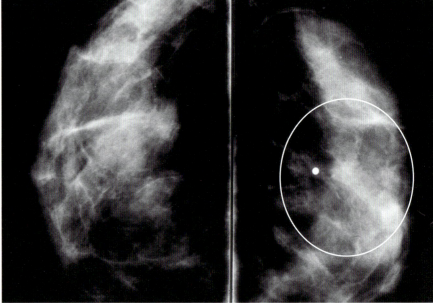

Ex. **7.11**-3

Ex.

Ex. **7.11**-5   Microfocus magnification image of the left breast in the lateromedial, horizontal projection. Several clusters of diverse type calcifications are demonstrated. The presence of clustered, powdery type calcifications is an indication for diagnostic surgery.

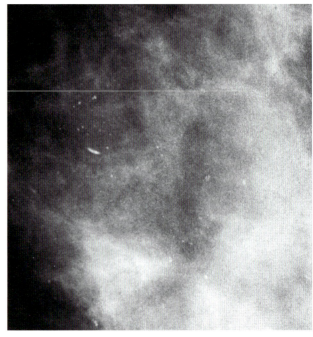

Ex.

Example 7.11

Ex. **7.11**-6 Radiograph of a 5 mm slice of the operative specimen. The diverse type calcifications are easily distinguishable, especially the tea cup–like (*a*) and the numerous clusters of powdery calcifications (*b*).

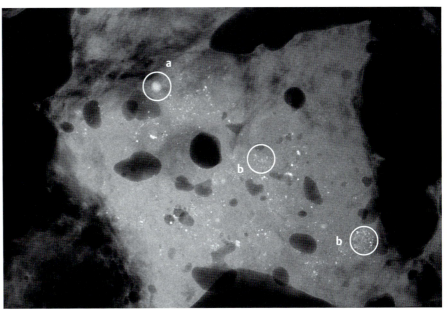

Ex. **7.11**-6

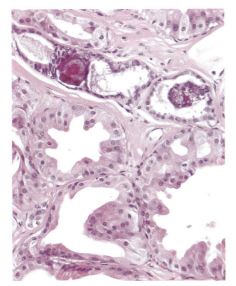

Ex. **7.11**-7

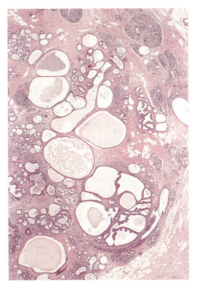

Ex. **7.11**-8

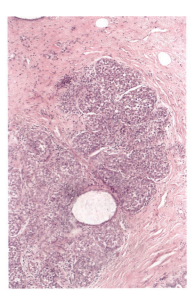

Ex. **7.11**-9

Ex. **7.11**-7 The psammoma body–like calcifications are associated with benign hyperplastic breast changes. This histological image shows apocrine metaplasia with calcification.

Ex. **7.11**-8 The clusters of cystically dilated and fluid-filled TDLUs and ducts, combined with dense fibrosis, account for the vague palpatory finding.

Ex. **7.11**-9 Mammographically and clinically occult LCIS was found at histological examination.

Ex. **7.11**-10 & 11   The continuation of this case serves to emphasize a basic rule in screening: Do not stop searching for additional lesions after having found the first one. When comparing the upper border of the fibroglandular tissue on the left side (concave, see Ex. **7.11**-17 & 18) with the corresponding, contralateral contour (convex), further work-up is indicated.

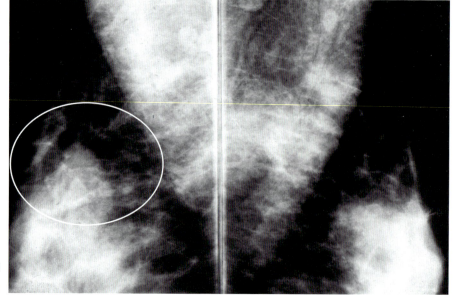

Ex. **7.11**-10

Ex. **7.11**-11

Ex. **7.11**-12 & 13   The mid-portion of the posterior contour of the fibroglandular tissue is protruding into the retroglandular clear space.

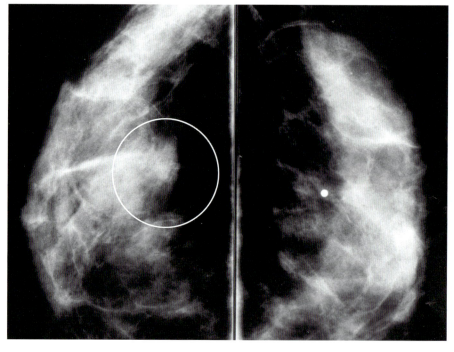

Ex. **7.11**-12

Ex. **7.11**-13

Ex. **7.11**-14   Microfocus magnification, MLO projection. The protruding lesion also has a radiating structure. As shown on page 197, 93% of all stellate lesions detected on the mammogram represent a malignant tumor.

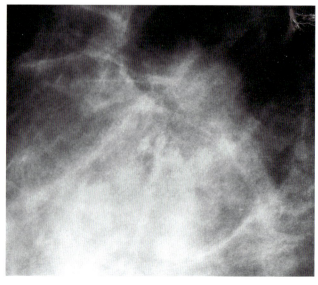

Ex. **7.11**-14

Example 7.11

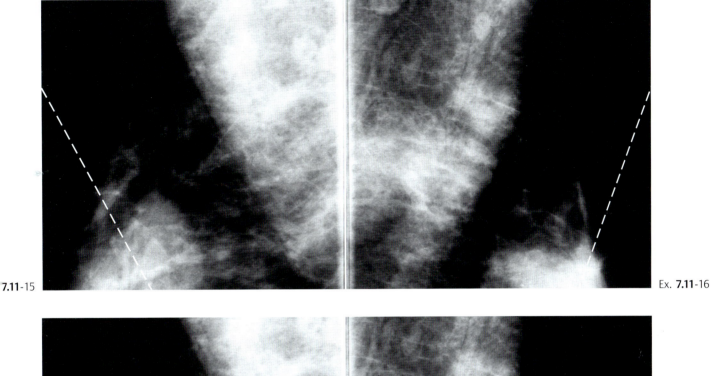

7.11-15

Ex. 7.11-16

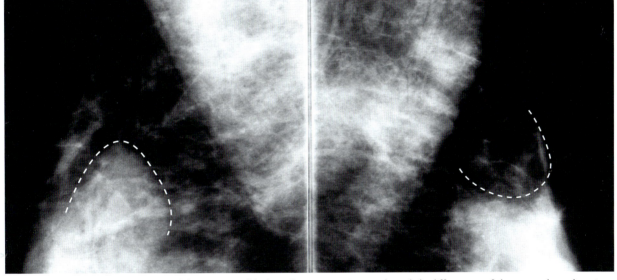

7.11-17

Ex. 7.11-18

Ex. 7.11-15 & 16 and 17 & 18   The use of the viewer will help to focus attention on the subtle differences of the parenchymal contours, facilitating perception of lesions that are difficult to perceive.

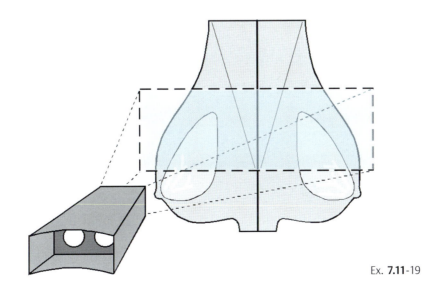

Ex. 7.11-19

Ex. **7.11**-20   Ultrasound examination is consistent with the mammographic diagnosis.

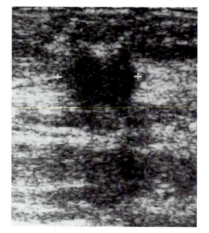

Ex. **7.11**-20

Ex. **7.11**-21   Ultrasound-guided fine-needle aspiration biopsy shows atypical cells.

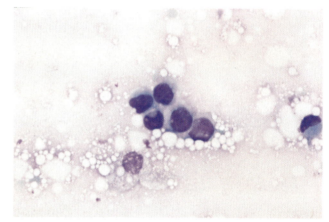

Ex. **7.11**-21

Ex. **7.11**-22 & 23   14-gauge core biopsy shows tubular carcinoma.

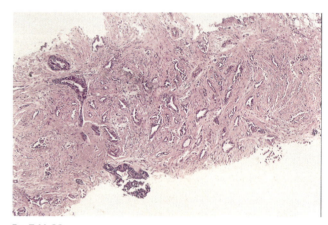

Ex. **7.11**-22

Comment
- Basic rule of screening: keep searching for additional lesions after having found the first one.
- The patient may present with a lesion that distracts attention from another, more subtle but malignant lesion.
- In the presence of powdery calcifications, open biopsy should be performed.

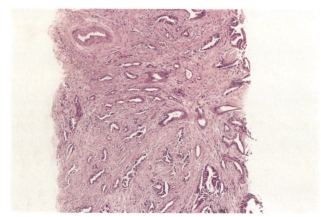

Ex. **7.11**-23

Example 7.11

Ex. **7.11**-24   Specimen radiograph shows that the tumor has been removed with a good margin. The use of the *bracketing technique* facilitated complete removal of the lesion. In the bracketing technique two or more hooked wires are placed preoperatively near the lesion borders to ensure complete surgical removal with adequate margins.

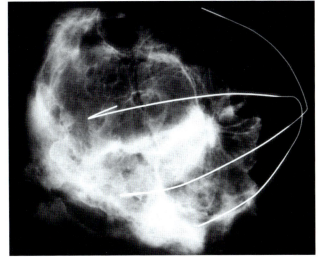

Ex. **7.11**-24

Ex. **7.11**-25   Large-section histology corresponding to the specimen radiograph.

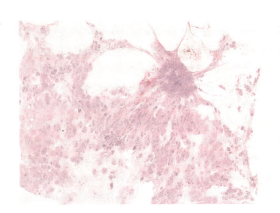

Ex. **7.11**-25

Ex. **7.11**-26   Low-power histological image of this 10 mm × 8 mm tubular carcinoma.

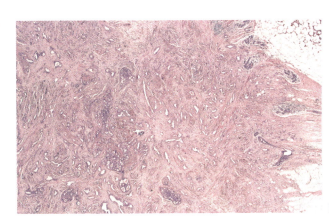

Ex. **7.11**-26

Ex. **7.11**-27   High-power histological image.

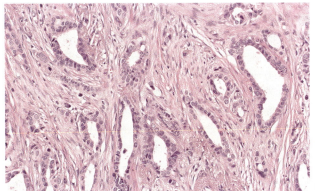

Treatment: Bilateral segmentectomy. Postoperative irradiation right breast.
Outcome: No signs of recurrence during the 4-year follow-up period.

Ex. **7.11**-27

285

Lesions Localized in the Upper Outer Quadrant

Example 7.12

A 66-year-old asymptomatic woman, screening case.

Ex. **7.12**-1 & 2   Right and left breasts, detailed image of the MLO projections. There is a nonspecific asymmetric density in the left breast, adjacent to the pectoral muscle.

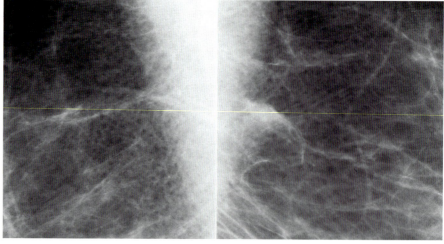

Ex. **7.12**-1   Ex.

Ex. **7.12**-3 & 4 and 5 & 6   These images demonstrate two different methods for enhancing perception of subtle lesions. In **7.12**-3 & 4 the lateral border of the "milky way" is outlined, serving to emphasize the presence of any asymmetric density; **7.12**-5 & 6 show the area seen through the viewer. Both methods lead to the detection of the nonspecific lesion in this particular case.

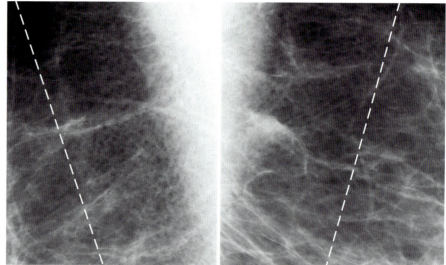

Ex. **7.12**-3   Ex.

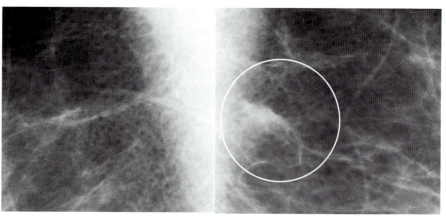

Ex. **7.12**-5   Ex.

Comment

- The reason for calling this patient back for further work-up is the convex upper border of this ill-defined density that is situated in one of the "forbidden areas" on the mammogram, the so-called "milky way." In fact, this particular region is home to more cancers than any other area on the mammogram.

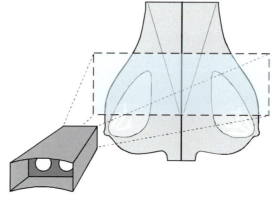

Ex. **7.12**-7

Example 7.12

Ex. **7.12**-8   The lesion is also well seen on this lateromedial, horizontal projection.

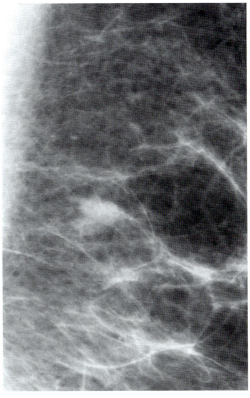

Ex. **7.12**-8

Ex. **7.12**-9   Microfocus magnification reveals the central tumor mass and ill-defined contours, characteristic of a mammographically malignant lesion.

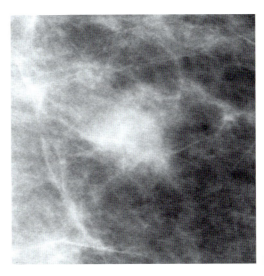

Ex. **7.12**-9

Lesions Localized in the Upper Outer Quadrant—Example 7.12

Ex. **7.12**-10 & 11   Right and left breasts, detail of the lateral aspect of the CC projections. The asymmetric density is encircled.

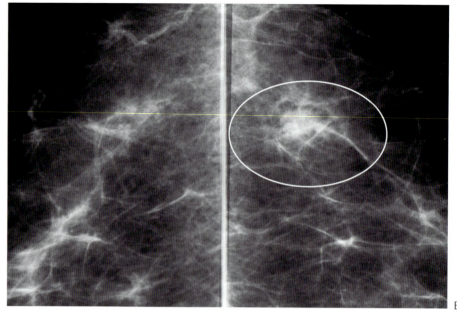

Ex. **7.12**-10

Ex.

Ex. **7.12**-12 & 13   The microfocus magnification images demonstrate a central tumor mass with lobulated, ill-defined contours characteristic of a mammographically malignant lesion.

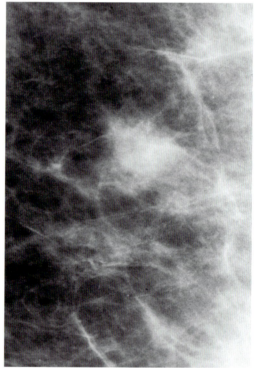

Ex. **7.12**-12

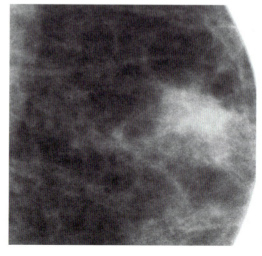

Ex. **7.12**-13

Example 7.12

Ex. **7.12**-14 Large-section histology image shows a 10 mm invasive carcinoma. This low-power histological image matches the microfocus magnification images (**7.12**-12 & 13).

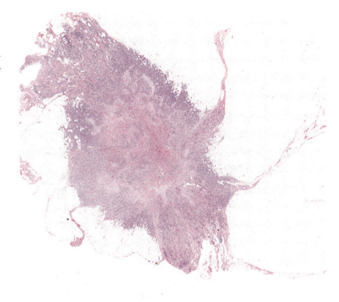

Ex. **7.12**-14

Ex. **7.12**-15 Further magnification of the histological image of this moderately differentiated invasive ductal carcinoma, showing the viable cancer cells at the periphery and the central fibrosis.

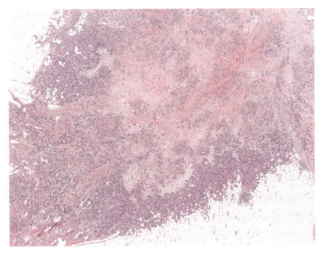

Ex. **7.12**-15

Ex. **7.12**-16 Higher-power histological image. Moderately differentiated invasive ductal carcinoma.

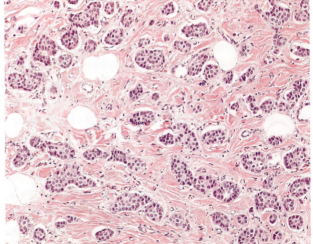

Lymph node status: Eight surgically removed axillary nodes showed no metastasis at histological examination.
Treatment: Segmentectomy and postoperative irradiation.
Outcome: Nine years and six months following treatment the patient developed skeletal metastases. Thirteen years following treatment there are no signs of local recurrence.

Ex. **7.12**-16

Lesions Localized in the Upper Outer Quadrant

Example 7.13

A 70-year-old asymptomatic woman, screening examination.

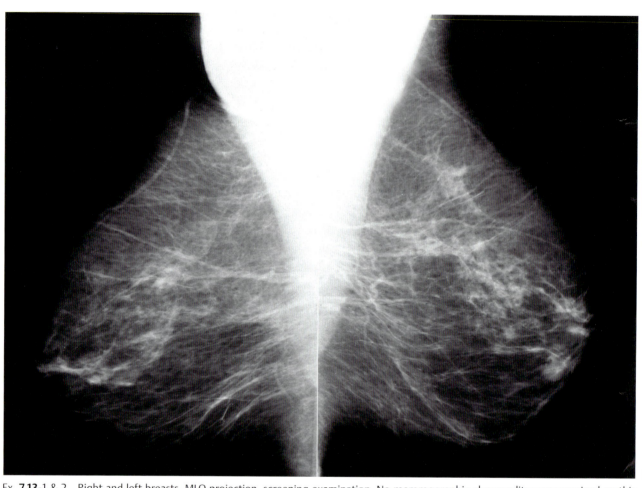

Ex. **7.13**-1

Ex.

Ex. **7.13**-1 & 2   Right and left breasts, MLO projection, screening examination. No mammographic abnormality was perceived on this occasion.

Ex. **7.13**-3   Left breast, CC projection, screening examination.

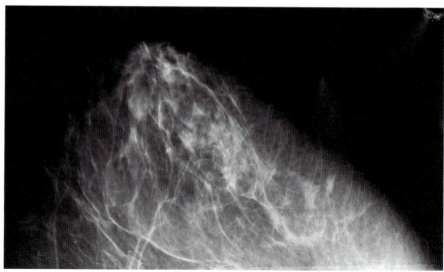

Ex. 7

Example 7.13

Ex. **7.13**-4 & 5   Same examination, demonstrating the use of the two perception enhancement methods described in the previous example (Ex. **7.12**-3 & 4), which might have resulted in detection of this extremely small tumor mass.

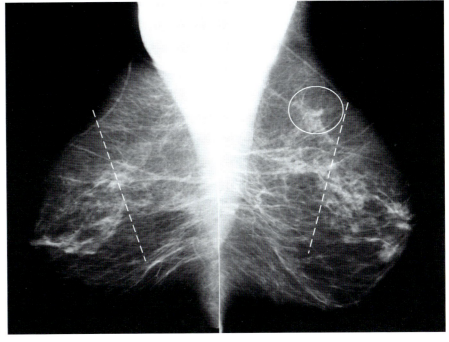

Ex. **7.13**-4   Ex. **7.13**-5

Ex. **7.13**-6 & 7   The mammography viewer facilitates careful comparison of corresponding areas on the right and left mammograms, and assists in the detection of subtle asymmetric densities, calcifications, etc. Use of the viewer might have helped detect the tiny lesion in this case.

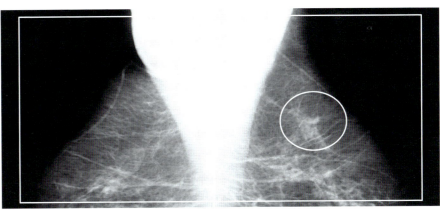

Ex. **7.13**-6   Ex. **7.13**-7

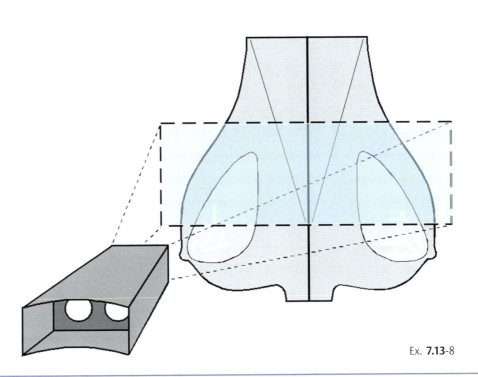

Ex. **7.13**-8

Lesions Localized in the Upper Outer Quadrant—Example 7.13

Ex. **7.13**-9 & 10   Next screening examination, two years later. The woman is now 72 years old and is still asymptomatic. The previously nonspecific tumor mass has developed to a more specific stellate lesion, although still small.

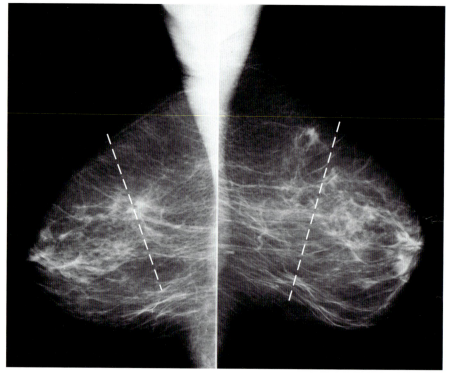

Ex. **7.13**-9   Ex. **7.13**-10

Ex. **7.13**-11   Left breast, CC projection. The tiny stellate lesion is localized in the upper outer quadrant (encircled).

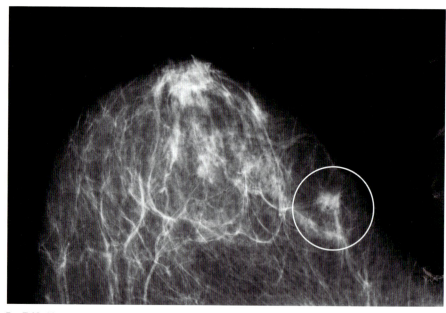

Ex. **7.13**-11

Example 7.13

Ex. **7.13**-12 & 13   Microfocus magnification images in the MLO and CC projections show a lobulated, central tumor mass surrounded by straight, individual spiculations, characteristic of a mammographically malignant tumor.

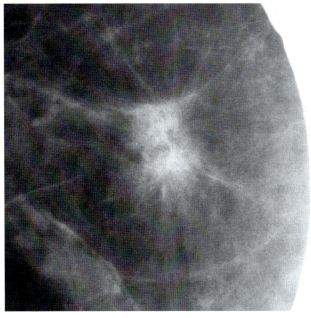

Ex. **7.13**-12

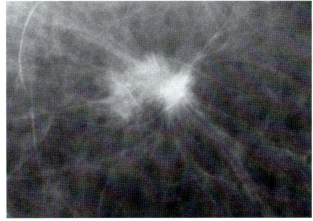

Ex. **7.13**-13

Ex. **7.13**-14   Ultrasound examination supports the mammographic diagnosis.

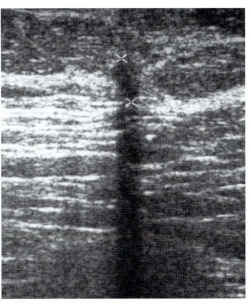

Ex. **7.13**-14

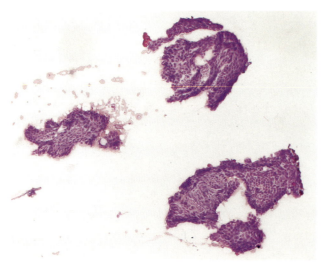

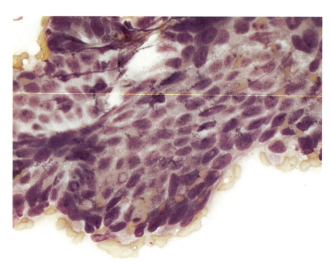

Ex. **7.13**-15

Ex. **7.13**-16

Ex. **7.13**-15 & 16   Cytology reveals atypical cells. However, cytology is not the recommended procedure in stellate tumors that are < 10 mm since about 90% of them are Grade 1 or Grade 2. The cytological diagnosis is too often indefinite, as in this case, and ultrasound-guided core biopsy is recommended.

Ex. **7.13**-17   Operative specimen radiograph. The lesion has been removed with wide margins.

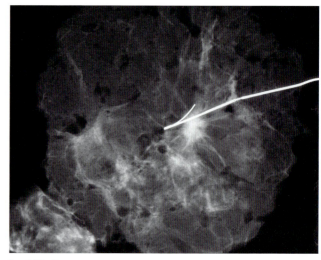

Ex. **7.13**-17

Ex. **7.13**-18   Large-section histology shows an 8 mm × 6 mm solitary, spiculated tumor.

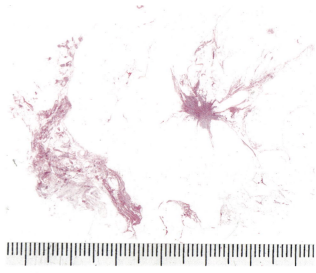

Ex. **7.13**-18

Example 7.13

Ex. **7.13**-19   Low-power histological image of the invasive tumor.

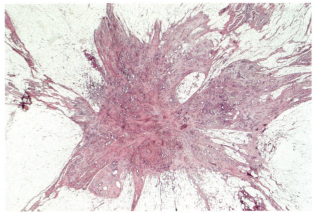

Ex. **7.13**-19

Ex. **7.13**-20 & 21   Moderate- and high-power histological images show a well-differentiated invasive ductal carcinoma.

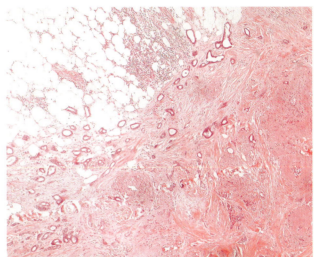

Ex. **7.13**-20

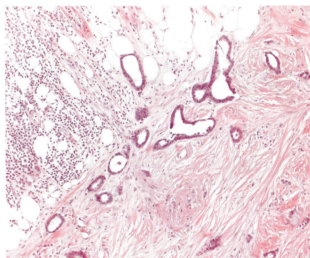

Treatment: The patient declined postoperative irradiation. She attended yearly follow-up examinations.

Ex. **7.13**-21

Follow-up: At the second annual postoperative mammographic examination, two *de novo* stellate lesions < 10 mm were detected in the medial half of the same breast, far from the site of the first operation. After her second breast-conserving surgery she once again declined adjuvant treatment and was symptom-free four years after the second operation.

Ex. **7.13**-22   Second follow-up examination, left breast, detail of the MLO projection. Two *de novo* stellate lesions are seen (rectangle). No associated calcifications are detected.

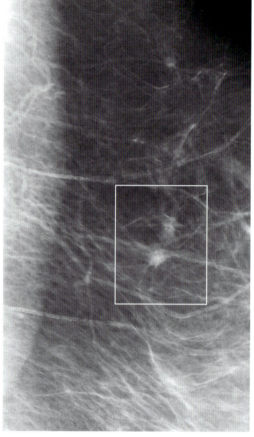

Ex. **7.13**-22

Ex. **7.13**-23   Left breast, CC projection. The area of the previous surgery in the lateral portion of the breast is encircled. The two newly developed, tiny densities are situated in the medial half of the breast, about 6.0 cm from the site of the previous biopsy.

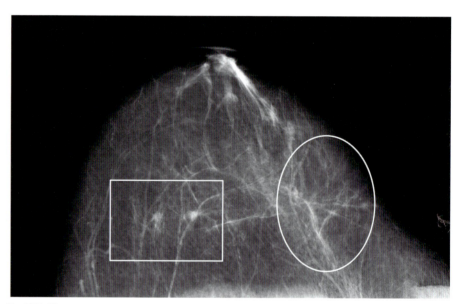

Ex. **7.13**-23

Example 7.13

Ex. **7.13**-24   Enlarged image of a detail of the left MLO projection with the two stellate tumors, which are mammographically malignant.

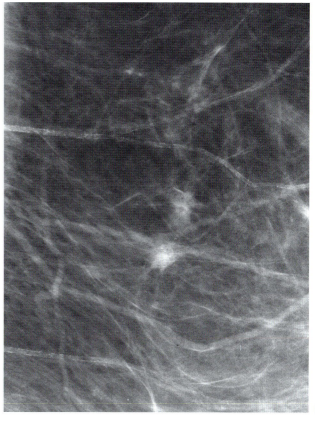

Ex. **7.13**-24

Ex. **7.13**-25 & 26   Ultrasound images of these two small tumors support the diagnosis of malignancy.

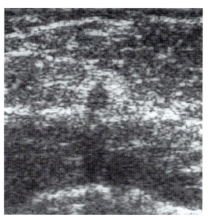

Ex. **7.13**-25

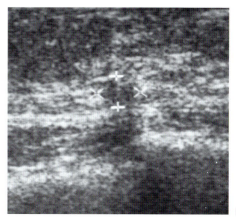

Ex. **7.13**-26

Ex. **7.13**-27 & 28   Fine-needle aspiration performed under ultrasound guidance shows malignant cells.

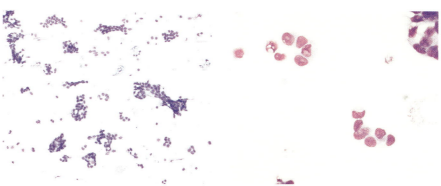

Ex. **7.13**-27

Ex. **7.13**-28

Lesions Localized in the Upper Outer Quadrant—Example 7.13

Ex. **7.13**-29   Microfocus magnification with spot compression in the CC projection shows the two tiny malignant tumors. The image can be directly correlated with the large-section histology image (Ex. **7.13**-30).

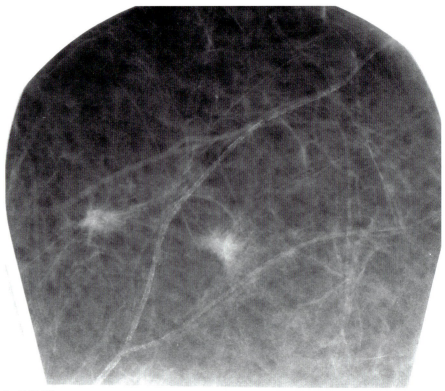

Ex. **7.13**-29

Ex. **7.13**-30   Large-section histology image demonstrating the two tubular carcinomas, each of them measuring < 10 mm.

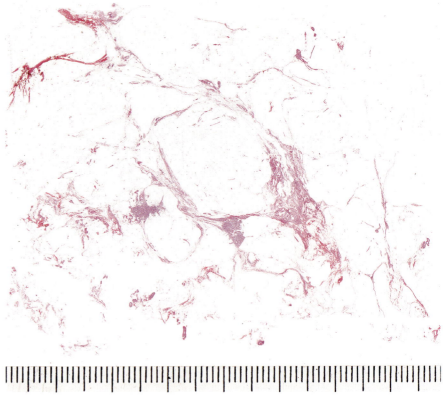

Ex. **7.13**-30

Example 7.13

Comment

- The nonspecific density in the upper outer quadrant of the left breast was not perceived at the initial examination. The reason for this oversight could have been its nonspecific appearance, which is characteristic of the very early phases of malignant, stellate lesions.
- However, the lesion had a convex contour and was situated in the "milky way."
- Although the cancer could have been detected two years earlier, using the above criteria, it was a slowly growing tumor with a long preclinical detectable phase in an older woman. The probability of her surviving from this breast cancer for the 24 years exceeds 99% (Ex. **7.13**-33).

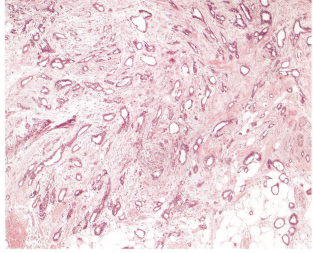

Ex. **7.13**-31

Ex. **7.13**-31 & 32   Medium-power histological images of the two tiny tubular carcinomas.

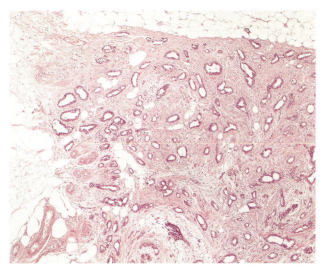

Ex. **7.13**-32

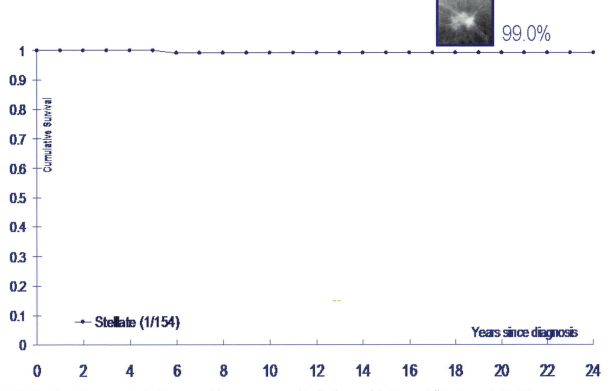

Ex. **7.13**-33

Ex. **7.13**-33   The 24-year survival of women with a mammographically detected 1–9 mm stellate tumor is 99.0%.

Example 7.14

A 41-year-old asymptomatic woman, first screening examination.

Ex. **7.14**-1 & 2   Right and left breasts, MLO projections.

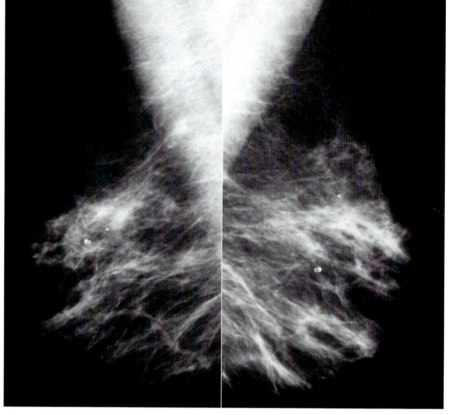

Ex. **7.14**-1

Ex.

Ex. **7.14**-3 & 4   Right and left breasts, detail of the CC projections.

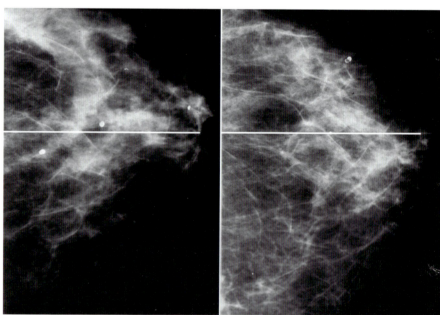

Ex. **7.14**-3

Ex. 7

Example 7.14

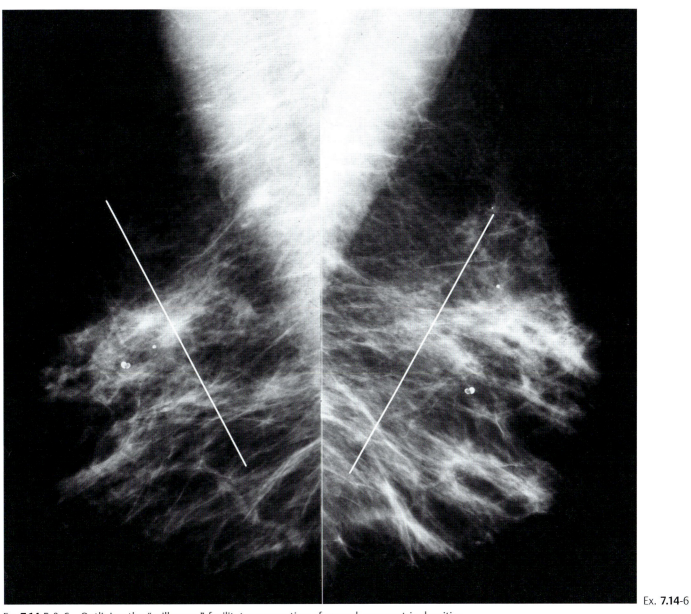

4-5

Ex. **7.14**-5 & 6   Outlining the "milky way" facilitates perception of several asymmetric densities.

Ex. **7.14**-6

Lesions Localized in the Upper Outer Quadrant—Example 7.14

Ex. **7.14**-7   The two asymmetric densities identified (arrows) are shown in greater detail in the microfocus magnification image (Ex. **7.14**-8).

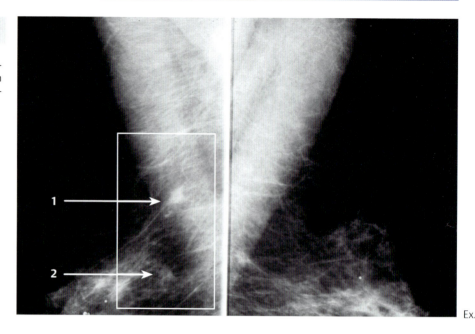

Ex. 7

Ex. 7

Ex. **7.14**-8   Density no. 1 appears to be focal fibroglandular tissue attached to a duct. Density no. 2 has a central tumor mass and an ill-defined contour, suggesting malignancy.

Example 7.14

Ex. **7.14**-9   Right breast, CC projection. The lesion labeled no. 2 in Ex. **7.14**-8 is encircled on the CC image.

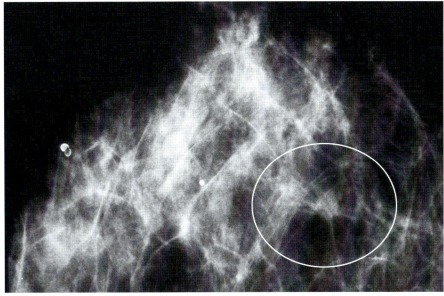

Ex. **7.14**-9

Ex. **7.14**-10   Microfocus magnification shows a lesion with a central tumor mass and straight spiculations, characteristic of a mammographically malignant lesion.

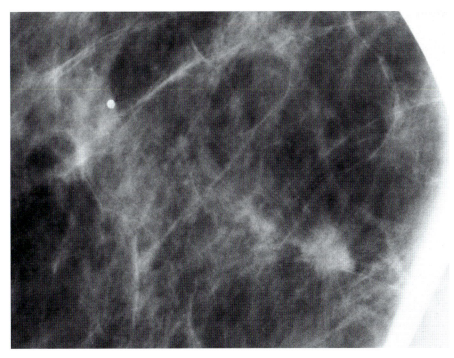

Ex. **7.14**-10

Ex. **7.14**-11   Ultrasound examination supports the mammographic diagnosis.

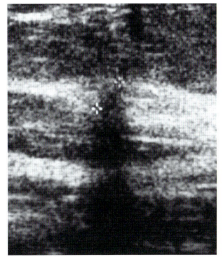

Comment
- Women are often called back from mammographic screening for asymmetric densities that turn out to be fibroglandular tissue at further work-up.
- Careful evaluation of other asymmetric densities may reveal a less obvious malignant tumor focus.

Ex. **7.14**-11

303

Lesions Localized in the Upper Outer Quadrant—Example 7.14

Ex. **7.14**-12 Ultrasound-guided fine-needle aspiration biopsy shows malignant cells.

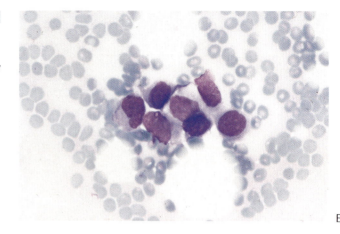

Ex.

Ex. **7.14**-13 Low-power histological image of the 14-gauge core biopsy specimen.

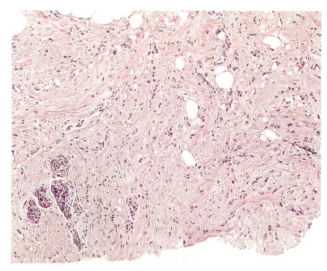

Ex.

Ex. **7.14**-14 High-power histological image: invasive lobular carcinoma.

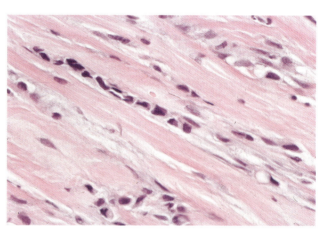

Ex.

Ex. **7.14**-15 Perforated-plate image taken in preparation for preoperative localization using the bracketing technique. The needles containing the hooked wires are inserted through the holes on either side of the lesion.

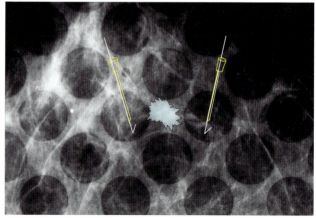

Ex.

Example 7.14

Ex. **7.14**-16   Specimen radiograph. The lesion is centrally located within the specimen, having been removed with wide margins.

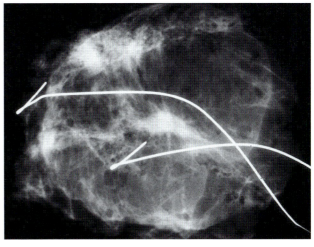

Ex. **7.14**-16

Ex. **7.14**-17   Large-section histology image corresponds closely to the specimen radiograph, showing the 9 mm × 4 mm invasive tumor.

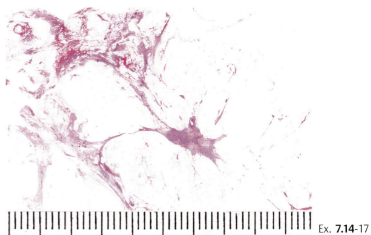

Ex. **7.14**-17

Ex. **7.14**-18   Microfocus magnification radiograph of a thin slice of the specimen.

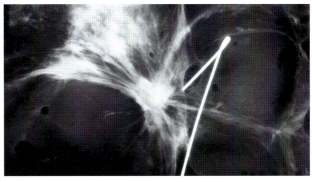

Ex. **7.14**-18

Ex. **7.14**-19   Low-power histological image of the moderately differentiated invasive lobular carcinoma, classic type. Higher-power histological examination also shows LCIS on an area measuring 50 mm × 50 mm.

Treatment: Segmentectomy and postoperative irradiation.
Outcome: No recurrence has been detected during the first three years following treatment.

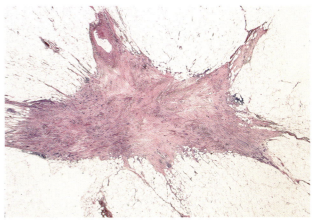

Ex. **7.14**-19

305

Example 7.15

A 67-year-old asymptomatic woman, screening examination.

Ex. **7.15**-1   Left breast, MLO projection. There is a nonspecific density projected over the pectoralis major muscle.

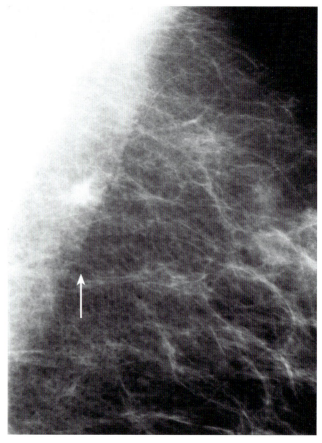

Ex.

Ex. **7.15**-2   Lateromedial horizontal projection. The nonspecific density is seen on the "milky way."

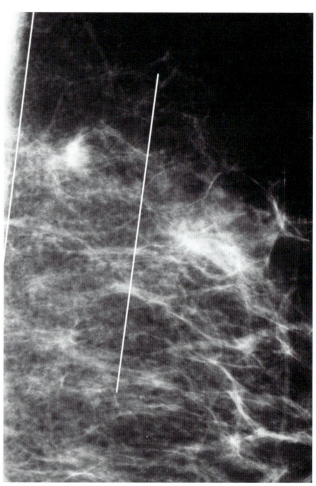

Ex.

Example 7.15

Ex. **7.15**-3 The nonspecific density is localized close to the chest wall.

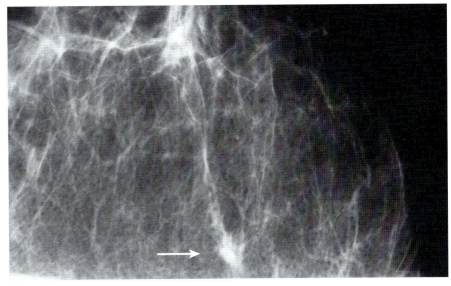

Ex. **7.15**-3

Ex. **7.15**-4 & 5 Microfocus magnification images in the CC (**7.15**-4) and MLO (**7.15**-5) projections. The small central tumor mass is surrounded by spiculations. The lesion is mammographically malignant.

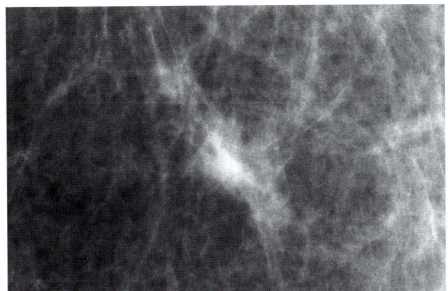

Ex. **7.15**-4

Comment
- The most commonly occurring mammographic feature of breast cancer is a stellate lesion, which has a characteristic appearance at sizes of 1 cm and larger. In the size-range 1–9 mm, when these tumors should be detected and removed, their mammographic image is often nonspecific.
- A nonspecific density is an asymmetric density that lacks the basic building blocks (absence of TDLUs, ducts, fibrosis with concave contours, adipose tissue), has a partially convex, ill-defined contour, and does not appear as a spiculated lesion on the screening mammogram.
- Nonspecific densities could represent a malignancy in its earliest detectable stage, especially when found in one of the "forbidden areas."

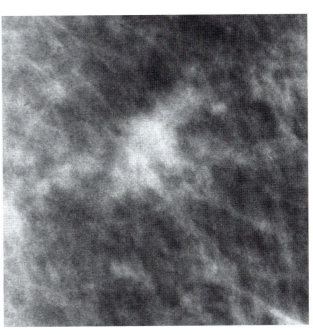

Ex. **7.15**-5

Ex. **7.15**-5 & 6   Preoperative stereotactic fine-needle aspiration biopsy.

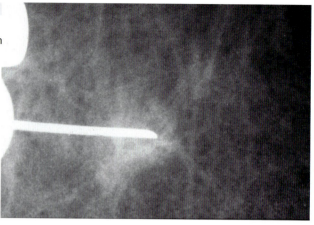

Ex. **7.1**

Ex. **7.15**-7   Cytological examination shows malignant cells.

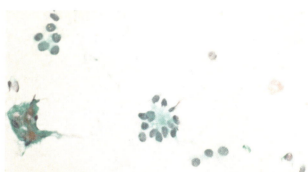

Ex. **7.15**

Ex. **7.15**-8   Specimen radiograph. The tumor has been excised.

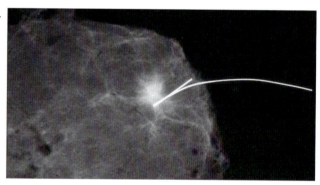

Ex. **7.15**

Ex. **7.15**-9   Specimen radiograph, axillary node dissection.

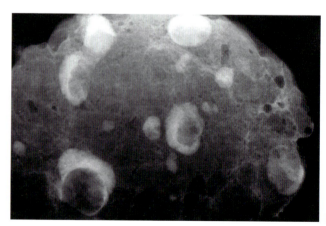

Ex. **7.15**

Example 7.15

Ex. **7.15**-10   Subgross, thick-section histology demonstrating the spiculated tumor.

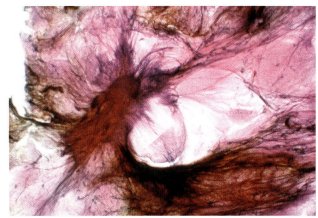

Ex. **7.15**-10

Ex. **7.15**-11   Low-power histological image of the 6 mm × 5 mm invasive carcinoma.

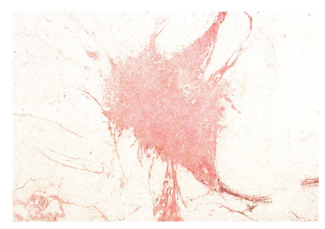

Ex. **7.15**-11

Ex. **7.15**-12 & 13   Higher-power magnification images show tubular cancer.

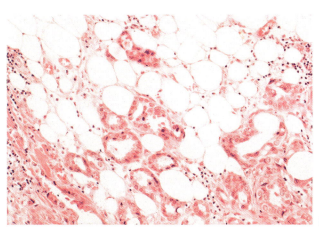

Ex. **7.15**-12

Lymph node status: No metastases were found at histological examination of 12 axillary lymph nodes.
Treatment: Segmentectomy. The final histological examination revealed several foci of low-grade DCIS and LCIS on a larger area in the breast; mastectomy was performed at the request of the patient.
Follow-up: Yearly follow-up examination showed no sign of recurrence during 10 years following treatment.

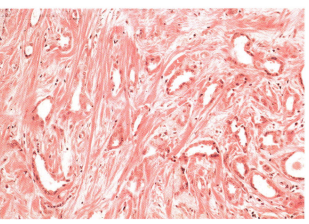

Ex. **7.15**-13

Example 7.16

A 74-year-old asymptomatic woman, screening examination.

Ex. **7.16**-1 & 2   Detail of the right and left MLO projections. The non-specific density in the left "milky way" was not perceived at screening.

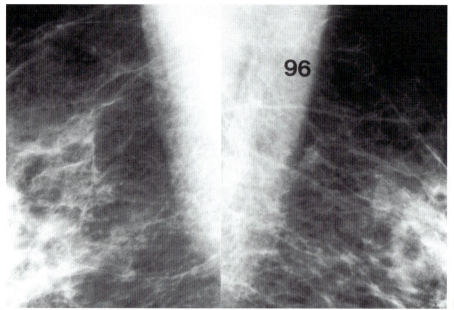

Ex. **7.16**-1

Ex.

Ex. **7.16**-4

Ex. **7.16**-3

Ex. 7.1

Ex. **7.16**-4 & 5   Proper use of the viewer should have led to the detection of this small lesion (encircled).

Ex. **7.16**-6 & 7   Detail of the right and left CC projections. The density (arrow) is difficult to distinguish from the surrounding parenchyma.

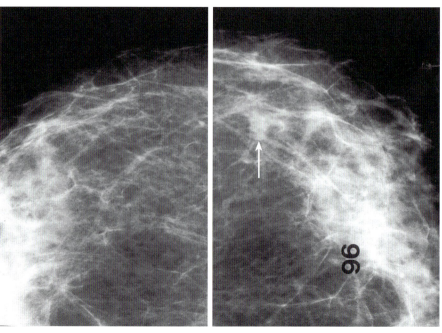

Ex. **7.16**-6

Ex.

Example 7.16

Ex. **7.16**-8 to 10   Comparison of the MLO projections from two successive screening examinations, using the masking technique to facilitate perception of the tiny tumor in the "milky way." Although the tumor has grown very little, it now has a more specific appearance, with a central tumor mass and surrounding spiculations (**7.16**-10 & 11).

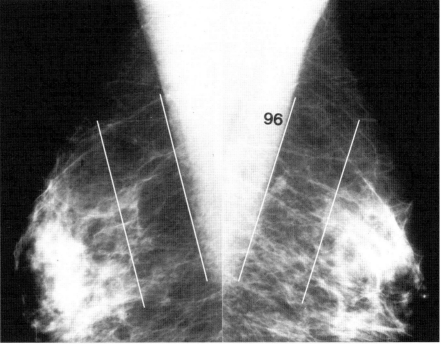

Ex. **7.16**-8

Ex. **7.16**-9

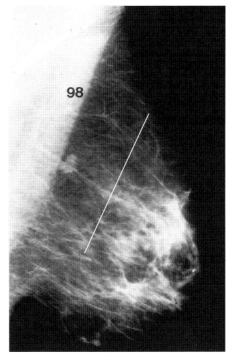

Ex. **7.16**-10

Ex. **7.16**-11   Microfocus magnification image in the MLO projection shows the characteristic mammographic appearance of a malignant tumor: a central tumor mass with lobulated contours and straight, individual spiculations.

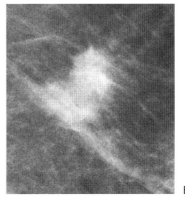

Ex. **7.16**-11

Lesions Localized in the Upper Outer Quadrant—Example 7.16

Ex. **7.16**-12   CC projection shows the small tumor in the retroglandular clear space.

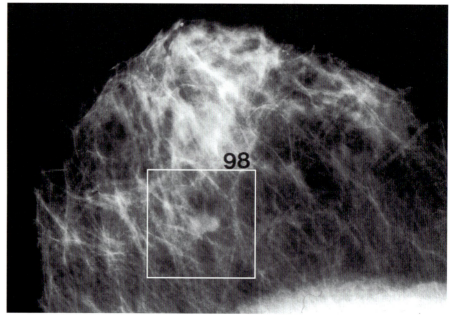

Ex. **7.16**-12

Ex. **7.16**-13   Microfocus magnification image shows the features of this stellate lesion more clearly.

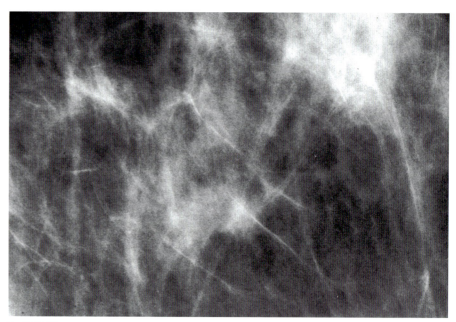

Ex. **7.16**-13

Ex. **7.16**-14   Ultrasound examination supports the mammographic diagnosis.

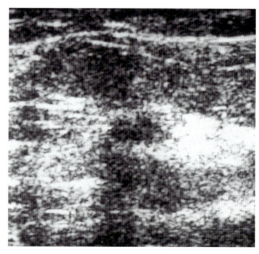

Comment
- This case serves to emphasize the comment for the previous case (Ex. **7.15**).

Ex. **7.16**-14

Example 7.16

Ex. **7.16**-15   Cytological examination: malignant cells.

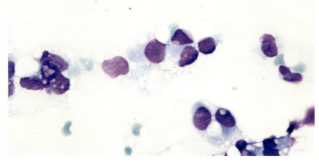

Ex. **7.16**-15

Ex. **7.16**-16   Large-section histological image. The 11 mm × 6 mm well-differentiated invasive carcinoma is solitary and has been removed with wide margins.

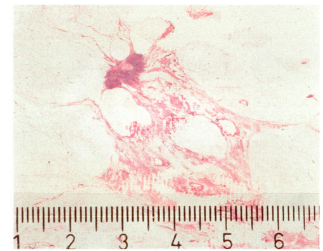

Ex. **7.16**-16

Ex. **7.16**-17   Subgross, thick-section image of this spiculated malignant tumor.

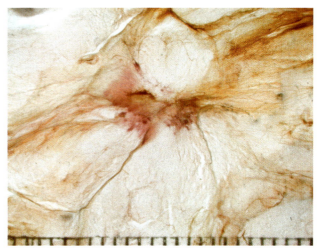

Ex. **7.16**-17

Ex. **7.16**-18   High-power histological image: well-differentiated invasive ductal carcinoma.

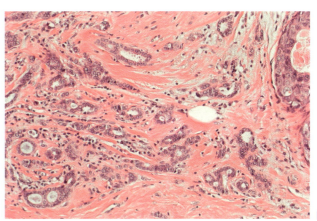

Treatment: Segmentectomy. No postoperative irradiation. No metastases found in sentinel nodes.
Follow-up: Recurrence-free during the 36 months following treatment.

Ex. **7.16**-18

313

Example 7.17

A 76-year-old asymptomatic woman, screening examination.

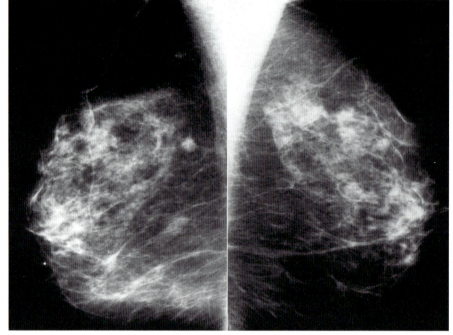

Ex. **7.17**-1 & 2   Right and left MLO projections. There is a small, asymmetric density with convex contours in the right "milky way."

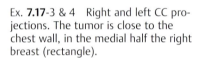

Ex. **7.17**-1

Ex. **7.17**-3 & 4   Right and left CC projections. The tumor is close to the chest wall, in the medial half the right breast (rectangle).

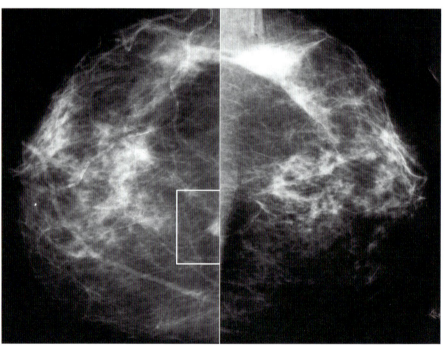

Ex. **7.17**-3

Ex.

Example 7.17

Ex. **7.17**-5 & 6   The "milky way" is outlined, simulating the masking technique to enhance perception.

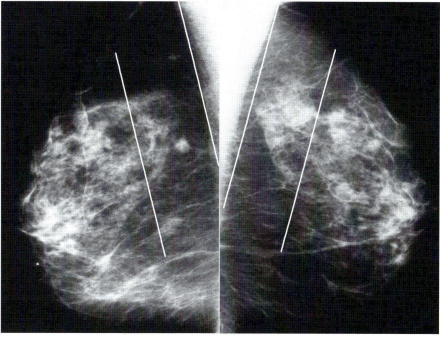

Ex. **7.17**-5

Ex. **7.17**-6

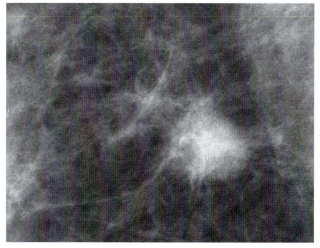

7-7

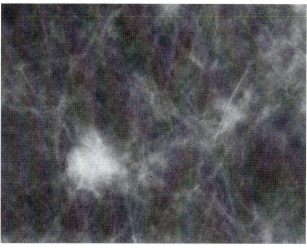

Ex. **7.17**-8

Ex. **7.17**-7 & 8   Microfocus magnification in the MLO (**7.17**-7) and CC (**7.17**-8) projections. There is a well-developed central tumor mass with ill-defined contours. The tumor is mammographically malignant.

Ex. **7.17**-9   Ultrasound examination supports the mammographic diagnosis.

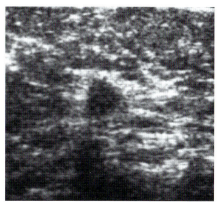

Ex. **7.17**-9

Lesions Localized in the Upper Outer Quadrant—Example 7.17

Ex. **7.17**-10   Specimen radiograph. The tumor has been excised.

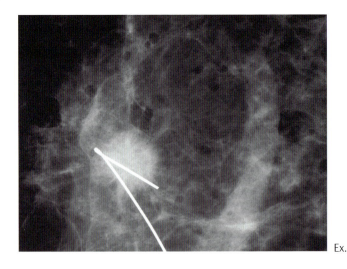

Ex.

Ex. **7.17**-11   Large-section histological image. There are four independent tumor foci (rectangles) at histological examination. Only the largest one was demonstrable on the mammogram.

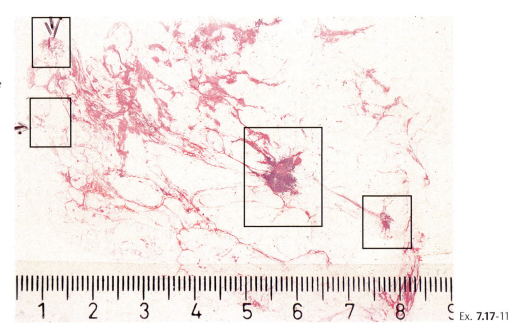

Ex. **7.17**-11

Ex. **7.17**-12   Low-power histological image of the mammographically detected invasive tumor. Histological size: 10 mm × 5 mm. Well-differentiated invasive ductal carcinoma.

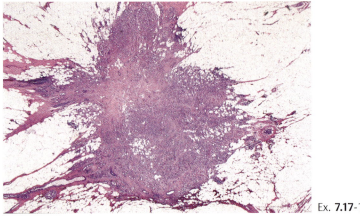

Ex. **7.17**-12

Example 7.17

Ex. **7.17**-13 to 15   Low- and medium-power histological images of the three smaller invasive tumors. Their **histological sizes** are: 8 mm × 6 mm; 3 mm × 2 mm; 1 mm × 2 mm.
Histological type: Invasive ductal carcinoma with invasive lobular component.
Histological grade: Well-differentiated.
Associated DCIS: Grade 1 **DCIS** on an area measuring 14 × 12 mm and 10 × 10 mm.

Ex. **7.17**-16   The largest tumor was examined for estrogen receptors using immunohistochemical staining and was found to be positive.

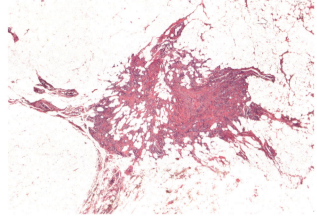

Ex. **7.17**-13

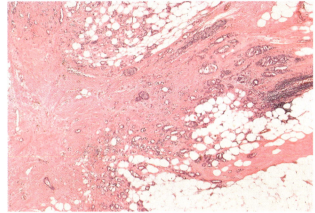

Ex. **7.17**-14

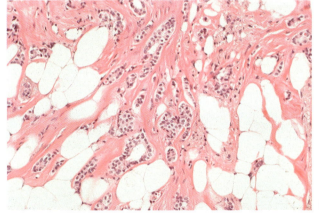

Ex. **7.17**-15

Comment
- Breast cancers are more often multifocal than unifocal.
- The radiologist should actively search for possible additional tumor foci during the diagnostic work-up.
- Large-section histology is most useful in demonstrating the presence of multiple tumor foci, even if the mammographic work-up fails to demonstrate all of them.

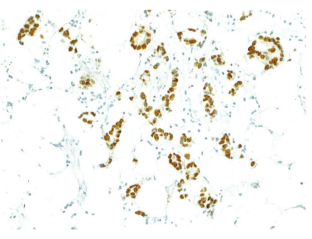

Lymph node status: No metastases were found in 13 surgically removed axillary lymph nodes.
Treatment: Mastectomy.
Follow-up: No signs of recurrence during the first 39 months of follow-up.

Ex. **7.17**-16

Lesions Localized in the Medial Half of the Breast

Twenty-eight percent of breast cancers develop in the medial half of the breast (Fig. **7.22**). Involution comes early to the medial half of the breast, facilitating detection of the lesion. The CC projection provides the best visualization of this region (shaded blue in Ex. **7.18**-5). Nonspecific asymmetric densities appearing in the medial half of the breast require further evaluation.

Example 7.18

A 45-year-old asymptomatic woman, screening examination.

Ex. **7.18**-1 & 2 and 3 & 4   Right and left breasts, MLO and CC projections. There is aberrant breast tissue in the left "milky way." An asymmetric density is demonstrable in the medial half of the left breast, as seen in the CC projection (rectangle).

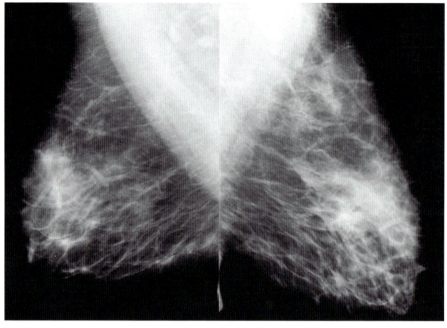

Ex. **7.18**-1   Ex. **7.18**-2

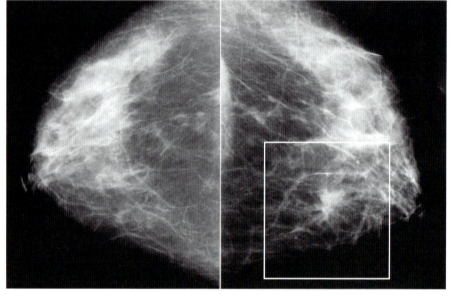

Ex. **7.18**-3   Ex. **7.18**-4

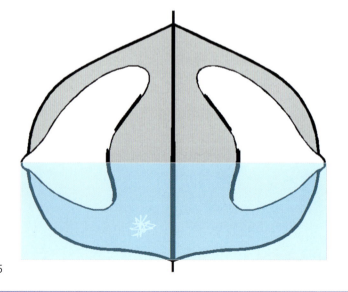

Ex. **7.18**-5

Example 7.18

Ex. **7.18**-6 to 8   Detail of the left and right CC projections. The asymmetric density in the medial half of the left breast has a radiating structure. Microfocus magnification (**7.18**-8) also shows nonspecific calcifications associated with this stellate lesion.

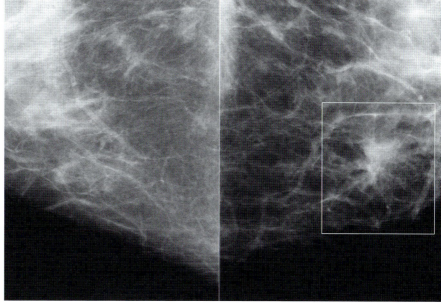

Ex. **7.18**-6

Ex. **7.18**-7

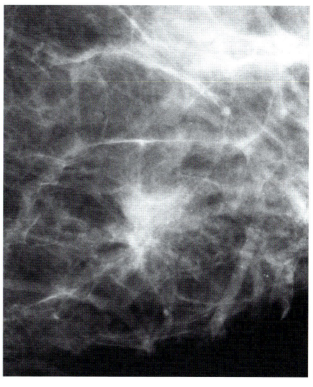

Ex. **7.18**-8

Ex. **7.18**-9   Histology: 15 mm tubular carcinoma surrounded by micropapillary DCIS on an area measuring > 65 mm.

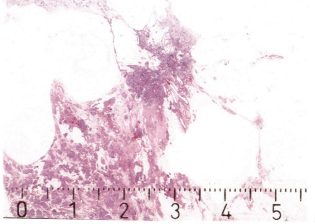

Ex. **7.18**-9

Comment
- Breast cancers are more often multifocal than unifocal.
- In this case, the presence of subtle, powdery calcifications was the only sign of the very extensive DCIS.

Ex. **7.18**-10   Detail of the specimen radiograph showing the invasive tumor. The nonspecific calcifications are seen both within the tumor and throughout much of the specimen.

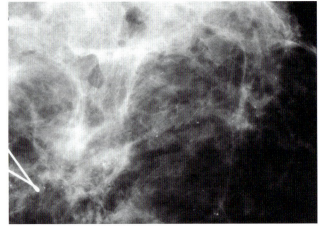

Ex. **7.18**-10

Ex. **7.18**-11   Detail of the specimen radiograph demonstrating several clusters of powdery calcifications, also seen at the resection margin.

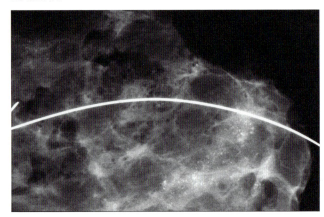

Ex. **7.18**-11

Ex. **7.18**-12   Low-power histological image of the tubular carcinoma.

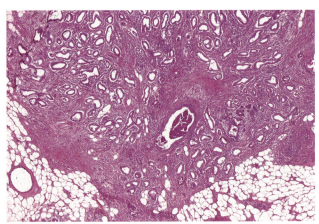

Ex. **7.18**-12

Ex. **7.18**-13   Histology of the associated Grade 1, predominantly micropapillary, ductal carcinoma in situ.

Lymph node status: One axillary lymph node had metastasis.
Treatment: Mastectomy. Postoperative irradiation and chemotherapy.
Outcome: At the most recent checkup, 15 years following treatment, the patient was recurrence-free.

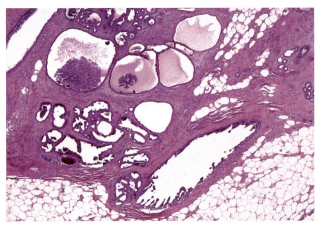

Ex. **7.18**-13

Example 7.19

A 58-year-old asymptomatic woman, screening examination.

Ex. **7.19**-1 & 2   Right and left breasts, MLO projections. An asymmetric density is seen in the lower half of the right breast (rectangle).

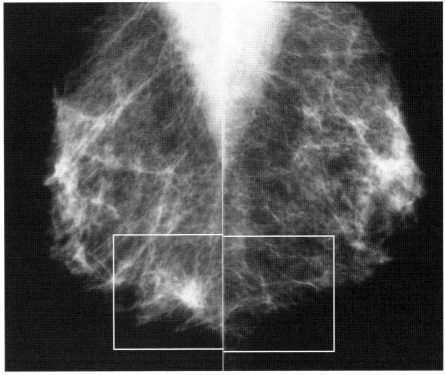

Ex. **7.19**-1   Ex. **7.19**-2

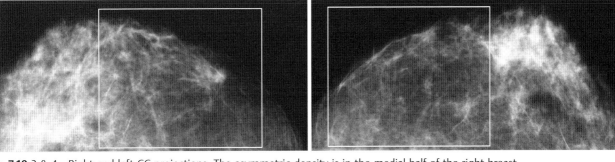

7.19-3   Ex. **7.19**-4

Ex. **7.19**-3 & 4   Right and left CC projections. The asymmetric density is in the medial half of the right breast.

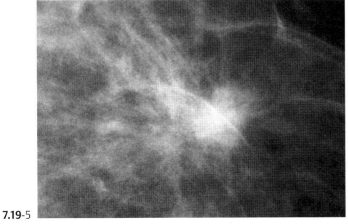

7.19-5   Ex. **7.19**-6

Ex. **7.19**-5   Right breast, microfocus magnification image in the CC projection. The ill-defined, stellate tumor is mammographically malignant.

Ex. **7.19**-6   Specimen radiograph. The tumor has been surgically removed with wide margins.

Histology: 5 mm × 5 mm well-differentiated ductal carcinoma, pN0/9.
Treatment: Segmentectomy and postoperative irradiation.

Outcome: No signs of recurrence during nine years and six months of follow-up.

Example 7.20

A 50-year-old asymptomatic woman, screening case.

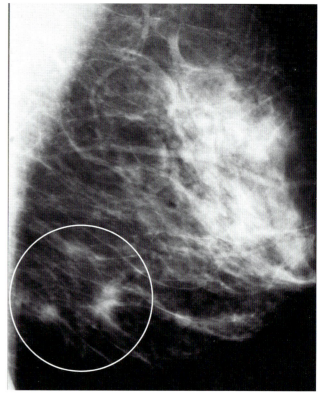

Ex. 7

Ex. **7.20**-1 & 2   Left breast, MLO and CC projections. There are several nonspecific densities in the lower inner quadrant (encircled).

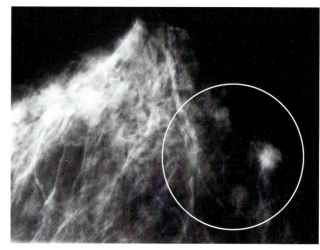

Ex. 7

Ex. **7.20**-3   Microfocus magnification image in the CC projection. The two high-density, ill-defined tumors appear to be interconnected. Additional ill-defined, low-density lesions surround these two tumors. The high-density, spiculated tumors are mammographically malignant.

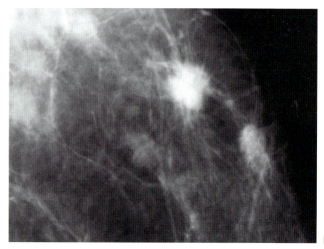

Ex. 7

Example 7.20

Ex. **7.20**-4   Specimen radiograph contains the two mammographically malignant, interconnected tumors. The surrounding circular/oval densities have also been removed.

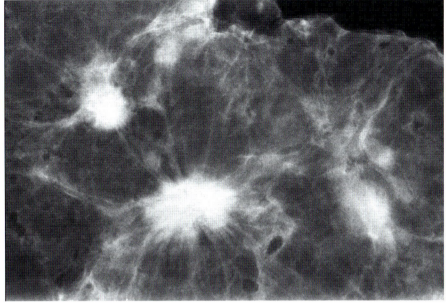

Ex. **7.20**-4

Ex. **7.20**-5   Subgross, thick-section histology demonstrates two invasive carcinomas. The interconnecting bridges between the two tumors consist of in-situ ductal carcinoma as well as fibrous strands.

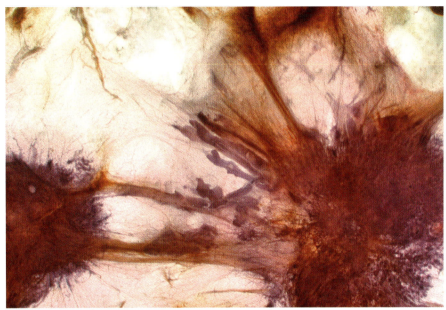

Ex. **7.20**-5

Ex. **7.20**-6   Low-power, conventional histological image of the interconnecting intraductal carcinoma.

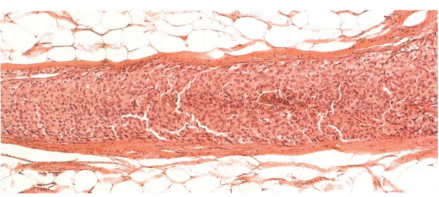

Ex. **7.20**-6

Lesions Localized in the Medial Half of the Breast—Example 7.20

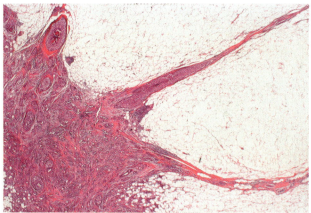

Ex. **7.20**-7

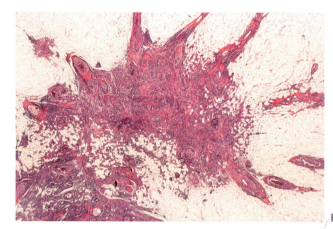

Ex.

Ex. **7.20**-7 & 8   Low-power histological images of the two adjacent invasive carcinomas. The larger one measures 10 mm.

Ex. **7.20**-9   High-power magnification image of one of the moderately differentiated invasive ductal tumors.

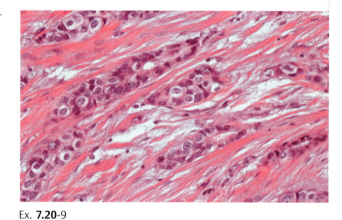

Ex. **7.20**-9

Ex. **7.20**-10 & 11   Medium- and high-power histological images of one of the associated in-situ components. Solid cell proliferation with central necrosis.

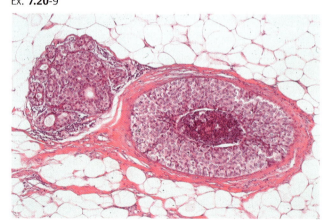

Ex. **7.20**-10

Comment
- Multifocality can appear in many ways on the mammogram. Once it consists of many individual foci of invasive carcinoma (pp. 314–317), in another case the solitary invasive carcinoma is seen among large numbers of DCIS foci, while in this case the DCIS was confined to the tissue bridging the space between the two invasive foci.

Lymph node status: The eight surgically removed axillary lymph nodes showed no metastasis at histological examination.

Treatment: Segmentectomy and postoperative irradiation.

Outcome: The yearly follow-up examinations showed no signs of recurrence during the first eight years after treatment.

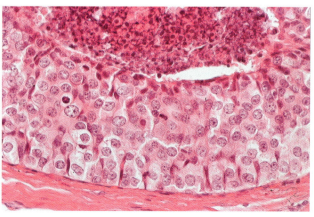

Ex. **7.20**-11

Example 7.21

A 55-year-old asymptomatic woman, screening examination.

Ex. **7.21**-1 & 2   Left breast, MLO and CC projections. A tiny lesion is barely perceptible in the MLO projection and is not visualized in the CC projection.

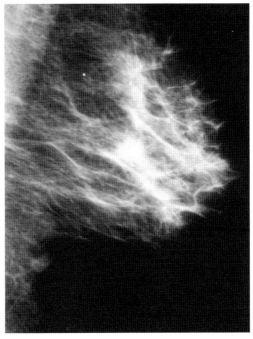

Ex. **7.21**-1

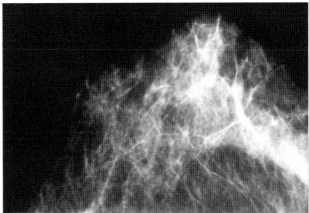

Ex. **7.21**-2

Lesions Localized in the Medial Half of the Breast—Example 7.21

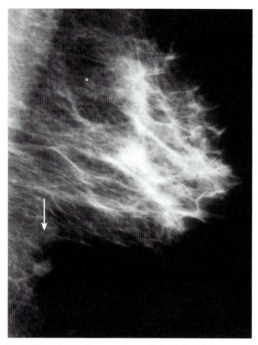 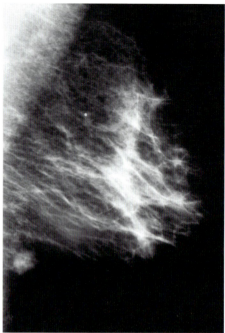

Ex. **7.21**-3   Ex. **7.21**-4

Ex. **7.21**-3 & 4   Comparison of the left MLO screening mammogram with the corresponding mammogram taken six months later, when the patient presented with a palpable lump below the inframammary fold of the left breast.

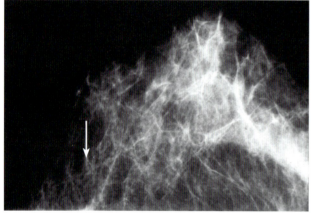 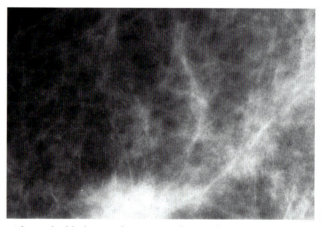

Ex. **7.21**-5   Ex. **7**

Ex. **7.21**-5 & 6   Comparison of the left CC screening mammogram with a magnified view of the palpable lesion in the left lower inner quadrant taken six months later when the patient presented

with a palpable lump. The arrow indicates the presumed site of the tumor. Lesions situated close to the inframammary fold cannot be fully visualized on the CC projection.

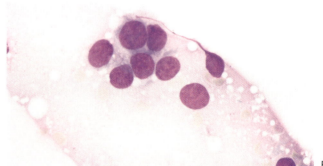

Ex. **7.21**-7   Fine-needle aspiration biopsy: malignant cells.   Ex. **7**

Example 7.21

Ex. **7.21**-8   Specimen radiograph. The tumor has been removed with wide margins.

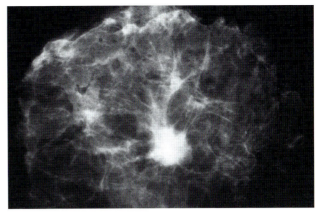

Ex. **7.21**-8

Ex. **7.21**-9   Large-section histology. The solitary tumor measures 11 × 10 mm.

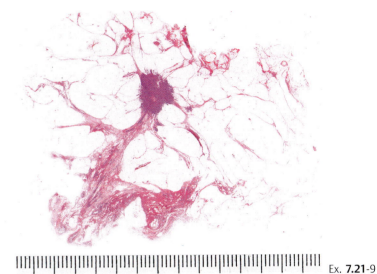

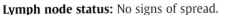

Ex. **7.21**-9

Ex. **7.21**-10   Low-power histological image: poorly differentiated invasive ductal carcinoma. There also is a 21 mm × 20 mm area with Grade 3 DCIS surrounding the tumor, occult on mammography.

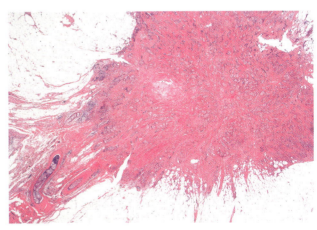

Ex. **7.21**-10

Ex. **7.21**-11   Histological examination of 14 axillary nodes showed no metastases.

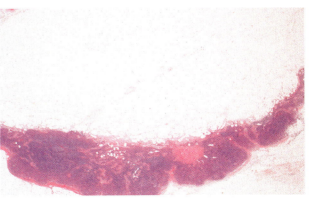

Lymph node status: No signs of spread.
Treatment: Segmentectomy and postoperative irradiation.
Outcome: Yearly follow-up examinations did not show recurrence during the period of seven years and two months after treatment.

Ex. **7.21**-11

Lesions Localized in the Retroglandular Clear Space on the CC Projection

Any abnormality developing behind the posterior border of the fibroglandular tissue (upper or lower part of the "milky way" in the MLO projection or the retroglandular clear space on the CC projection) will be readily visible because of the surrounding adipose tissue.

Example 7.22

A 65-year-old asymptomatic woman, first screening examination.

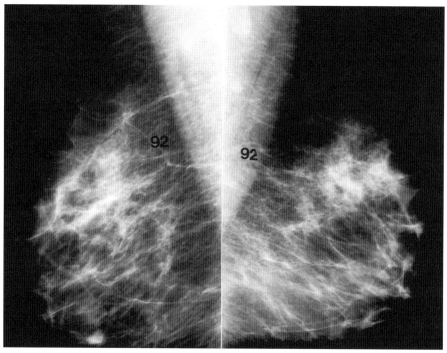

Ex. **7.22**-1

Ex. 7.22-1 & 2 and 3 & 4   Right and left breasts, MLO and CC projections. No mammographic abnormality was perceived.

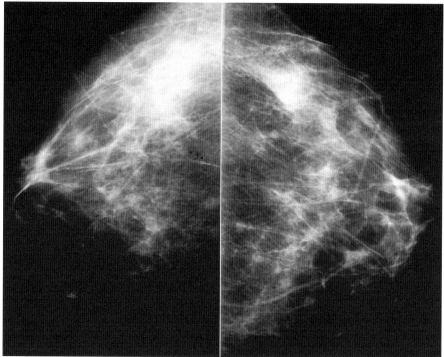

Ex. **7.22**-3

Ex. 7

Example 7.22

Ex. **7.22**-5 & 6 and 7 & 8 Second screening examination, right and left breasts, MLO and CC projections. A tiny, de-novo density is seen both on the left MLO projection on the "milky way" (rectangle) and on the CC projection in the retroglandular clear space (rectangle).

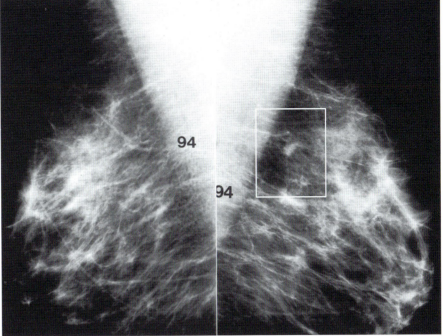

Ex. **7.22**-5   Ex. **7.22**-6

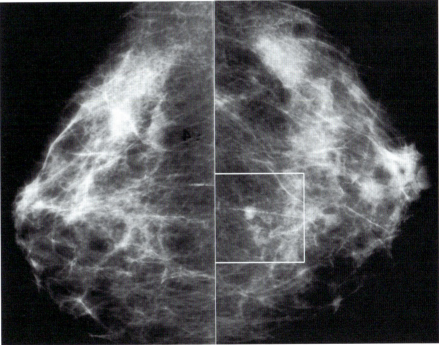

Ex. **7.22**-7   Ex. **7.22**-8

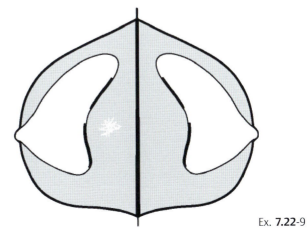

Ex. **7.22**-9 Schematic representation of a lesion in the left retroglandular clear space in the CC projection.

Ex. **7.22**-9

329

Ex. **7.22**-10   The borders of the "milky way" are outlined.

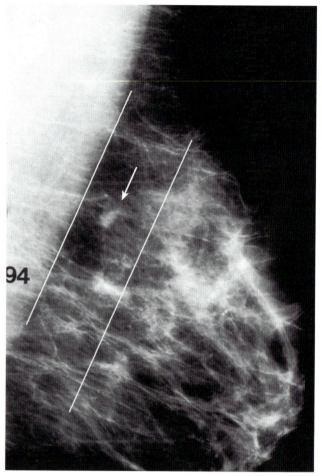

Ex. **7.22**-10

Ex. **7.22**-11   Microfocus magnification, MLO projection. The high-density, ill-defined lesion is mammographically malignant.

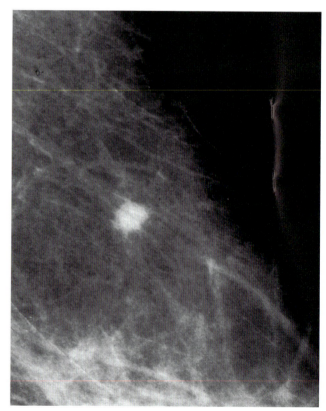

Comment
- Any *de novo* asymmetric density, specific or nonspecific, should be worked up, especially when localized in one of the "forbidden areas."
- Careful comparison with the previous mammograms is essential.

Ex. **7.22**-11

Example 7.22

Ex. **7.22**-12   The *de novo* lesion is located in the medial half of the breast, within the retroglandular clear space.

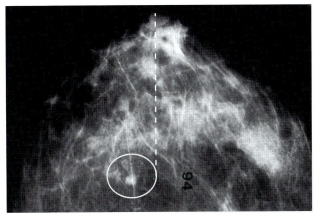

Ex. **7.22**-12

Ex. **7.22**-13   Subgross, thick-section histological image of the solitary, 6 mm × 6 mm invasive breast cancer.

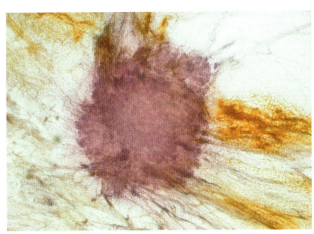

Ex. **7.22**-13

Ex. **7.22**-14   Histology (H&E). Well-differentiated invasive cribriform carcinoma.

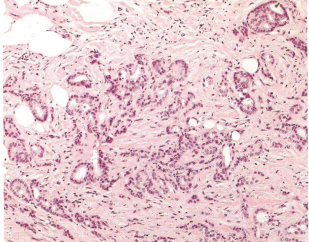

Lymph node status: No metastasis shown at histological examination of six surgically removed axillary lymph nodes.
Treatment: Segmentectomy and postoperative irradiation.
Outcome: No sign of recurrence shown at the yearly follow-up examinations during the nine-year follow-up period.

Ex. **7.22**-14

Example 7.23

A 77-year-old asymptomatic
woman, screening case.

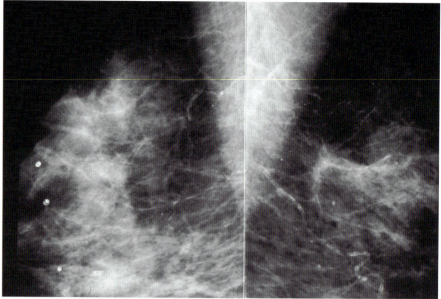

Ex. **7.23**-1

Ex.

Ex. **7.23**-1 & 2 and 3 & 4   Right and
left breasts, details of the MLO and
CC projections.

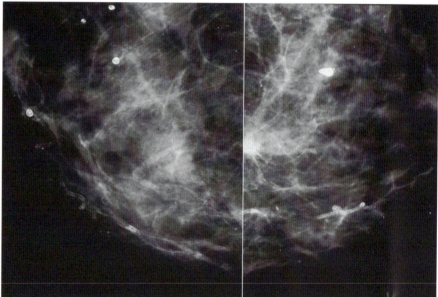

Ex. **7.23**-3

Ex.

Comment
- The subtle asymmetric density representing the earliest detectable phase of breast cancer is often seen in more than one of the "forbidden areas" on the mammograms.
- In this case the density is obvious on the retroglandular clear space, and although also visible on the "milky way," it is more difficult to perceive.
- One should not be misled when a density suspicious for malignancy is seen on only one view.
- Work-up should begin in the projection where the lesion is best seen.

Example 7.23

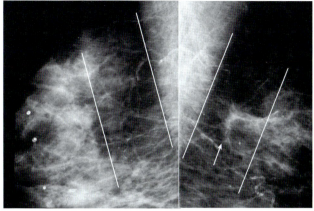

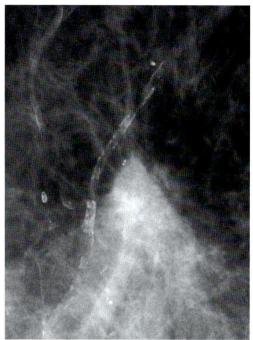

Ex. **7.23**-5 & 6   The borders of the "milky way" are outlined. The arrow points to an asymmetric density within the "milky way."

Ex. **7.23**-9

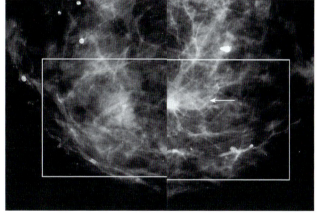

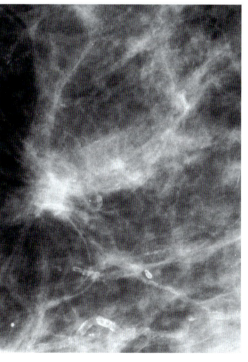

Ex. **7.23**-7 & 8   Use of the viewer emphasizes the asymmetric density in the retroglandular clear space of the left breast (arrow).

Ex. **7.23**-9 & 10   Microfocus magnification views clearly demonstrate a small, spiculated, mammographically malignant lesion.

Ex. **7.23**-10

Ex. **7.23**-11   Histology (H&E stain): 9 mm well-differentiated invasive ductal carcinoma.

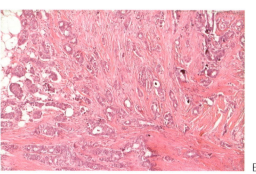

Lymph node status: No metastasis was found at histological examination of four axillary lymph nodes.
Treatment: Segmentectomy, no postoperative irradiation.
Outcome: Yearly follow-up examinations during 11 years after treatment showed no signs of recurrence.

Ex. **7.23**-11

Example 7.24

A 55-year-old asymptomatic
woman, screening examination.

Ex. **7.24**-1 & 2   Right and left
breasts, detail of the MLO projections.

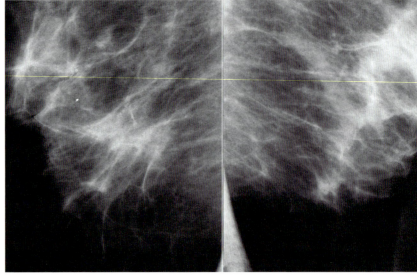

Ex. **7.24**-1

Ex. **7.24**-2

Ex. **7.24**-3 & 4   Right and left
breasts, detail of the CC projections.

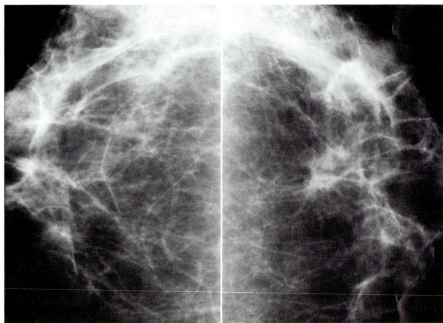

Ex. **7.24**-3

Ex. 7

Example 7.24

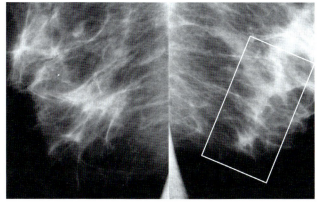

24-5
24-6

Ex. **7.24**-5 & 6   The rectangle outlines an area of asymmetric density with subtle architectural distortion in the left breast. The asymmetric density in the left retroglandular clear space is far easier to perceive (Ex. **7.24**-3, 4, 8).

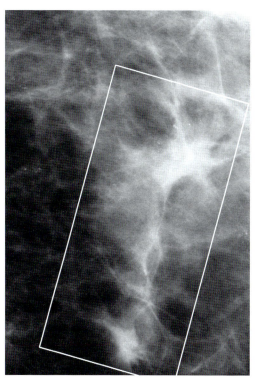

Ex. **7.24**-7   The microfocus magnification image demonstrates several stellate lesions with associated nonspecific calcifications.

Ex. **7.24**-7

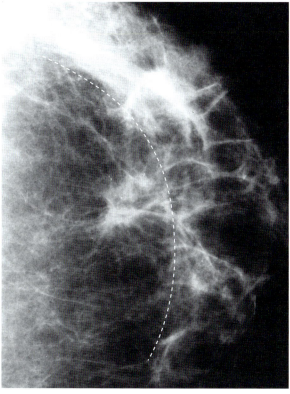

x. **7.24**-8

Ex. **7.24**-8   Left breast, CC projection. The density with architectural distortion is in the retroglandular clear space.

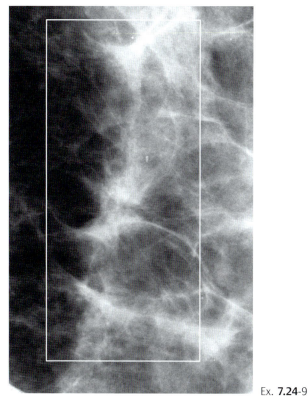

Ex. **7.24**-9

Ex. **7.24**-9   Left breast, CC projection, microfocus magnification with spot compression. The multiple stellate lesions have been spread out by compression.

Ex. **7.24**-10   Specimen radiograph showing multiple tumor foci. The microcalcifications are widely distributed.

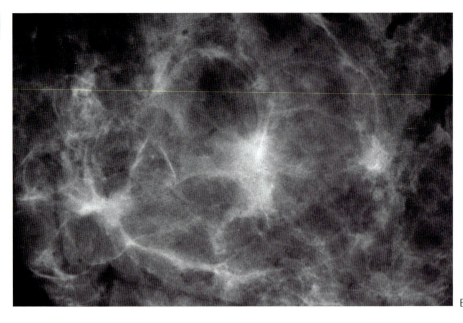

Ex. 7

Ex. **7.24**-11 to 13   High- and medium-power histological images of the three invasive tumor foci. Corresponding to the nonspecific calcifications seen on the mammogram, low-grade cribriform and micropapillary DCIS are demonstrated.

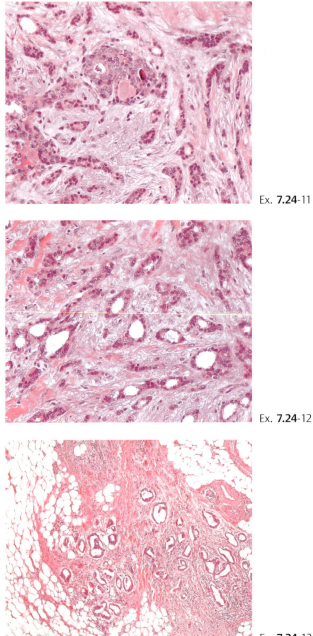

Ex. **7.24**-11

Ex. **7.24**-12

Lymph node status: No metastasis was found in the two surgically removed lymph nodes (pN0/2).
Treatment: Segmentectomy and postoperative irradiation.
Outcome: No recurrence detected during the 14 years and 3 months of follow-up.

Ex. **7.24**-13

Example 7.25

A 68-year-old woman, asymptomatic screening case.

Ex. **7.25**-1 & 2   Comparison of detail images of the left breast in the MLO projection from two consecutive screening examinations 25 months apart. During the interscreening interval a nonspecific density (encircled) has arisen on the "milky way."

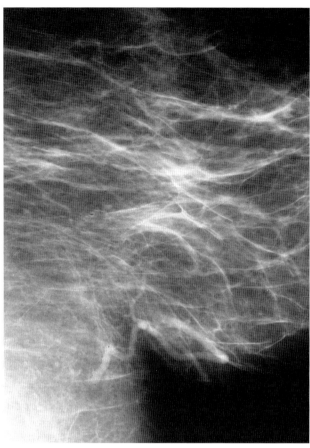

Ex. **7.25**-1

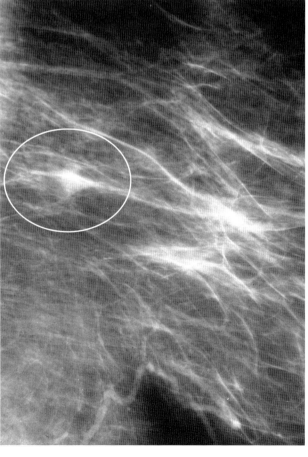

Ex. **7.25**-2

Lesions Localized in the Retroglandular Clear Space—Example 7.25

Ex. **7.25**-3   Left breast, detail of the CC projection. The *de novo* < 10 mm tumor mass (arrow) has no associated calcifications.

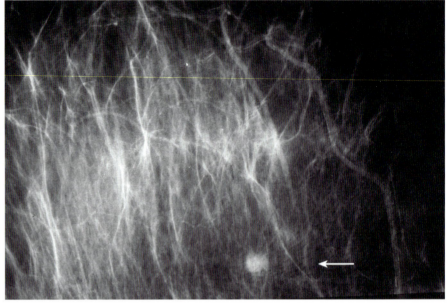

Ex. **7.25**-3

Ex. **7.25**-4   Microfocus magnification view, CC projection. The circular, high-density tumor, adjacent to a calcified artery, has ill-defined contours and is mammographically malignant.

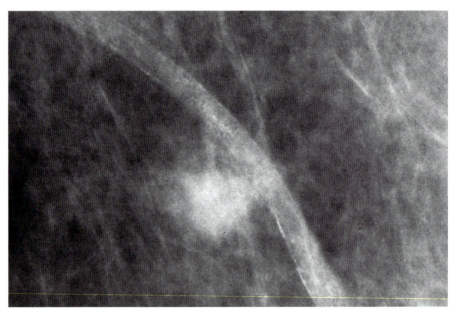

Ex. **7.25**-4

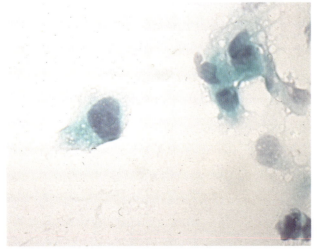

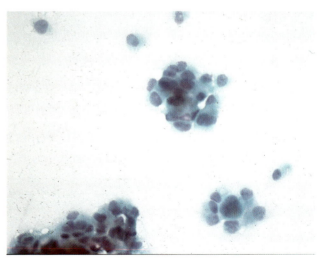

Ex. **7.25**-5

Ex. **7.25**-6

Ex. **7.25**-5 & 6   Preoperative cytology shows malignant cells and confirms the mammographic diagnosis.

Example 7.25

Ex. **7.25**-7 Preoperative localization. The hooked wire is placed "beside and beyond" the lesion instead of through the tumor, in order to avoid displacement of the cancer cells.

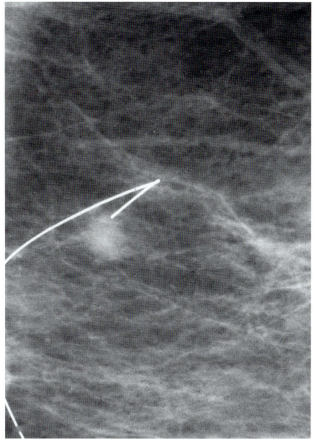

Ex. **7.25**-7

Ex. **7.25**-8 Specimen radiograph showing that the mammographically solitary lesion has been removed with a wide margin.

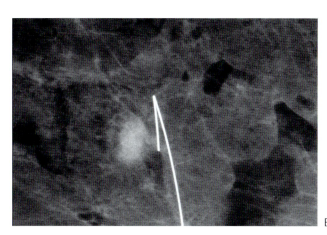

Ex. **7.25**-8

Ex. **7.25**-9 Specimen radiograph of the tissue slice containing the tumor.

Comment
- The extensive high-grade DCIS in this case was not mammographically demonstrable despite ideal imaging circumstances, not even on the magnification image of the thin specimen slice.
- The value of large-section and subgross, thick-section histology in detecting and mapping the extent of the disease is well demonstrated.

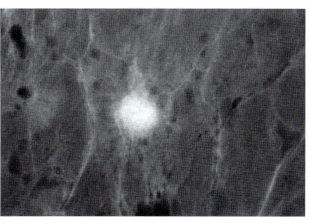

Ex. **7.25**-9

339

Ex. **7.25**-10 Large-section histology demonstrates the 8 mm moderately differentiated invasive carcinoma, but also shows three areas with mammographically occult in-situ carcinoma (rectangles B–D). The disease extends over a 40 × 40 mm area.

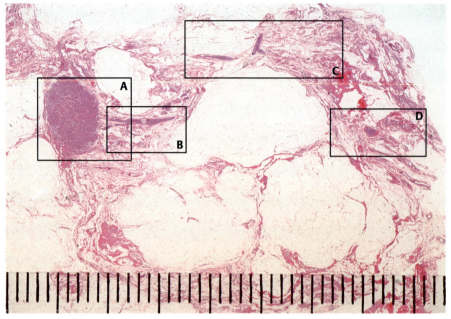

Ex. **7.25**-10

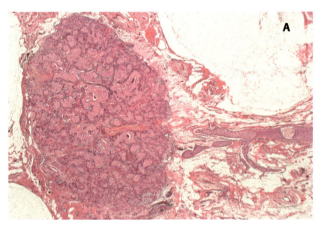

Ex. **7.25**-11

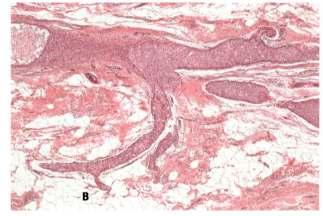

Ex. **7.25**-12

Ex. **7.25**-11 Low-power histological image showing the invasive carcinoma and the adjacent in-situ cancer (rectangle A in Ex. **7.25**-10).

Ex. **7.25**-12 Low-power magnification of the tissue within rectangle B in Ex. **7.25**-10, demonstrating the cancerous ducts containing noncalcified DCIS.

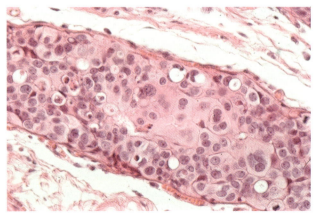

Ex. **7.25**-13

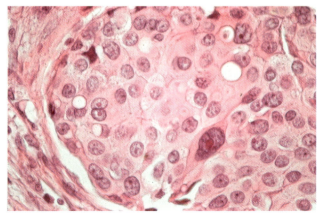

Ex. **7.25**-14

Ex. **7.25**-13 & 14 High-power histological images of the high nuclear grade DCIS without associated necrosis or calcification.

Example 7.25

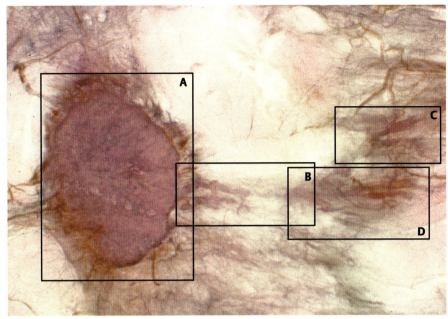

Ex. **7.25**-15   Subgross, thick-section histological image showing both the invasive carcinoma (A) and the extensive, mammographically occult DCIS component (rectangles B–D).

Ex. **7.25**-15

Ex. **7.25**-16   Portion of the invasive tumor and the adjacent large area with in-situ carcinoma from rectangles B–D.

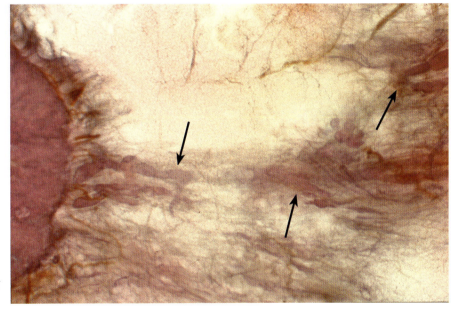

Lymph node status: No demonstrable metastases in 16 surgically removed axillary nodes (pN0/16).
Treatment: Segmentectomy and postoperative irradiation.
Outcome: No demonstrable signs of recurrence during nine years of follow-up.

Ex. **7.25**-16

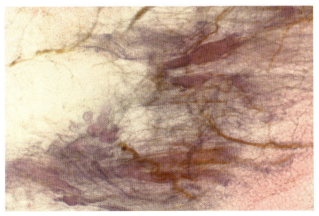

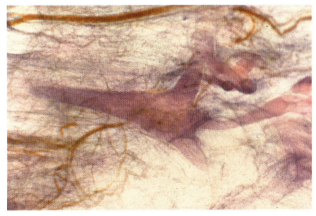

Ex. **7.25**-17

Ex. **7.25**-18

Ex. **7.25**-17 & 18   Subgross, thick-section histological images of the in-situ component (4 mm-free margin).

Example 7.26

A 65-year-old asymptomatic woman, screening case.

Ex. **7.26**-1 & 2   Right and left breasts, detail of the MLO projections, first screening examination. There is a tiny, circular, asymmetric density (rectangle) in the right "milky way." The left breast is normal. Mammographic Pattern II.

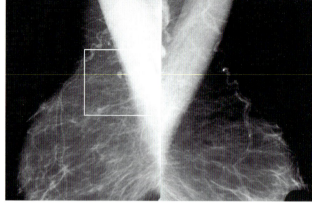

Ex. **7.26**-1

Ex. **7**

Ex. **7.26**-3   Microfocus magnification image. The asymmetric density corresponds to a lymph node.

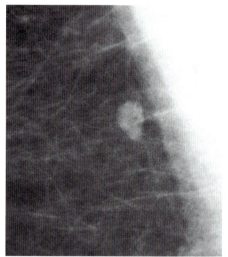

Ex. **7.26**-3

Ex. **7.26**-4 & 5   Next screening examination. The lesion in the right breast is unchanged (rectangle), but there is a *de novo* tiny tumor mass in the left "milky way" (encircled).

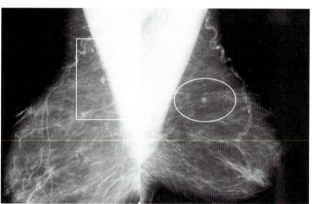

Ex. **7.26**-4

Ex. **7**

Ex. **7.26**-6 & 7   Right and left CC projections. The *de novo* tumor in the left breast is encircled.

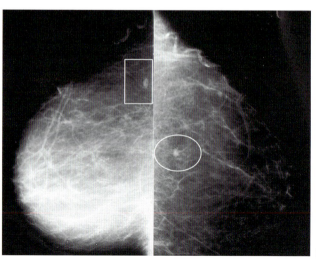

Ex. **7.26**-6

Ex. **7.**

Example 7.26

Ex. **7.26**-8 Microfocus magnification image. The tiny, ill-defined tumor mass is mammographically malignant.

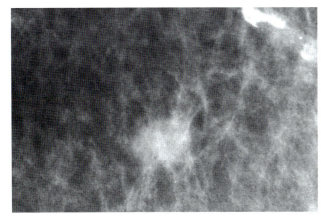

Ex. **7.26**-8

Ex. **7.26**-9 & 10 Specimen radiograph. The lesion has been removed with wide margins.

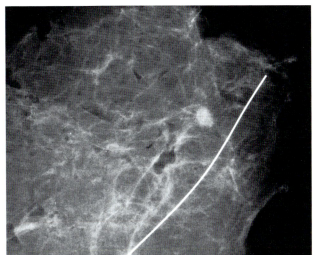

Ex. **7.26**-9

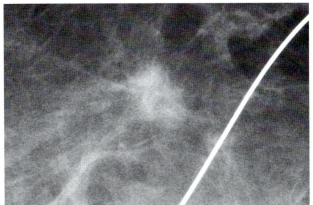

Ex. **7.26**-10

Ex. **7.26**-11 Subgross, thick-section histological image of the solitary, 3 mm × 3 mm well-differentiated invasive ductal carcinoma.

Comment
- Benign lesions outnumber breast cancer by a few orders of magnitude. Their distracting influence should not be underestimated.

Lymph node status: Ten surgically removed axillary nodes showed no metastasis at histological examination.
Treatment: Segmentectomy and postoperative irradiation.
Outcome: Yearly follow-up examination during 11 years 4 months after treatment showed no sign of recurrence or *de novo* breast tumor.

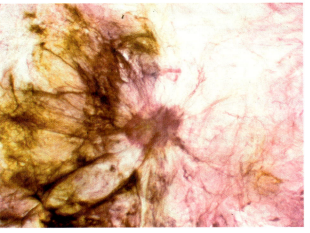

Ex. **7.26**-11

Example 7.27

A 59-year-old woman, asymptomatic screening case.

Ex. **7.27**-1 & 2   Right and left breasts, MLO projections, first screening examination. There is a tiny, circular, asymmetric density (rectangle) in the lower part of the left "milky way."

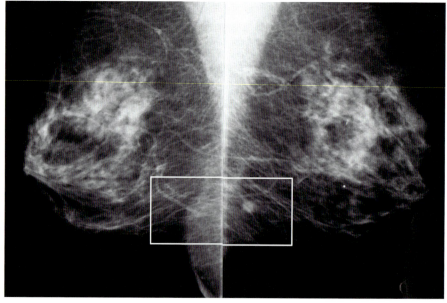

Ex. **7.27**-1

Ex. **7**

Ex. **7.27**-3 & 4   Right and left breasts, CC projections. The tiny lesion is easily visible in the left retroglandular area.

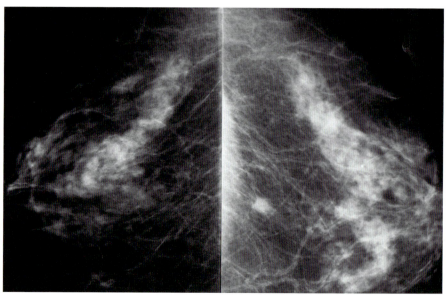

Ex. **7.27**-3

Ex. **7**

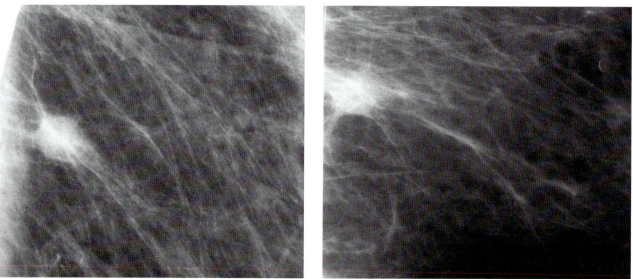

Ex. **7.27**-5

Ex. **7.**

Ex. **7.27**-5 & 6   Left breast, microfocus magnification images (CC and MLO projections) demonstrating the high-density tumor with ill-defined margins, mammographically malignant.

Example 7.27

Ex. **7.27**-7   Specimen radiograph. The abnormality has been removed with wide margins.

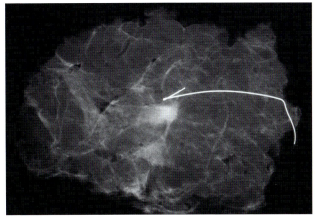

Ex. **7.27**-7

Ex. **7.27**-8   Large-section histology. The solitary lesion measures 8 mm × 6 mm in diameter. The tumor-free margin is 20 mm.

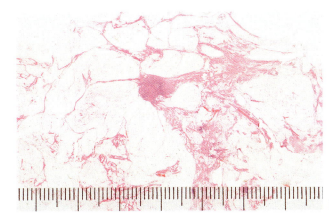

Ex. **7.27**-8

Ex. **7.27**-9   Low-power histological image of the well-differentiated carcinoma.

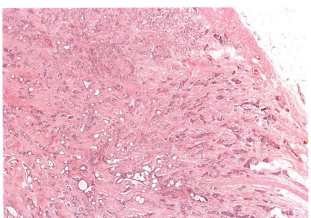

Ex. **7.27**-9

Ex. **7.27**-10   High-power histological image of this tubular carcinoma.

Comment
- The patient with this solitary breast cancer measuring < 10 mm in diameter will have a 99 % probability of surviving this disease at 24 years of follow-up.

Lymph node status: No axillary nodes removed.
Treatment: Segmentectomy and postoperative irradiation.
Outcome: Yearly follow-up examination during the first four years after treatment has not shown any sign of recurrence.

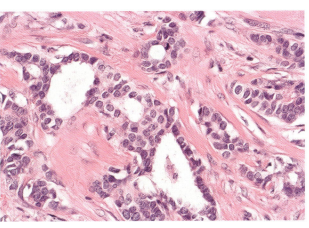

Ex. **7.27**-10

Lesions Localized in the Retroareolar Area

Breast cancer is localized to the nipple and retroareolar area in 1–2% of all cases (Fig. **7.22**). Retroareolar fibrosis can impair detection of abnormalities in this location. The rich lymphatics of the retroareolar Sappey plexus facilitate the early metastatic spread of breast cancer. This may explain why women with tumors localized behind the nipple have a poorer prognosis.[4] Breast cancer in men frequently occurs in the retroareolar region, is more frequently metastatic, and has a higher case fatality rate than breast cancer in women.

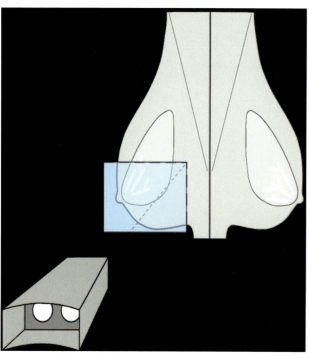
7.24-1

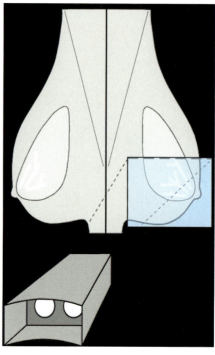
7.24-2

Fig. **7.24** Schematic representation of viewing the retroareolar areas.

Example 7.28

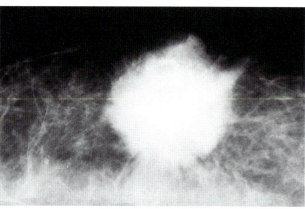
Ex. **7.28**

Ex. **7.28** This male breast cancer extends from the nipple to the chest wall and infiltrates the underlying pectoralis major muscle.

Example 7.29

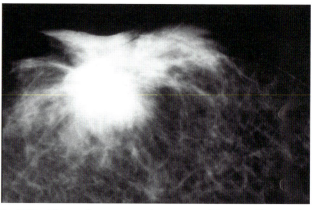
Ex. 7

Ex. **7.29** This stellate tumor of a 72-year-old man infiltrates the nipple and surrounding retroareolar tissues, causing nipple retraction and skin thickening.

Example 7.30

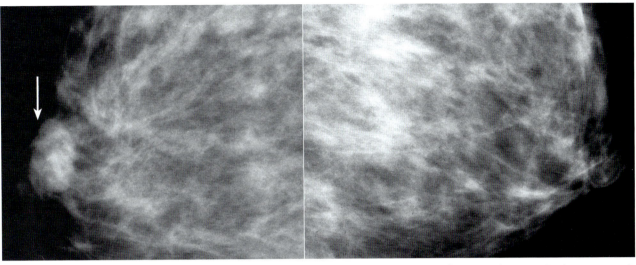

Ex. **7.30**-1 Ex. **7.30**-2

Ex. **7.30**-1 & 2   Right and left breasts, detail of MLO projections, demonstrating the retroareolar areas. There is a circular, asymmetric density (arrow) behind the right nipple.

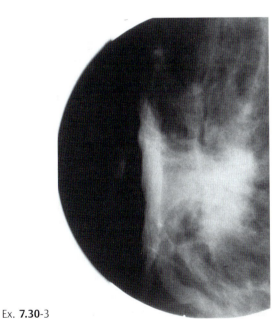

Ex. **7.30**-3

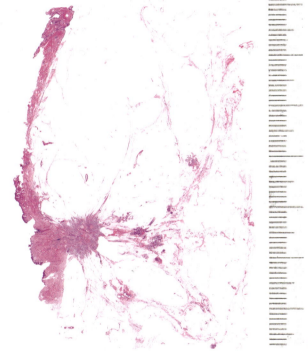

Ex. **7.30**-4

Ex. **7.30**-3   Microfocus magnification with spot compression over the right retroareolar region shows a spiculated, mammographically malignant tumor that infiltrates the nipple.

Ex. **7.30**-4   Large-section histology of the retroareolar tumor.

Example 7.31

A 64-year-old woman who underwent left mastectomy eight years earlier for advanced breast cancer.

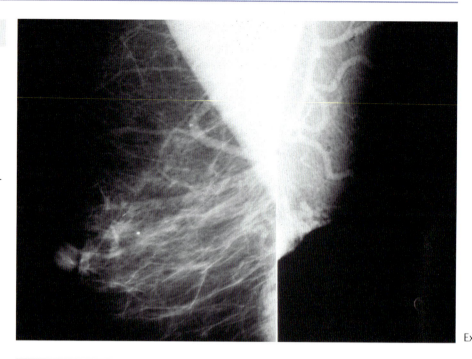

Ex. **7.31**-1   Right breast, MLO projection and MLO projection of the subcutaneous tissue on the mastectomy side (left).

Ex. **7.31**-2 & 3   Right breast, microfocus magnification images, MLO and CC projections. Slight nipple retraction is seen in **7.31**-2 and a retroareolar stellate lesion is seen in **7.31**-3 (rectangle).

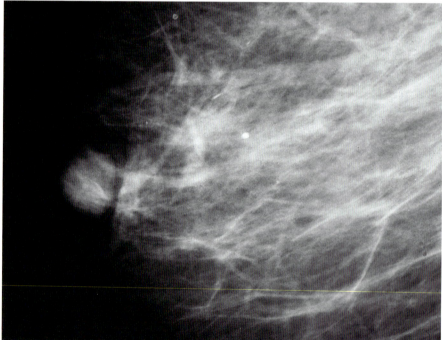

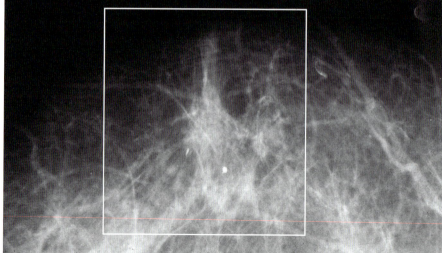

Comment
- Retroareolar tumors are uncommon and are easily missed.
- Detection is facilitated by comparing the left retroareolar area with the right.
- After unilateral mastectomy, the opportunity for contralateral comparison is lost, and mistakes can easily follow.

Ex.

Ex. 7

Ex. 7.

Example 7.31

Ex. **7.31**-4   Specimen radiograph showing the stellate lesion.

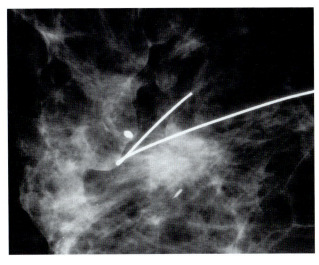

Ex. **7.31**-4

Ex. **7.31**-5   Large-section histological image of this invasive lobular carcinoma measuring 20 mm × 18 mm.

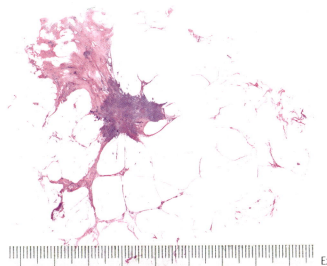

Ex. **7.31**-5

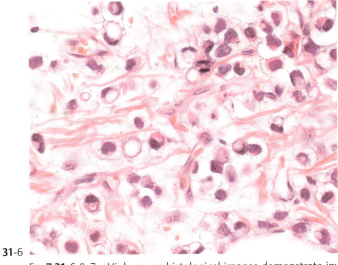

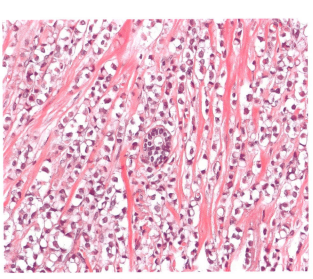

31-6

Ex. **7.31**-7

Ex. **7.31**-6 & 7   High-power histological images demonstrate invasive lobular carcinoma of the classic type.

Lesions Localized in the Retroareolar Area

Example 7.32

An 81-year-old woman who felt a retroareolar tumor for three years.

Ex. **7.32**-1 & 2 and 3 & 4   Right and left breasts, MLO and CC projections. The left nipple and areola are thickened and there is an asymmetric density in the left retroareolar region. Additionally, a lymph node is seen in the left axillary tail (sentinel node).

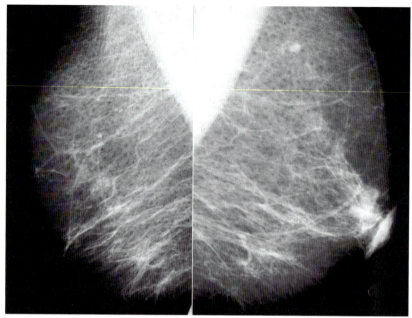

Ex. 7.32-1

Ex. 7

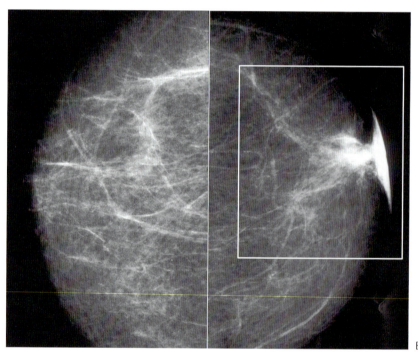

Ex. 7.32-3

Ex. 7

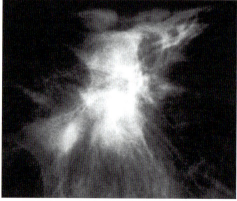

Ex. 7.32-5

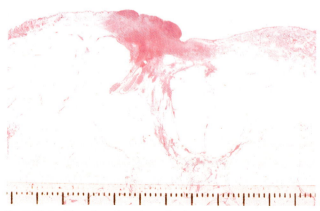

Ex. 7

Ex. **7.32**-5   Microfocus magnification image showing the nipple–areolar complex with a mammographically malignant stellate tumor.

Ex. **7.32**-6   This thin slice through the complex tumor demonstrates the retroareolar involvement.

Example 7.32

Ex. **7.32**-7 & 8   Low-power histological images of the nipple–areolar area showing multiple foci of invasive lobular cancer. Classic and solid invasive lobular carcinoma foci are seen in an area measuring 21 mm × 14 mm.

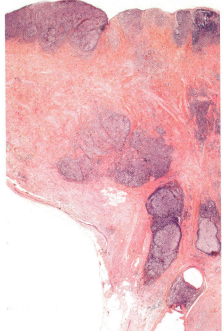

Ex. **7.32**-7

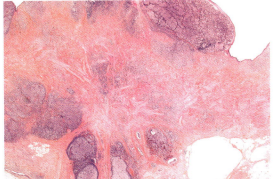

Ex. **7.32**-8

Ex. **7.32**-9 & 10   High-power histological images of solid invasive lobular carcinoma.

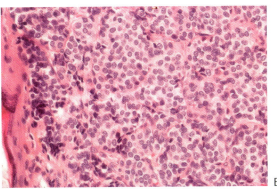

Ex. **7.32**-9

Treatment: Modified radical mastectomy.
Outcome: No signs of recurrence during the first three years after surgery.

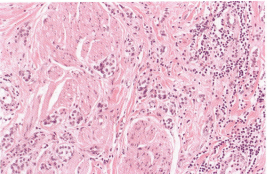

Ex. **7.32**-10

Example 7.33

This 45-year-old man felt a lump adjacent to his right nipple.

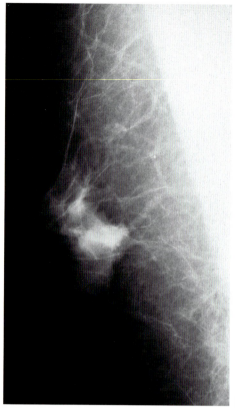

Ex. **7.33**-1 & 2   Right breast, MLO and CC projections. There is a lobulated, ill-defined tumor in the medial half of the right breast. An additional tiny, circular lesion is posterior to this tumor mass (rectangle).

Ex. **7.33**-1

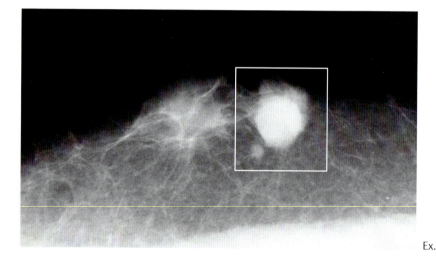

Ex. **7**

Ex. **7.33**-3   Large-section histology. There is good correlation between the mammographic and low-power histological images.

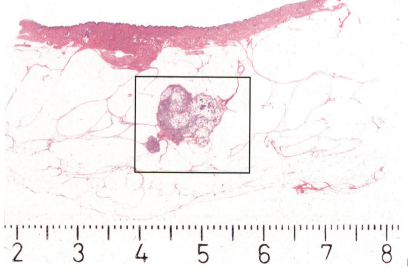

Ex. **7**

Example 7.33

Ex. **7.33**-4 Radiograph of the mastectomy specimen. The tumors and the adjacent retroareolar fibrosis have been removed with a wide margin.

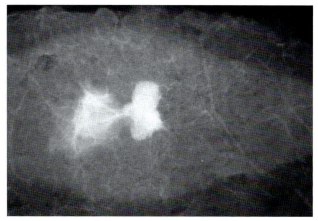

Ex. **7.33**-4

Ex. **7.33**-5 Detail of the large-section histology image, demonstrating the two adjacent tumors.

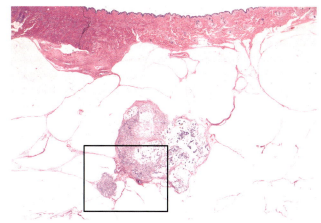

Ex. **7.33**-5

Ex. **7.33**-6 The two tumors are interconnected with a narrow tissue bridge. The smaller tumor (rectangle) is magnified in Ex. **7.33**-7.

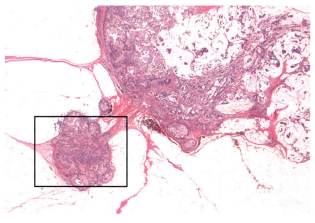

Ex. **7.33**-6

Ex. **7.33**-7 The smaller tumor is histologically invasive ductal carcinoma measuring < 5 mm.

Comment
- Breast cancer in men is rare, especially in younger and middle-aged men.
- Its retroareolar location near the lymphatic plexus leads to early and frequent metastases.
- The case fatality rate of breast cancer is worse for men than for women.

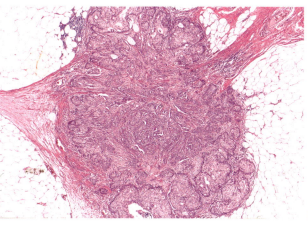

Ex. **7.33**-7

Ex. **7.33**-8 Low-power histological image of the larger tumor measuring 14 mm, which is an invasive ductal carcinoma with a mucinous (colloid) component.

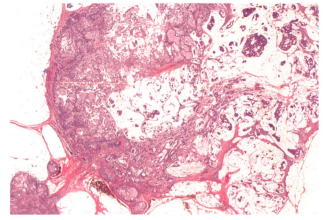

Ex. **7.33**-8

Ex. **7.33**-9 Medium-power histological image of both the invasive ductal (A) and the mucinous carcinoma component (B).

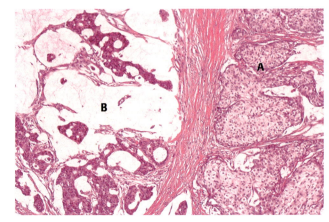

Ex. **7.33**-9

Ex. **7.33**-10 High-power histological image of the mucinous carcinoma component.

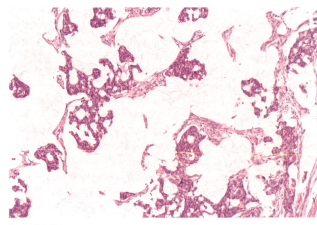

Ex. **7.33**-10

Ex. **7.33**-11 Radiograph of the axillary specimen with lymph nodes, some of which are high density and lack a hilus, suggesting metastases. Histological examination of 17 nodes showed no metastases.

Treatment and outcome: The patient underwent mastectomy. Three years later the patient underwent chemotherapy for suspected lung metastases. He is currently asymptomatic seven years after operation.

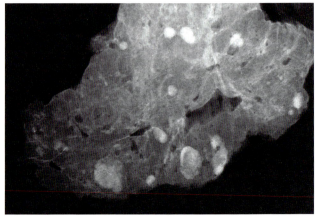

Ex. **7.33**-11

Example 7.34

This 72-year-old woman had a right mastectomy six years earlier for a 32-mm invasive ductal carcinoma. She is currently asymptomatic.

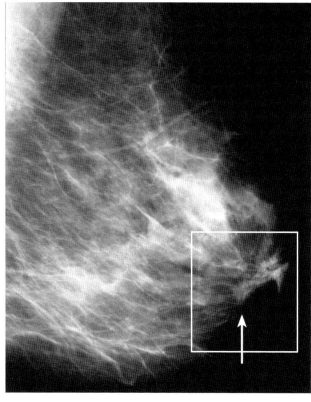

Ex. **7.34**-1 & 2   Left breast, MLO and CC projections. There is a tiny, stellate tumor in the lower inner quadrant of the breast (arrow).

Ex. **7.34**-1

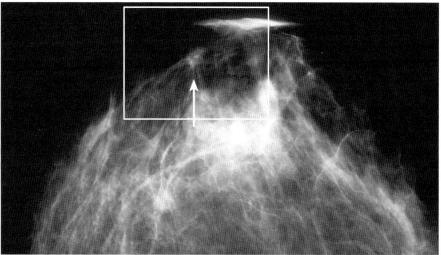

Ex. **7.34**-2

Ex. **7.34**-3   Microfocus magnification spot image in the CC projection shows a < 10 mm spiculated, mammographically malignant tumor.

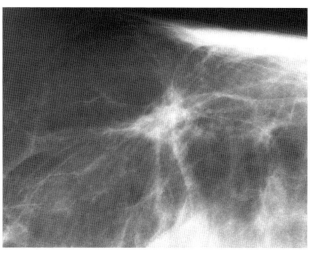

Ex. **7.34**-3

Ex. **7.34**-4   Breast ultrasound examination supports the mammographic diagnosis.

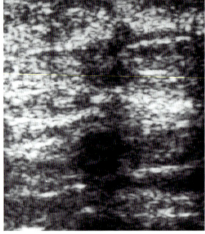

Ex. **7.34**-4

Ex. **7.34**-5   Specimen radiograph. The tumor mass has been surgically removed with wide margins.

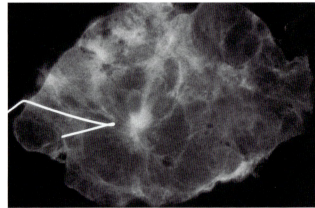

Ex. **7.**

Ex. **7.34**-6   Microfocus magnification image of one of the specimen slices, demonstrating the tumor with a solid, central tumor mass and straight spiculations.

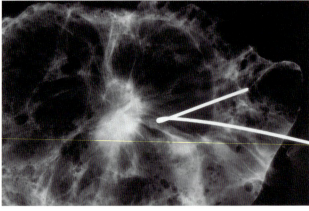

Ex. **7.**

Ex. **7.34**-7   Large-section histology image, H&E stain. The tumor is solitary and measures 7 mm × 6 mm.

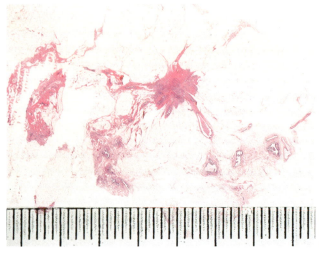

Ex. **7.**

Example 7.34

Ex. **7.34**-8   Low-power histological image of the invasive tumor.

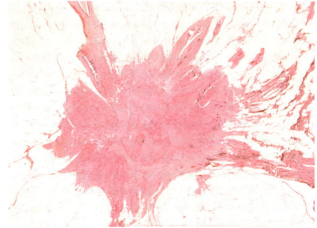

Ex. **7.34**-8

Ex. **7.34**-9   Immunohistochemical staining of E-cadherin shows absence of reaction within the structures of the invasive tumor, indicating its tubulolobular character.

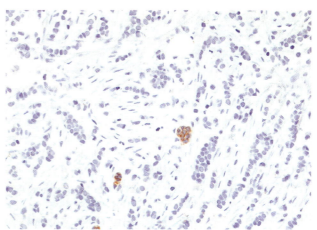

Ex. **7.34**-9

Ex. **7.34**-10   High-power magnification of this tubulolobular carcinoma, H&E stain.

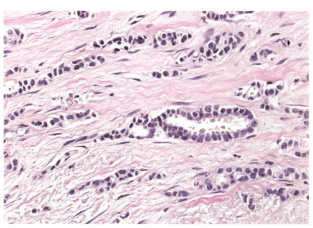

Ex. **7.34**-10

Ex. **7.34**-11   Immunohistochemical staining: estrogen receptor-positive tumor.

Comment
- Women with a breast cancer diagnosis are at the highest risk of developing another breast cancer.
- Careful annual life-long follow-up using physical examination, mammography, and often breast ultrasound is mandatory to find metachronous breast cancers as early as possible.
- Retroareolar breast cancer can be difficult to find.

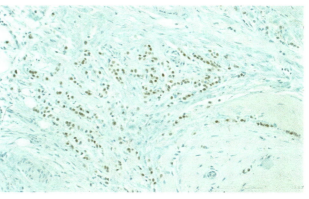

Ex. **7.34**-11

■ Characteristics of Lesions Regardless of Location

Lesions Causing Architectural Distortion

Example 7.35

A 52-year-old asymptomatic woman, screening examination.

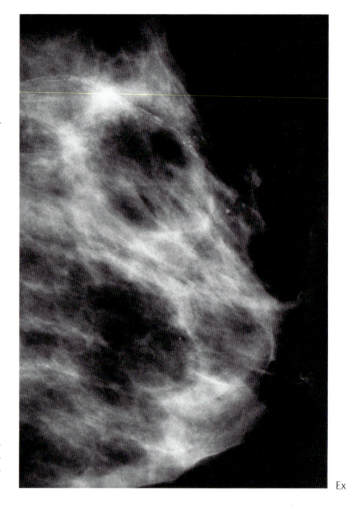

Ex. **7.35**-1 & 2   Left breast, details of the MLO and CC projections. This case demonstrates some of the complexities encountered when screening a Pattern I-type breast that is undergoing involution.

Ex. 7

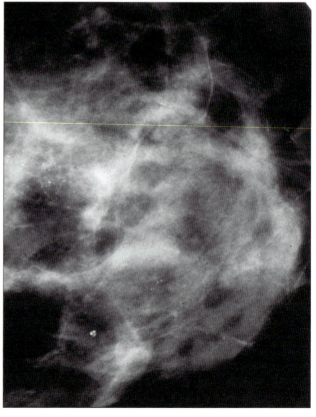

Ex. 7.

Example 7.35

Ex. **7.35**-3 & 4   Left breast, microfocus spot images in the MLO projection. There are multiple foci of calcification (upper rectangles, **7.35**-3) and subtle architectural distortion in the retroareolar region (lower rectangle in **7.35**-3, enlarged in **7.35**-4).

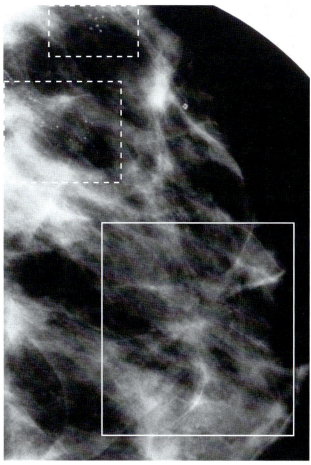

Ex. **7.35**-3

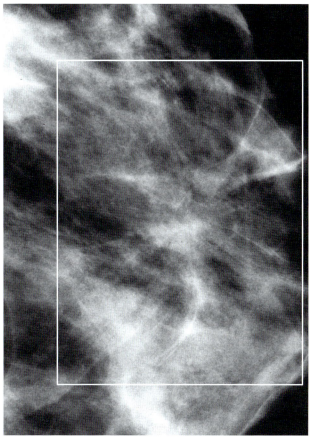

Ex. **7.35**-4

Lesions Causing Architectural Distortion—Example 7.35

Ex. **7.35**-5   Left breast, CC projection, same as Ex. **7.35**-2. In this view the retroareolar architectural distortion appears to be a tumor mass (solid rectangle). The multiple foci of calcifications are within the dashed rectangles.

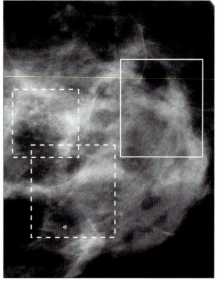

Ex. **7.35**-5

Ex. **7.35**-6 & 7   These microfocus magnification images demonstrate an ill-defined, mammographically malignant, retroareolar tumor and the crushed stone–like calcifications closer to the chest wall.

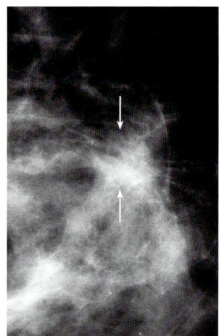

Ex. **7.35**-6

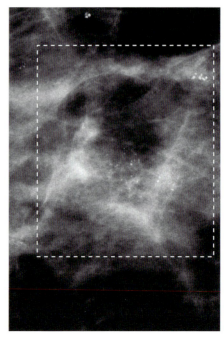

Ex. **7.35**-7

Example 7.35

Ex. **7.35**-8 Ultrasound examination of the retroareolar tumor supports the mammographic diagnosis.

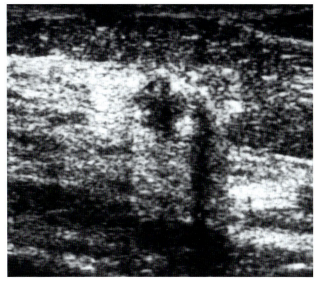

Ex. **7.35**-8

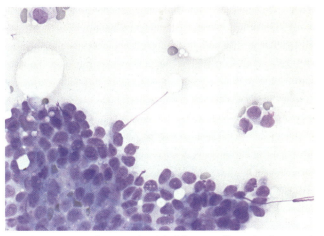

Ex. **7.35**-9

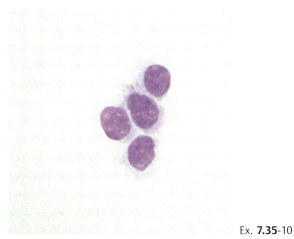

Ex. **7.35**-10

Ex. **7.35**-9 & 10 Ultrasound-guided fine-needle aspiration cytology shows malignant cells.

Ex. **7.35**-11 Specimen radiograph following hooked wire localization using the bracketing technique with multiple wires.

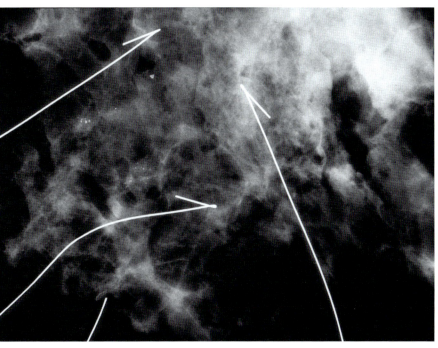

Ex. **7.35**-11

Comment
- Calcifications are easier to perceive than subtle architectural distortion.
- When detection and removal of architectural distortion reveals an invasive cancer in its preclinical stage, a process is arrested that would have progressed to an advanced stage.
- Although it is more difficult to detect architectural distortion than calcifications, the benefit of finding small invasive cancers is many times greater than the benefit of finding DCIS (calcifications).

Lesions Causing Architectural Distortion—Example 7.35

Histology (Ex. **7.35**-12)**:** One focus of well-differentiated invasive ductal cancer measures 7 mm × 6 mm, surrounded by innumerable foci of Grade II DCIS, LCIS over an area measuring 60 mm × 40 mm. In addition, hyperplastic breast changes such as papilloma, radial scar, and sclerosing adenosis are intermixed within the area with DCIS. Left mastectomy. LCIS foci in the mastectomy specimen.

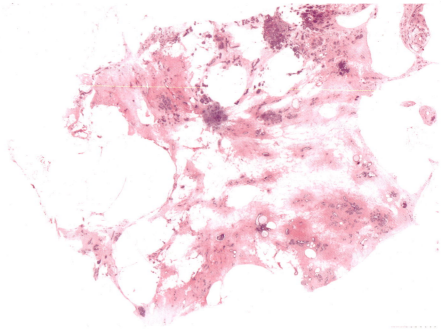

Ex. **7.35**-12

Ex. **7.35**-13 Radiograph of a specimen slice demonstrating the spiculated tumor (rectangle).

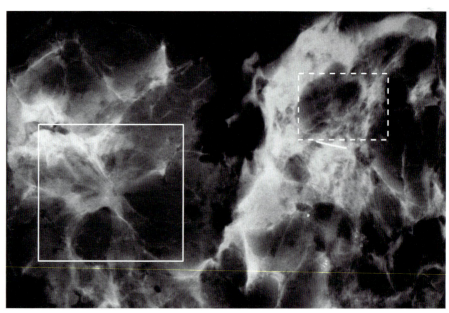

Lymph node status: pN0/14. **Treatment**: Mastectomy and reconstruction. **Outcome**: Yearly follow-up with mammography, ultrasound, and MRI. No signs of recurrence during the first five years after mastectomy.

Ex. **7.35**-13

Example 7.35

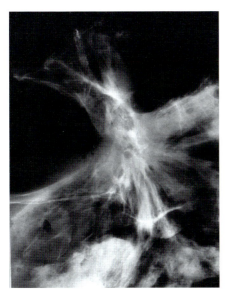

Ex. **7.35**-14

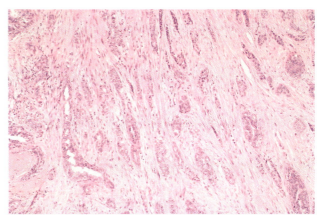

Ex. **7.35**-15

Ex. **7.35**-14 & 15   One of the sliced specimen radiographs shows the spiculated tumor, corresponding to a Grade 2 invasive carcinoma at histology (**7.35**-15).

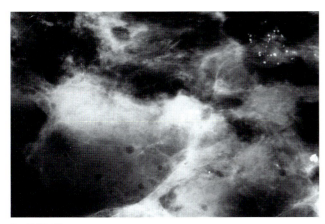

Ex. **7.35**-16

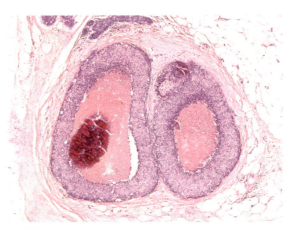

Ex. **7.35**-17

Ex. **7.35**-16 & 17   In another specimen slice, the microcalcifications are seen (**7.35**-16). Histological examination reveals Grade 2 DCIS with calcifications (**7.35**-17).

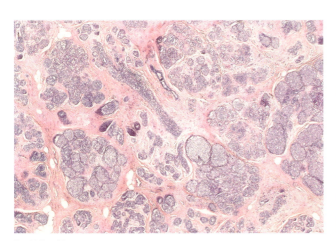

Ex. **7.35**-18

Ex. **7.35**-18   Noncalcified LCIS shown on histology over an area of 60 mm × 40 mm (not detectable on the mammogram).

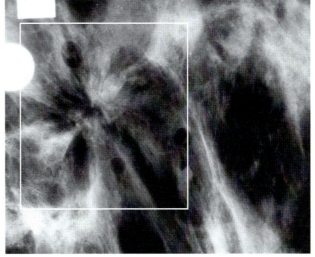

Ex. **7.35**-19

Ex. **7.35**-19   In a third specimen slice (dashed rectangle in Ex. **7.35**-13) a small radiating structure is revealed (not visible on the mammograms). This corresponds to a radial scar at histological examination.

Example 7.36

A 61-year-old asymptomatic woman, screening examination.

Ex. **7.36**-1 & 2   Right breast. Two images in the MLO projection were required for full coverage of this large breast. There is a lesion with a convex contour in the lower portion of the breast, requiring further work-up.

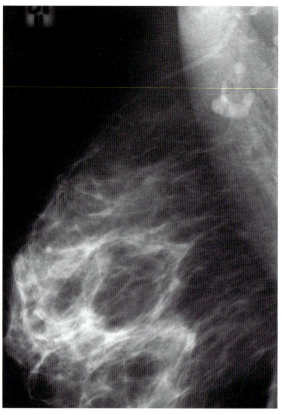

Ex. **7.36**-1

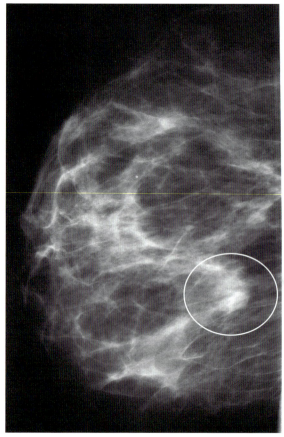

Ex. **7.36**-2

Example 7.36

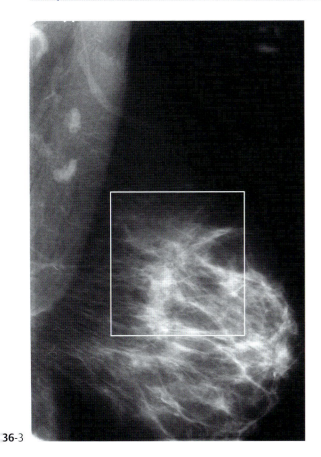

Ex. **7.36**-3 & 4   Left breast, two images in the MLO projection. There is architectural distortion in the upper portion of the breast (rectangle).

36-3

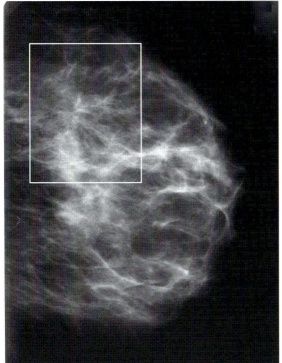

36-4

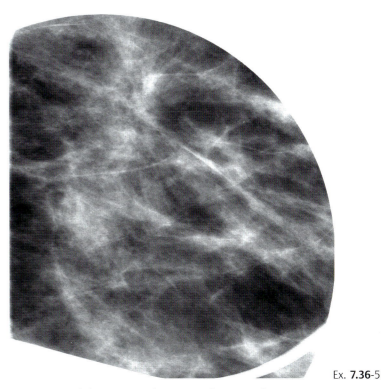

Ex. **7.36**-5

Ex. **7.36**-5   Left breast, microfocus magnification and spot compression view in the MLO projection.

Lesions Causing Architectural Distortion—Example 7.36

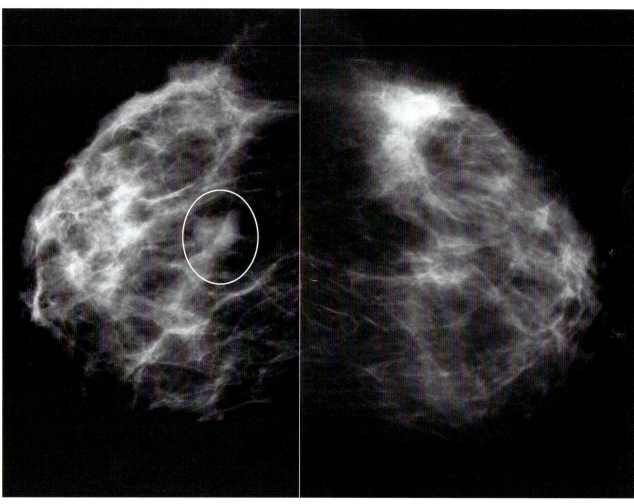

Ex. **7.36**-6

Ex. **7**

Ex. **7.36**-6   Right breast, CC projection. The oval-shaped lesion was shown to be a simple cyst at ultrasound examination and was aspirated.

Ex. **7.36**-7   Left breast, CC projection, screening examination.

Lesions Causing Architectural Distortion—Example 7.36

Example 7.36

Ex. **7.36**-8   Left breast, CC projection: the presence of a tent sign (straight borders of the fibroglandular tissue) suggests a pathological lesion.

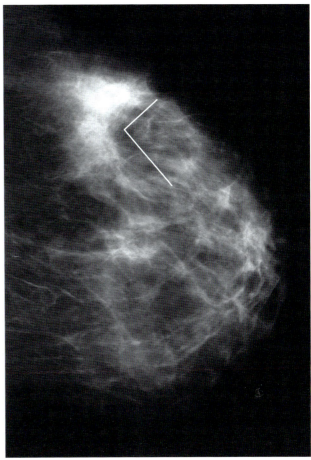

Ex. **7.36**-8

Ex. **7.36**-9   Left breast, microfocus magnification and spot compression view shows a spiculated, mammographically malignant lesion.

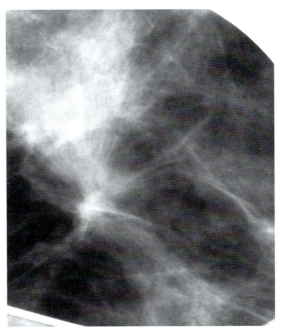

Ex. **7.36**-9

Ex. **7.36**-10 Specimen radiograph showing the surgically removed stellate tumor.

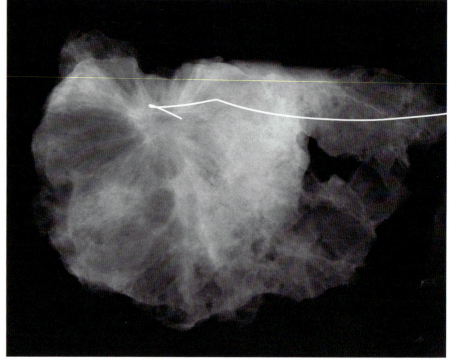

Ex. **7.36**-10

Ex. **7.36**-11 Large-section histology demonstrates the 18 mm × 14 mm spiculated malignant tumor partially embedded within the dense fibroglandular tissue.

Comment
- It is easier to detect masses with a convex contour on the mammogram than lesions with architectural distortion.
- The vast majority of lesions having a convex contour are benign, as in this case.
- More than 90% of the lesions with radiating structure on the mammogram (stellate tumors/architectural distortion) represent a malignant process, as in this case.

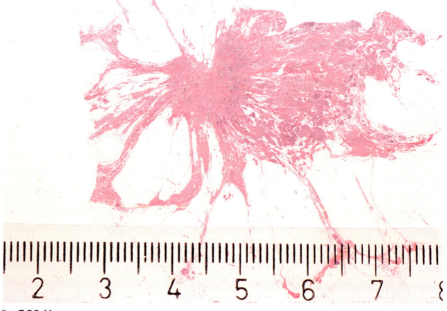

Ex. **7.36**-11

Example 7.36

Ex. **7.36**-12 **Histology:** tubular carcinoma.

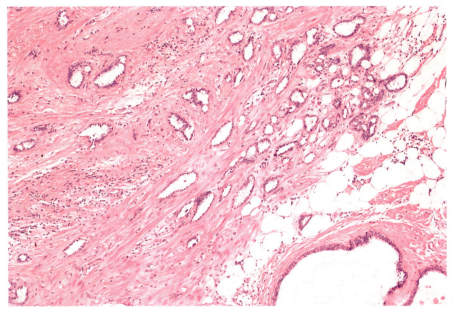

Ex. **7.36**-12

Ex. **7.36**-13 Anti-actin immuno-staining. The lack of a myoepithelial cell layer supports the histological diagnosis of invasive tubular carcinoma. The myoepithelial layer is only preserved around ducts and vessels.

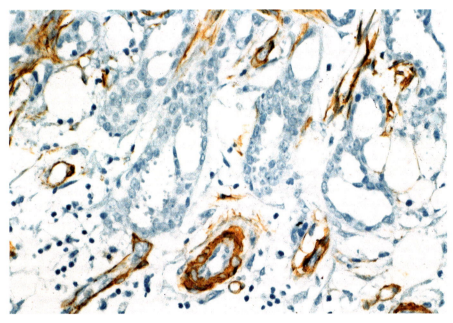

Ex. **7.36**-13

Lymph node status: Histological examination did not show metastases in the nine surgically removed axillary lymph nodes.

Treatment: Segmentectomy and postoperative irradiation.
Outcome: No signs of recurrence were detected during the first four years of follow-up.

Lesions Causing Architectural Distortion

Example 7.37

A 58-year-old woman felt a "thickening" in the lateral portion of her left breast (year 2000). Her two previous mammograms are also shown for comparison (years 1997 and 1999).

Ex. **7.37**-1 & 2   Left breast, MLO and CC projections. Pattern II breast (fatty replaced). No mammographic abnormality is demonstrable (year 1997).

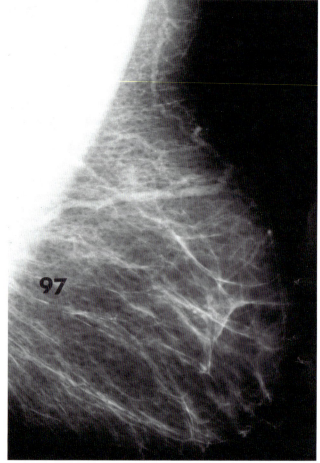

Ex. 7

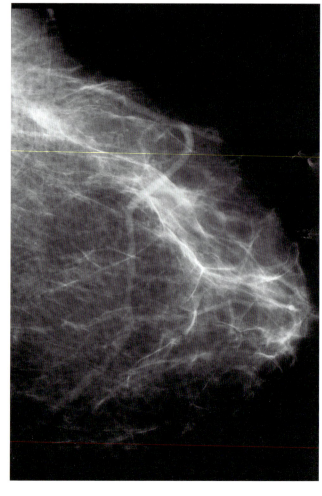

Ex. 7

Example 7.37

Ex. **7.37**-3   Second examination two years later (year 1999), still asymptomatic. Left breast, MLO projection. Normal mammogram.

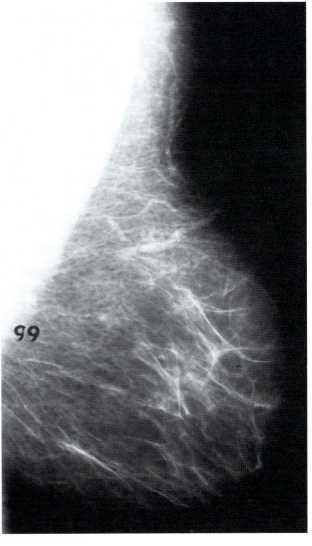

Ex. **7.37**-3

Ex. **7.37**-4 & 5   Second examination (year 1999), detail of the lateral portion of the right and left CC projections. No mammographic abnormality is demonstrable.

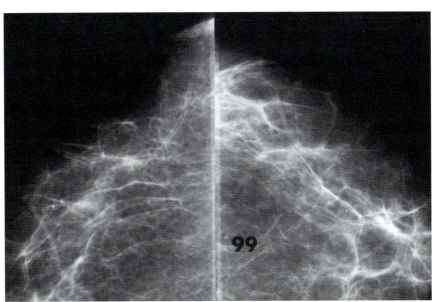

Ex. **7.37**-4

Ex. **7.37**-5

371

Lesions Causing Architectural Distortion—Example 7.37

Ex. **7.37**-6 & 7   Third examination (year 2000). The patient complains about a vague thickening in the upper-outer portion of her left breast. Right and left MLO projections.

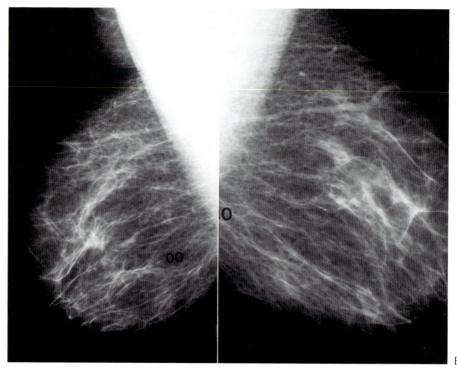

Ex. **7.37**-6

Ex. "

Ex. **7.37**-8 & 9   Third examination (year 2000). Detail of the right and left CC projections. Corresponding to the vague thickening in the lateral portion of the left breast, a non-specific asymmetric density has developed.

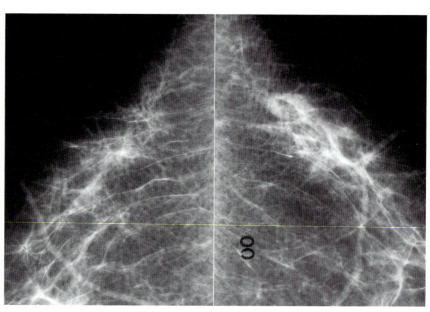

Ex. **7.37**-8

Ex. **7.37**

Example 7.37

Ex. **7.37**-10 & 11 Comparison of the CC projections from the first and third examinations shows the development of a nonspecific density (encircled).

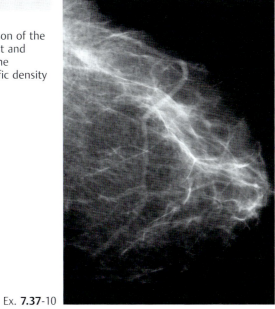
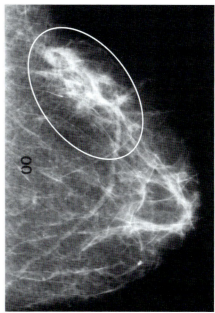

Ex. **7.37**-10

Ex. **7.37**-11

Ex. **7.37**-12 & 13 Comparative right and left CC projections from the second examination show no abnormality.

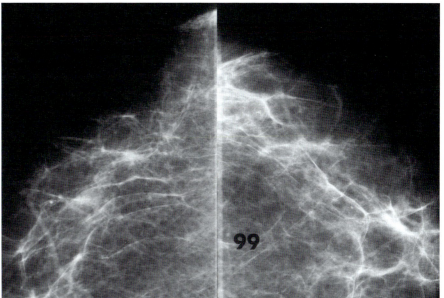

Ex. **7.37**-12

Ex. **7.37**-13

Ex. **7.37**-14 & 15 Comparative right and left CC projections from the third examination demonstrate that the nonspecific density has evolved over a large area.

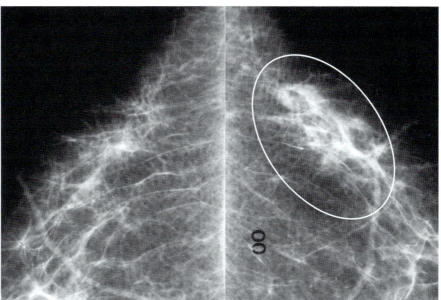

Ex. **7.37**-14

Ex. **7.37**-15

373

Lesions Causing Architectural Distortion—Example 7.37

Ex. **7.37**-16 & 17   Comparative left CC projections from the second and third examinations.

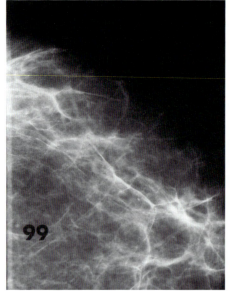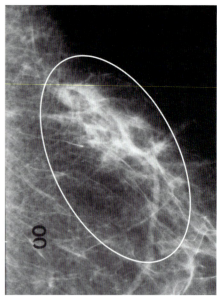

Ex. **7.37**-16   Ex. **7.37**-17

Ex. **7.37**-18   Spot magnification of the area with thickening, left breast, MLO projection. See comment below.

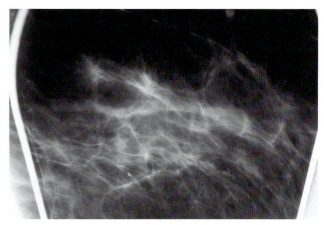

Ex. **7.37**-18

Ex. **7.37**-19   Spot magnification of the area with thickening, left breast, CC projection. See comment below.

Comment
- Whenever there is a developing, nonspecific mammographic density associated with a palpable lesion, one of the differential diagnostic options is invasive lobular carcinoma. The magnification-spot images may be misleading, because the classic form of invasive lobular carcinoma infiltrates the preexisting normal breast structure (fibrous strands and ducts) instead of forming a central tumor mass. Breast ultrasound examination can quickly lead to the correct diagnosis.

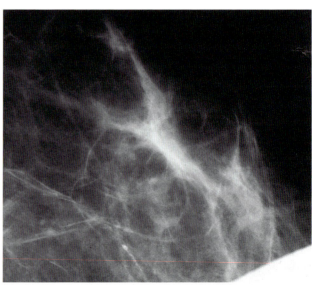

Ex. **7.37**-19

Example 7.37

Ex. **7.37**-20   Breast ultrasound shows several foci of malignant tumors.

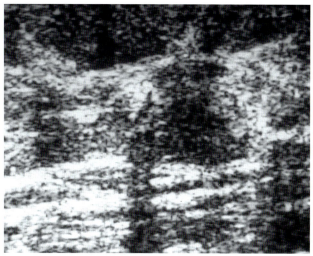

Ex. **7.37**-20

Ex. **7.37**-21   Ultrasound-guided FNAB: atypical cells.

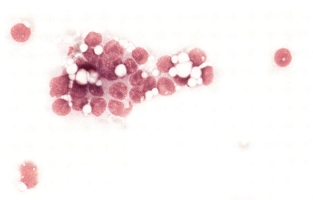

Ex. **7.37**-21

Ex. **7.37**-22   14-gauge core biopsy: invasive lobular carcinoma.

Comment
- When there is a palpable tumor corresponding to a subtle asymmetric density with slight architectural distortion on the mammogram, thorough breast ultrasound and large-core needle biopsy are indicated because of a suspicion for invasive lobular carcinoma. FNAB may lead to a misleading result and is not the procedure of choice in these cases.

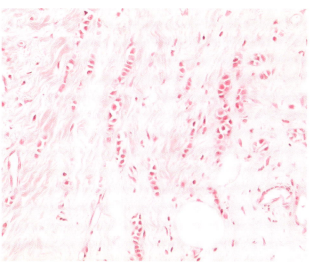

Ex. **7.37**-22

Lesions Causing Architectural Distortion—Example 7.37

Ex. **7.37**-23   Radiograph of one of the specimen slices. Even at this level of detail, one cannot distinguish with certainty the remaining fibroglandular tissue from malignancy.

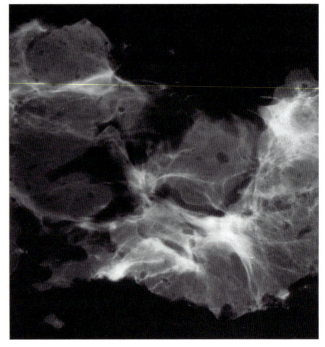

Ex. **7.37**-23

Ex. **7.37**-24   Large-section histology demonstrates multiple foci of invasive lobular carcinoma (ink circles). The extent of the disease has been estimated at 30 mm × 26 mm. Direct comparison with the corresponding specimen radiograph (Ex. **7.37**-23) demonstrates how similar the mammographic appearance of the classic invasive lobular carcinoma and remnants of fibroglandular tissue can be.

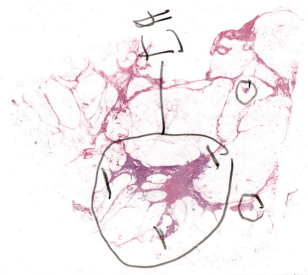

Ex. **7.37**-24

Example 7.37

Ex. **7.37**-25 **Histology**: Invasive lobular carcinoma, classic type, showing periductal "targetoid" infiltration.

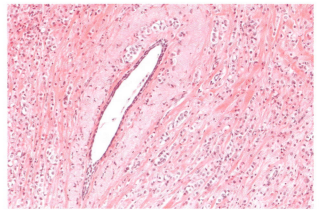

Ex. **7.37**-25

Ex. **7.37**-26 Immunohistochemical staining. The tumor is estrogen receptor-positive.

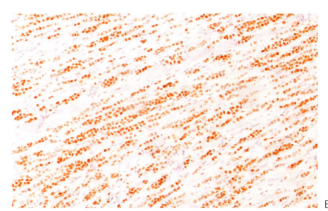

Ex. **7.37**-26

Ex. **7.37**-27 Associated lobular carcinoma in situ.

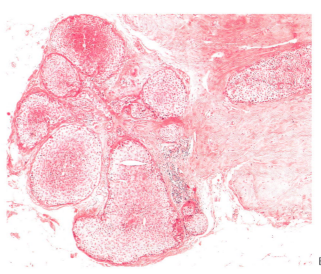

Ex. **7.37**-27

Ex. **7.37**-28 **Lymph node status:** Examination of two sentinel nodes and an additional nine axillary lymph nodes did not reveal metastases.

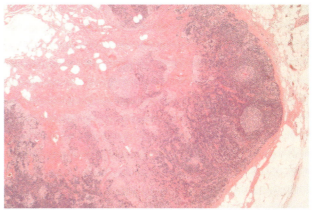

Treatment: Segmentectomy and postoperative irradiation.
Outcome: The patient has remained recurrence-free for the first three postoperative years.

Ex. **7.37**-28

Example 7.38

A 55-year-old asymptomatic woman, screening examination.

Ex. **7.38**-1 & 2   Detail of the right and left MLO projections.

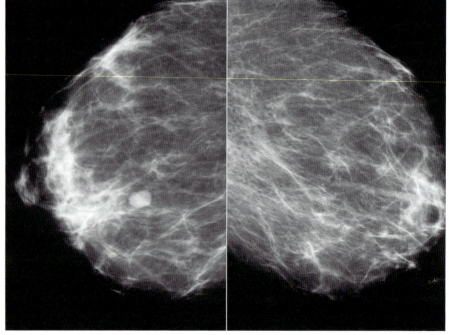

Ex. **7.38**-1   Ex. **7.38**-2

Ex. **7.38**-3 & 4   Detail of the right and left CC projections.

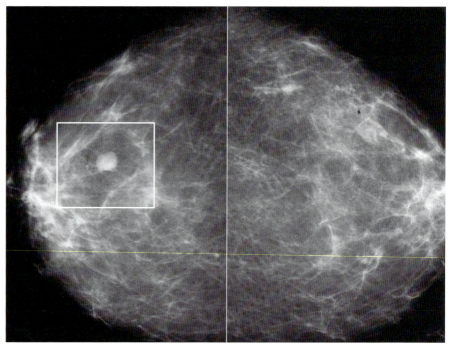

Ex. **7.38**-3   Ex. **7.38**-4

Example 7.38

Ex. **7.38**-5   The solitary, oval lesion in the central portion of the right breast has low density and is sharply outlined on this microfocus magnification image. Mammographic diagnosis: benign lesion.

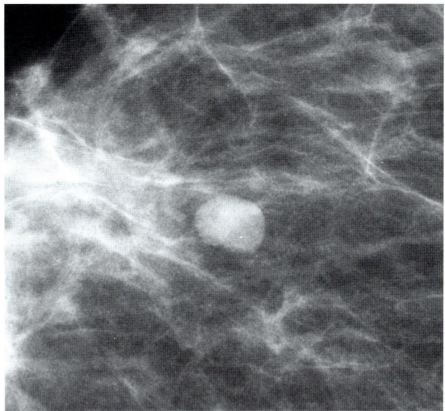

Ex. **7.38**-5

Ex. **7.38**-6   Ultrasound examination shows a simple cyst, which was aspirated under ultrasound guidance.

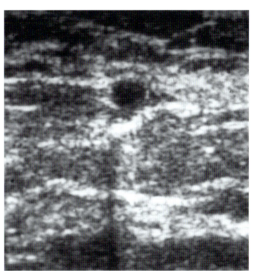

Ex. **7.38**-6

Lesions Causing Architectural Distortion—Example 7.38

Ex. **7.38**-7   Left breast, detail of the MLO projection.

Ex. **7.38**-8   Photographic magnification shows no tumor mass, but hints at faint calcifications.

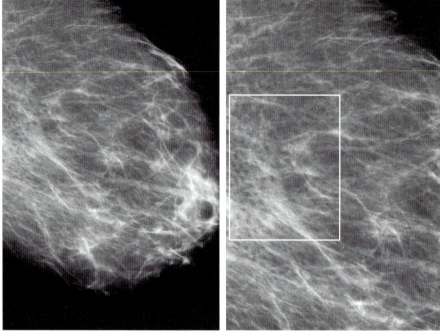

Ex. **7.38**-7

Ex. **7.38**-8

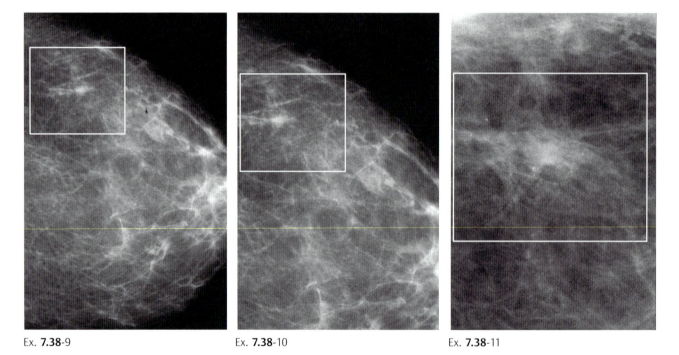

Ex. **7.38**-9

Ex. **7.38**-10

Ex. **7.38**-11

Ex. **7.38**-9 to 11   Left breast. CC-projection (**7.38**-9) and detail of the lateral portion of the CC projection (**7.38**-10) demonstrate a tiny tumor mass with very faint associated calcifications. The microfocus magnification image (**7.38**-11) reveals that both the ill-defined tumor and the associated calcifications are mammographically malignant.

Example 7.38

Ex. **7.38**-12   Preoperative localization using the bracketing technique.

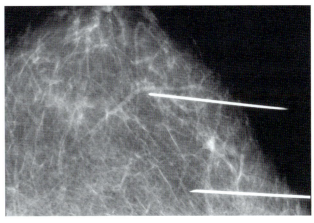

Ex. **7.38**-12

Ex. **7.38**-13   Specimen radiograph. The areas within rectangles are magnified in Ex. **7.38**-14 & 15.

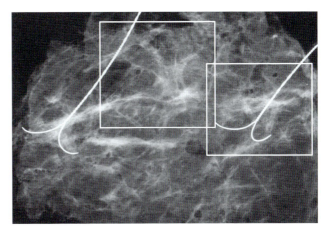

Ex. **7.38**-13

Ex. **7.38**-14 & 15   Detailed images of the specimen radiograph reveal clusters of calcifications as well as ill-defined densities.

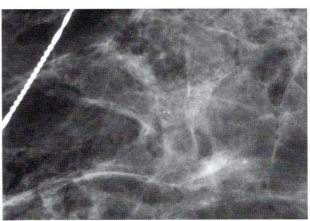

Ex. **7.38**-14

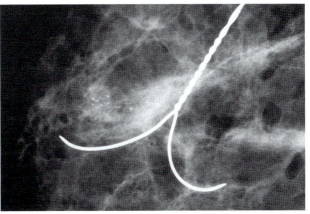

Ex. **7.38**-15

Lesions Causing Architectural Distortion—Example 7.38

Ex. **7.38**-16   Radiograph of one of the specimen slices (4 × magnification). There are numerous distended branching ducts containing the malignant type calcifications (continuous rectangle). Only a few of these are seen on the thin histological section within the continuous rectangles on Ex. **7.38**-17. A lobulated, ill-defined tumor is associated with these dilated ducts (dashed rectangle) corresponding to the invasive carcinoma on large-section histology (dashed rectangle in Ex. **7.38**-17).

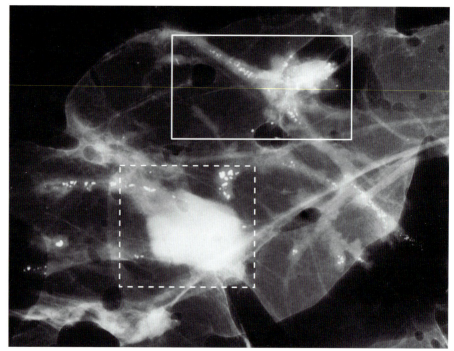

Ex. **7.38**-16

Ex. **7.38**-17   Large-section histology, showing the small invasive tumor (dashed rectangle). The ducts within the continuous rectangles correspond to some of the many ducts within the continuous rectangle in the specimen radiograph.

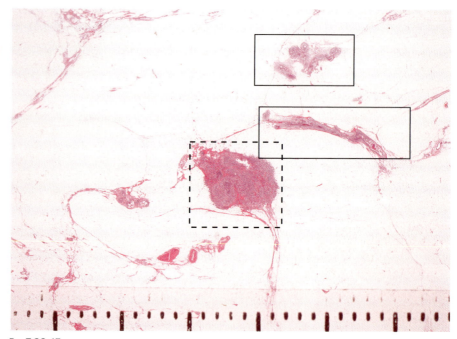

Ex. **7.38**-17

Example 7.38

Ex. **7.38**-18 Histological image of the associated high-grade ductal carcinoma in situ (area within the longer rectangle in Ex. **7.38**-17).

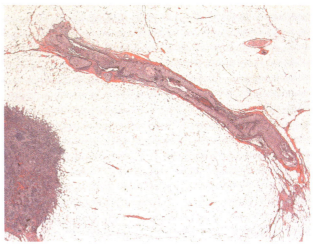

Ex. **7.38**-18

Ex. **7.38**-19 Grade 3 in-situ carcinoma was found on an area measuring 30 mm × 20 mm. The solid and cribriform DCIS was associated with central necrosis, amorphous calcifications, and periductal lymphocytic infiltration.

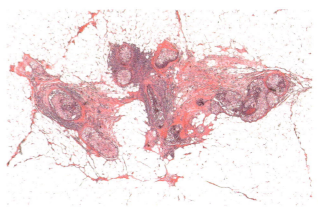

Ex. **7.38**-19

Ex. **7.38**-20 Higher-power histological image of the solid carcinoma in situ with necrosis and amorphous calcifications.

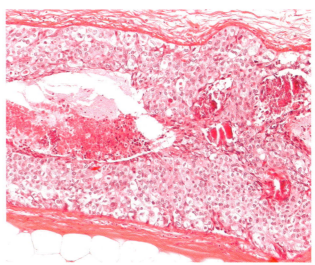

Ex. **7.38**-20

**Lesions Causing Architectural
Distortion—Example 7.38**

Ex. **7.38**-21   The invasive tumor as
seen on the specimen radiograph
(rectangle). The corresponding histology is demonstrated in Ex. **7.38**-22.

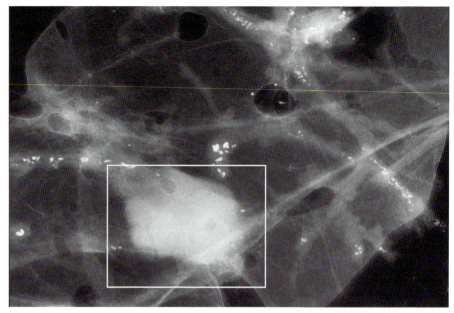

Ex. **7.38**-21

Ex. **7.38**-22   Low-power magnification histological image of the 7 mm ×
5 mm invasive carcinoma.

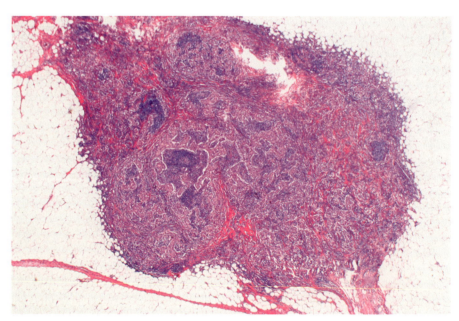

Ex. **7.38**-22

Example 7.38

Ex. **7.38**-23 & 24   Higher-power histological images show a poorly differentiated atypical medullary carcinoma.

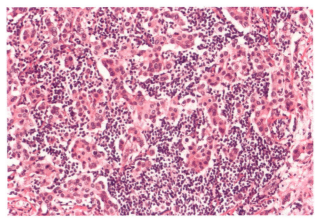

Ex. **7.38**-23

Comment
- This case emphasizes again how easy it is to detect a lesion with a convex contour, and how this may distract from a far more important malignant lesion elsewhere.
- The primary goal of mammographic screening is to find those cancers early that would soon have developed to poorly differentiated, advanced carcinoma, as demonstrated by this case.

Lymph node status: Ten axillary nodes showed no metastases at histological examination.
Treatment: Segmentectomy and postoperative irradiation.
Follow-up: The patient was recurrence-free at the most recent follow-up 64 months following treatment.

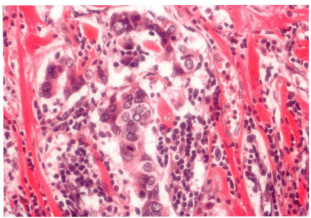

Ex. **7.38**-24

Example 7.39

A 45-year-old woman who has been treated for recurring abscesses and fistulas in the lower central portion of her right breast.

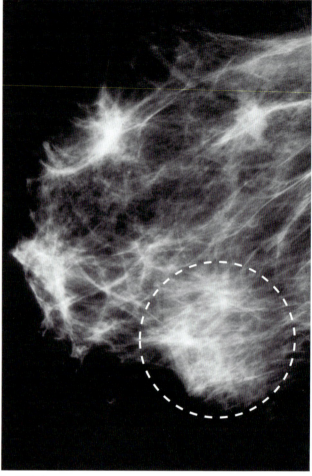

Ex. **7.39**-1 & 2   Right breast, detail of the MLO and CC projections. The postinflammatory fibrosis is encircled.

Ex. **7.39**-1

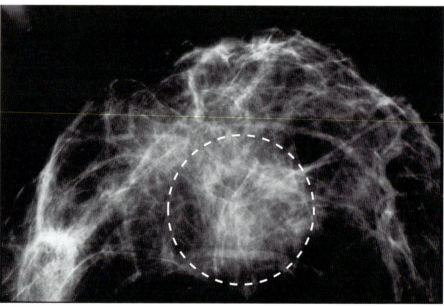

Ex. **7.39**-2

Example 7.39

Ex. **7.39**-3 Right breast, CC projection, same mammographic image as Ex. **7.39**-2. Perception of pathological findings is always facilitated by first visualizing the background of adipose tissue (yellow outlines). The remaining density with an irregular contour can then be more readily detected (density filled in with orange).

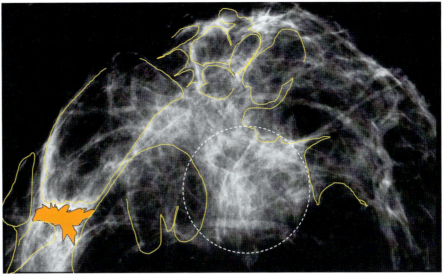

Ex. **7.39**-3

Ex. **7.39**-4 Spot compression and microfocus magnification demonstrate a mammographically malignant stellate tumor mass surrounded by nonspecific densities.

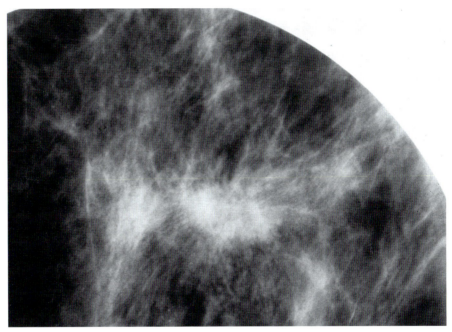

Ex. **7.39**-4

Ex. **7.39**-5 Ultrasound examination supports the mammographic diagnosis.

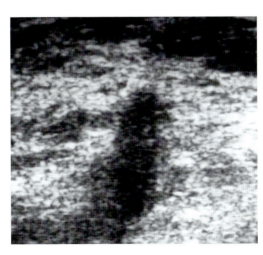

Ex. **7.39**-5

Ex. **7.39**-6   Specimen radiograph of the postinflammatory fibrosis and abscess cavity (arrow).

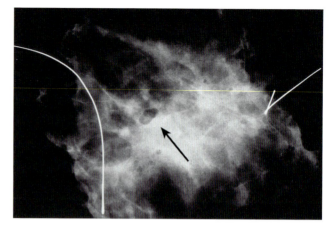

Ex. **7.39**-6

Ex. **7.39**-7   Specimen radiograph of the stellate tumor and its surroundings.

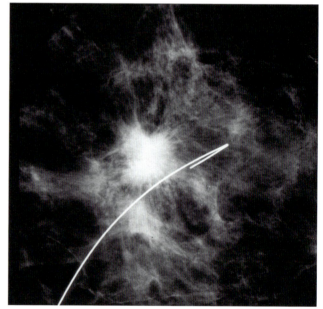

Ex. **7.39**-7

Comment
- When a mammographically malignant lesion is surrounded by nonspecific densities or calcifications, a wide excision is necessary to remove potential additional tumor foci.
- Involution may occur in a haphazard fashion. Emphasizing the radiolucent background pattern of the adipose tissue by outlining the interfacing fibroglandular and adipose tissue heightens perception of any abnormality and enables the reader to better differentiate pathological lesions from the remnants of fibroglandular tissue.

Example 7.39

Ex. **7.39**-8 Radiograph of one of the specimen slices containing the stellate tumor. An elongated, nonspecific density is adjacent to the tumor.

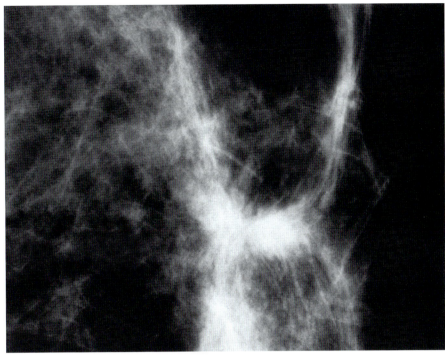

Ex. **7.39**-8

Ex. **7.39**-9 Large-section histological image of the tissue demonstrated in Ex. **7.39**-8.

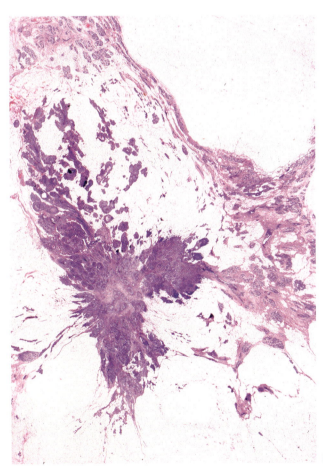

Ex. **7.39**-9

Lesions Causing Architectural Distortion—Example 7.39

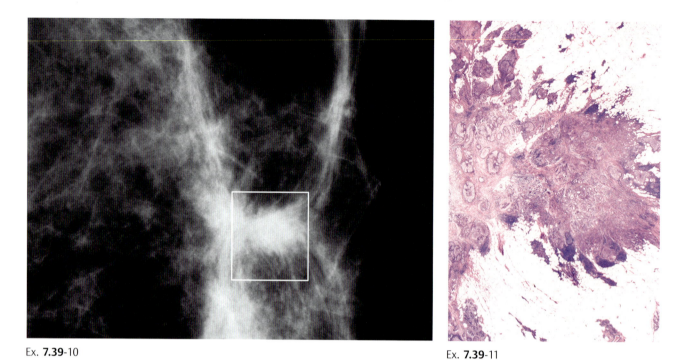

Ex. **7.39**-10

Ex. **7.39**-11

Ex. **7.39**-10 & 11   Mammographic–histological comparison of the spiculated lesion (rectangle). The moderately differentiated invasive ductal carcinoma measures 14 mm × 12 mm.

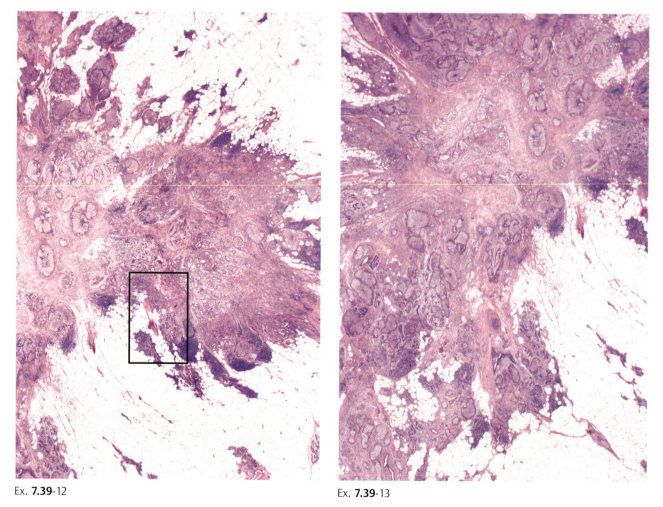

Ex. **7.39**-12

Ex. **7.39**-13

Ex. **7.39**-12 & 13   Low- and higher-power histological images: invasive ductal carcinoma associated with in-situ cancer.

Example 7.39

Ex. **7.39**-14   The nonspecific density adjacent to the spiculated lesion is encircled.

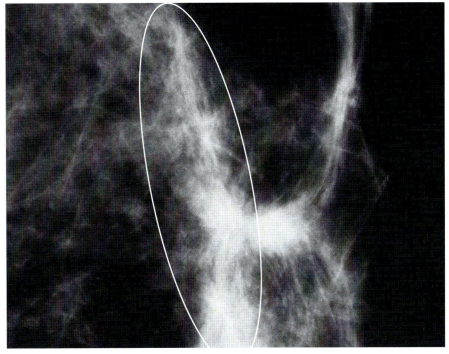

Ex. **7.39**-14

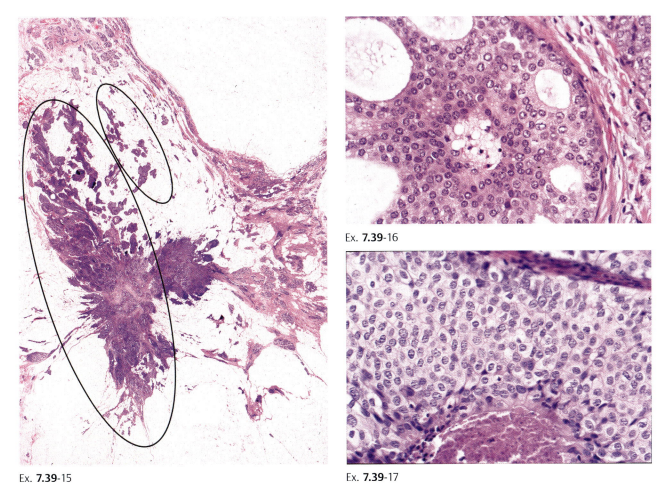

Ex. **7.39**-15

Ex. **7.39**-16

Ex. **7.39**-17

Ex. **7.39**-15 to 17   Low- and higher-power histological images. The nonspecific density seen on the mammogram corresponds at histological examination to multiple foci of DCIS over a large area.

Lymph node status: One of 10 surgically removed axillary nodes showed metastasis at histological examination.
Treatment: Segmentectomy, postoperative irradiation, chemotherapy, hormonal therapy.

Follow-up: The patient had no signs of recurrence at the most recent follow-up examination, five years after treatment.

Lesions Causing Architectural Distortion

Example 7.40

A 45-year-old asymptomatic woman, screening examination.

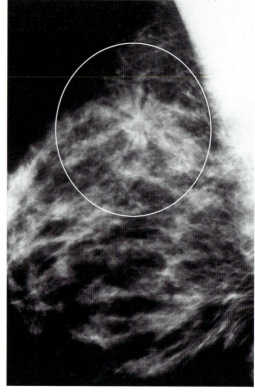

Ex. **7.40**-1

Ex. **7.40**-1 & 2 Right breast, MLO and CC projections. A region with architectural distortion in the upper outer quadrant is encircled.

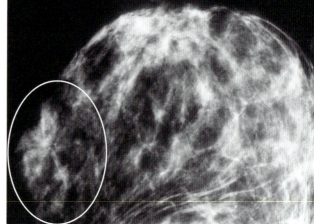

Ex. **7.**

Ex. **7.40**-3 Spot compression and microfocus magnification demonstrate further details of the architectural distortion. The lack of straight, individual spiculations and the lack of a palpable abnormality despite its superficial location suggest that the radiating structure consists of a radial scar. For this reason preoperative needle biopsy is not indicated.

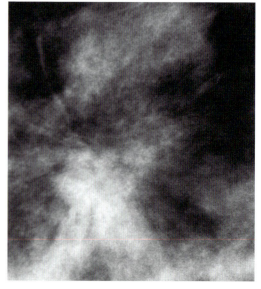

Ex. **7.40**-3

Example 7.40

Ex. **7.40**-4   Specimen radiograph. The lesion has been removed with good margins.

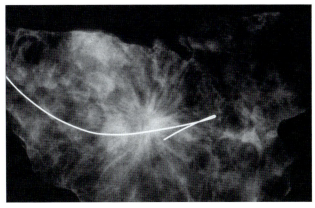

Ex. **7.40**-4

Ex. **7.40**-5   Low-power histological image shows the central fibroelastic core surrounded by proliferating ducts arranged in a radiating fashion.

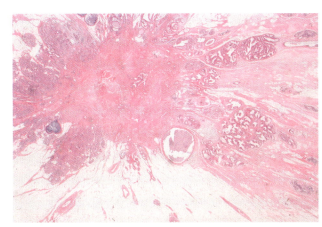

Ex. **7.40**-5

Ex. **7.40**-6 & 7   Higher-power histological images confirm the diagnosis of a radial scar. There is no associated malignancy.

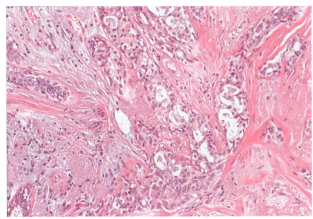

Ex. **7.40**-6

Comment
- Architectural distortion can occasionally be caused by a benign lesion. The most frequent cause is a surgical scar, which seldom leads to diagnostic difficulties. Radial scar accounts for 7 % of the cases of surgically removed architectural distortion (see Chapter 6, page 197).
- The considerable difference in the underlying histology of invasive carcinoma and radial scar results in dissimilar mammographic appearance, often making differential diagnosis possible. While preoperative needle biopsy is recommended in lesions suspicious for malignancy, needle biopsy carries a high risk of over- and underdiagnosis in radial scar. Open surgical biopsy is the procedure of choice for a suspected radial scar.

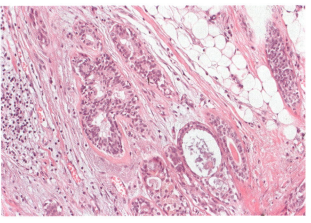

Ex. **7.40**-7

Lesions Causing Parenchymal Contour Changes

Example 7.41

A 67-year-old asymptomatic woman, screening examination.

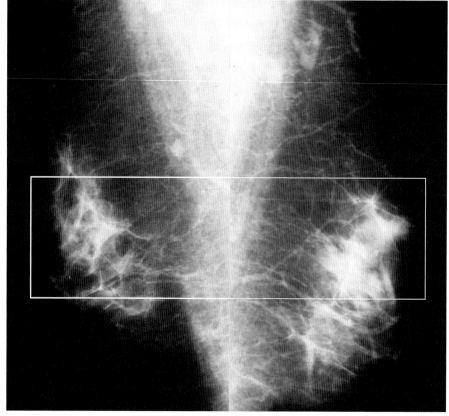

Ex. **7.41**-1 & 2   Right and left breasts, MLO projections. The considerable difference in the outline of the parenchymal contour is an indication for further work-up.

Ex. **7.41**-1   Ex. **7.41**-2

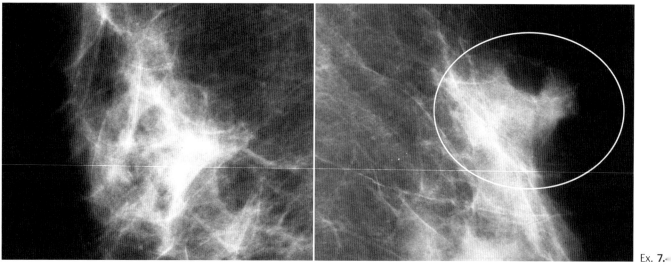

Ex. **7.41**-3   Ex. **7.**

Ex. **7.41**-3 & 4   Magnified images of the area outlined in Ex. **7.41**-1. An ill-defined asymmetric density protrudes from the fibroglandular tissue, greatly altering the parenchymal contour.

Example 7.41

Ex. **7.41**-5 Microfocus magnification view, left MLO projection. The lesion is lobulated, ill-defined, mammographically malignant.

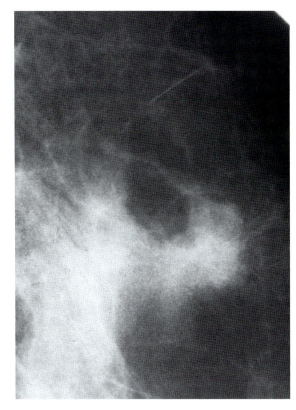

Ex. **7.41**-5

Ex. **7.41**-6 Operative specimen radiograph, showing the solitary, ill-defined tumor.

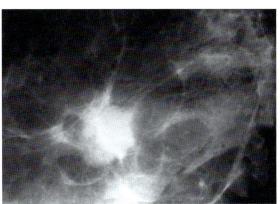

Ex. **7.41**-6

Ex. **7.41**-7 **Large-section histology:** 9 mm × 7 mm poorly differentiated invasive ductal carcinoma with Grade 3 in-situ components on an area measuring 25 mm × 15 mm.

Comment
- The contour of the fibroglandular tissue is most frequently scalloped and symmetric. Use of the side-by-side viewing technique will facilitate detection of alterations in the parenchymal contour such as protrusion or retraction. These should be worked up using spot-compression images and breast ultrasound.

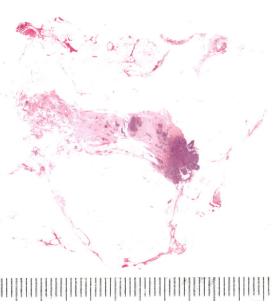

Treatment: Mastectomy.
Outcome: One year following operation the patient died of pancreatic cancer (verified by autopsy).

Ex. **7.41**-7

Example 7.42

A 68-year-old asymptomatic woman, screening examination.

Ex. **7.42**-1 & 2   Right and left breasts, MLO projections.

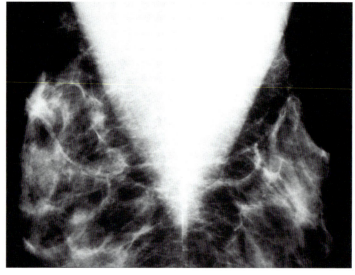

Ex. **7.42**-1

Ex. **7.42**-2

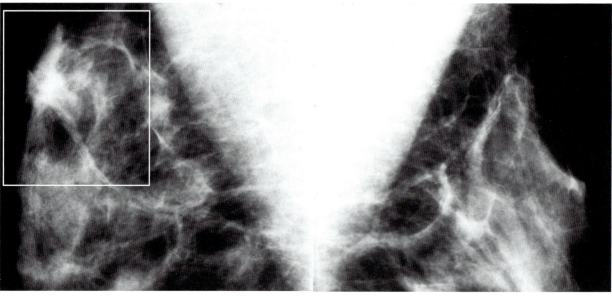

Ex. **7.42**-3

Ex. **7.42**

Ex. **7.42**-3 & 4   Right and left breasts, detail of the MLO projections, showing a change in the contour (rectangle) relative to the corresponding area in the contralateral breast.

Ex. **7.42**-5   Microfocus magnification image of the area in the rectangle in Ex. **7.42**-3. The ill-defined, irregular lesion is mammographically malignant.

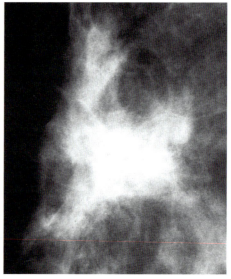

Ex. **7.42**-5

Example 7.42

Ex. **7.42**-6 & 7 Detail of the lateral portions of the right and left breasts, CC projection. The tent sign on the right CC-projection points at the malignant tumor hidden in the dense fibroglandular tissue.

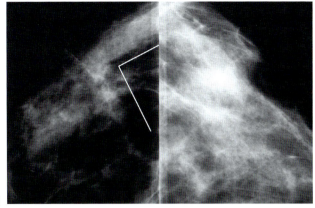

Ex. **7.42**-6   Ex. **7.42**-7

Ex. **7.42**-8 Microfocus magnification image of the lateral portion of the right breast, CC projection. The tent sign is more obvious and points to the ill-defined malignant tumor.

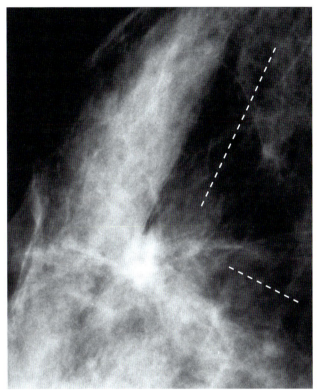

Ex. **7.42**-8

Ex. **7.42**-9 & 10 Histological examination of both the large-core needle biopsy specimen (**7.42**-9) and the surgical specimen (**7.42**-9) shows invasive lobular carcinoma.

Comment
- A stellate lesion near the parenchymal contour can straighten the regular, scalloped outline, pointing at the tumor hidden in the dense tissue. This is called the "tent-sign" when it occurs along the posterior parenchymal contour.

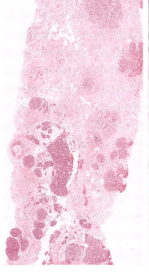
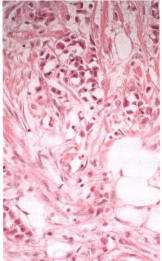

Ex. **7.42**-9   Ex. **7.42**-10

Lesions Causing Parenchymal Contour Changes

Example 7.43

A 70-year-old asymptomatic woman, screening examination.

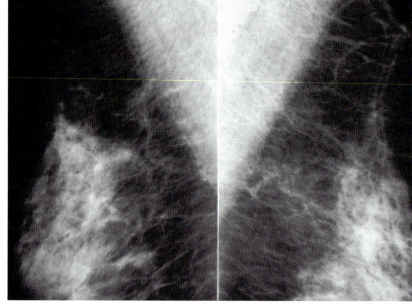

Ex. **7.43**-1 & 2   Right and left breasts, details of the MLO projections.

Ex. **7.43**-1   Ex. **7.43**-2

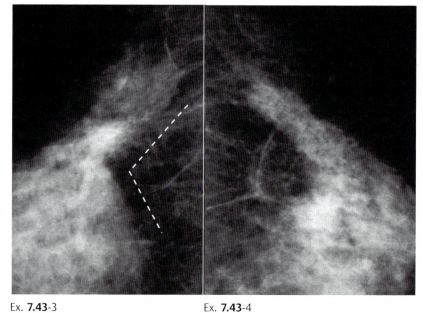

Ex. **7.43**-3 & 4   Right and left breasts, details of the CC projections. A tent sign is seen at the interface of the fibroglandular and adipose tissue in the right breast. This tent sign can be contrasted with the arcadelike posterior contour in the opposite breast in Ex. **7.43**-7 & 8.

Ex. **7.43**-3   Ex. **7.43**-4

Ex. **7.43**-5   Right breast, detail of the lateromedial horizontal projection. The contour protrudes, indicating the presence of a pathological lesion (rectangle).

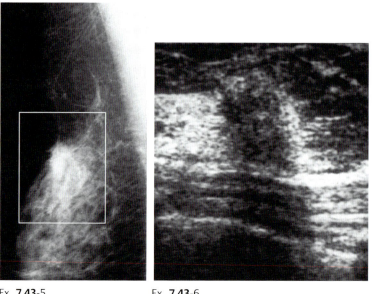

Ex. **7.43**-6   Breast ultrasound demonstrates a malignant breast tumor that is hidden in the dense fibroglandular tissue on the mammogram.

Ex. **7.43**-5   Ex. **7.43**-6

Example 7.43

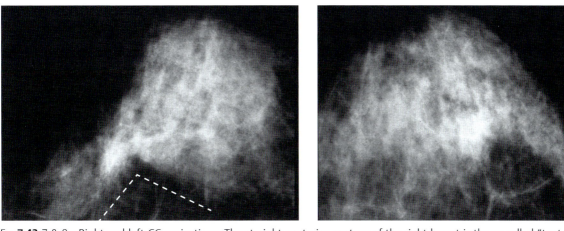

Ex. **7.43**-7   Ex. **7.43**-8

Ex. **7.43**-7 & 8   Right and left CC projections. The straight posterior contour of the right breast is the so-called "tent sign."

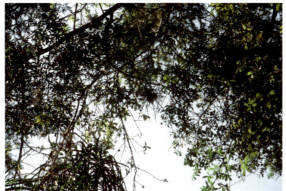

Ex. **7.43**-9

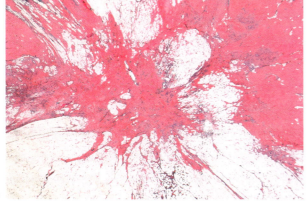

7.43-10

Ex. **7.43**-10   Large-section histological image of the 13 mm invasive lobular carcinoma.

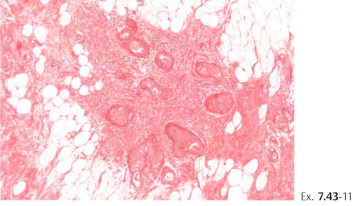

Ex. **7.43**-11

Ex. **7.43**-11   Medium-power histological image showing invasive and in-situ carcinoma.

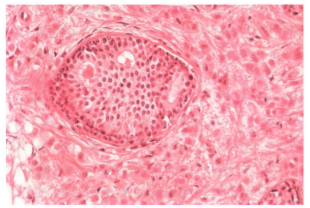

7.43-12

Ex. **7.43**-12   Higher magnification of Ex. **7.43**-11.

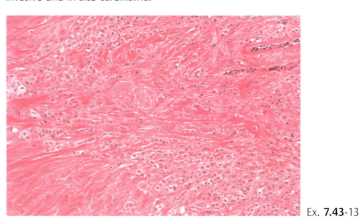

Ex. **7.43**-13

Ex. **7.43**-13   High-power histology of the invasive part of the tumor.

Lesions Causing Parenchymal Contour Changes

Example 7.44

A 49-year-old asymptomatic woman, screening examination.

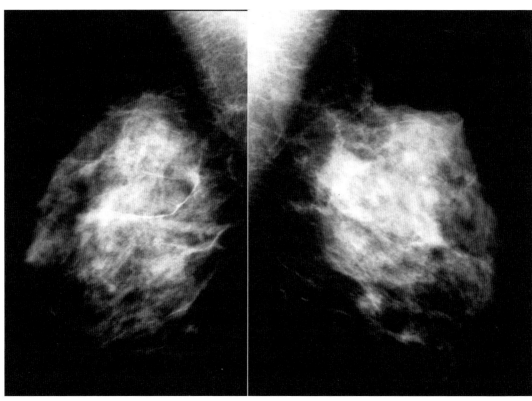

Ex. **7.44**-1

Ex. **7.44**-2

Ex. **7.44**-1 & 2   Right and left breasts, MLO projections. Dense fibroglandular tissue is seen in both breasts. Comparison of the upper portions of the two mammograms reveals an alteration in the contour of the left breast, the "ellbow sign", which is reminiscent of the angle of a flexed elbow.

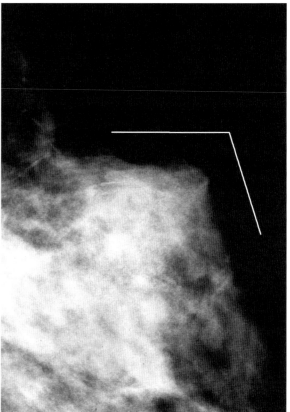

Ex. **7.44**-3   The contour change, the only sign leading to the detection of an abnormality, is better seen.

Ex. **7.44**-3

Example 7.44

Ex. **7.44**-4 Ultrasound examination clearly demonstrates a malignant tumor in this dense breast.

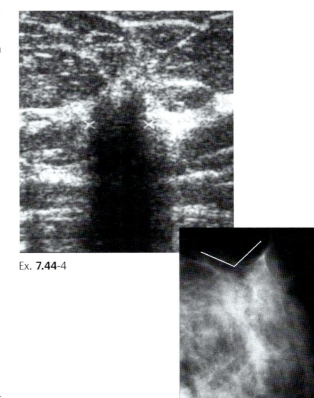

Ex. **7.44**-4

Ex. **7.44**-5 An additional microfocus magnification image shows a V-shaped contour change, pointing to the site of the tumor.

Ex. **7.44**-5

Ex. **7.44**-6 Large-section histological image of this tubular carcinoma, partially hidden in the dense fibrous stroma.

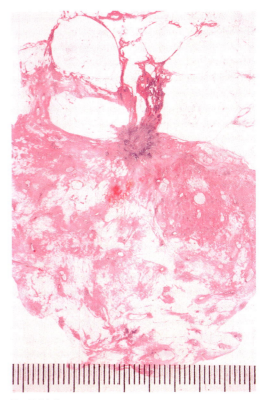

Ex. **7.44**-6

Lesions Causing Parenchymal Contour Changes

Example 7.45

A 68-year-old asymptomatic woman, screening examination.

Ex. **7.45**-1 & 2   Right and left breasts, MLO projections.

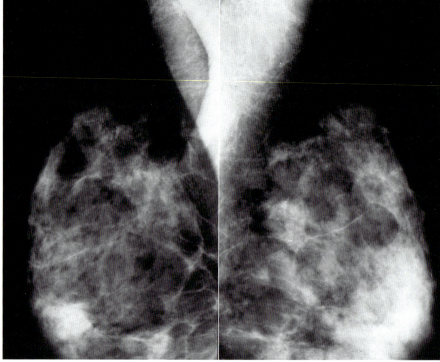

Ex. **7.45**-1

Ex. **7.4**

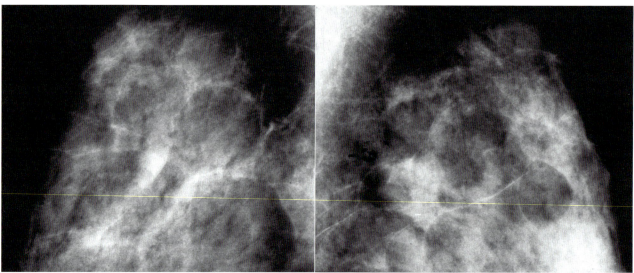

Ex. **7.45**-3

Ex. **7.4**

Ex. **7.45**-3 & 4   Photographic magnification and comparison of the upper portions of the right and left breasts, as seen through a mammography viewer. Although the breasts are dense, all four building blocks of the normal fibroglandular tissue can be discerned. No contour change or other pathological abnormality can be seen.

Example 7.45

Ex. **7.45**-5 & 6 The images of the right and left breasts from the next screening examination are displayed in the same layout as in Ex. **7.45**-1 & 2. There is now a bulge in the contour in the upper portion of the left breast.

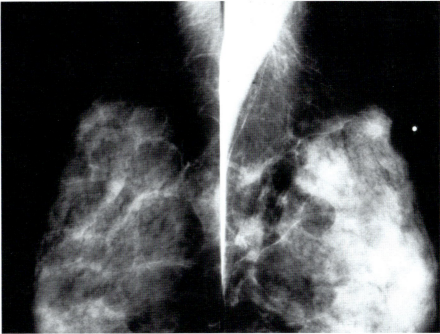

Ex. **7.45**-5   Ex. **7.45**-6

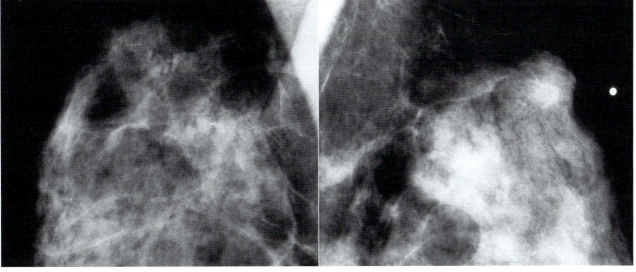

.45-7   Ex. **7.45**-8

Ex. **7.45**-7 & 8 Photographic magnification and comparison of the upper portions of the right and left breasts, as seen through a mammography viewer, show the lobulated, ill-defined bulge that gives the suspicion of malignancy on this mammogram.

Lesions Causing Parenchymal Contour Changes—Example 7.45

Ex. **7.45**-9 Microfocus magnification confirms that the bulge is caused by a spiculated, mammographically malignant tumor.

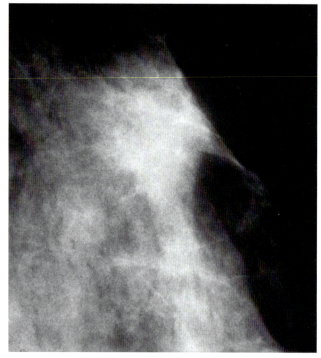

Ex. **7.45**-9

Ex. **7.45**-10 Low-power histological image of this 13 mm Grade 1 invasive cribriform carcinoma.

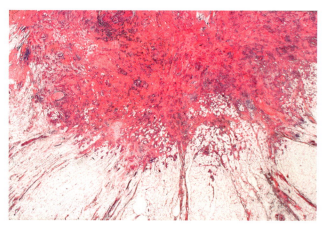

Ex. **7.45**-10

Ex. **7.45**-11 Higher-magnification histological image. Invasive cribriform carcinoma with a Grade 1 in-situ component.

Treatment: Segmentectomy and postoperative irradiation.

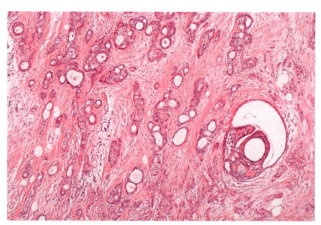

Ex. **7.45**-11

Chapter 8: Large-Section Histology of the Breast

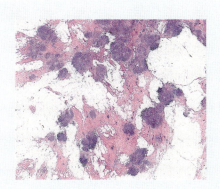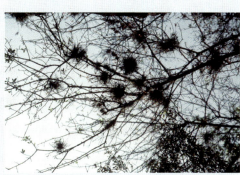

Introduction

Mammographic screening has shifted the spectrum of breast pathology away from mostly large tumors, easily seen and readily palpable, toward ever smaller and frequently noninvasive tumors. As larger and larger numbers of asymptomatic women undergo mammography screening at regular intervals, impalpable tumors are no longer the exception and are gradually becoming the rule.

This is a new era for all specialties involved in breast care. This challenging clinical environment affects the pathologist as well. Tissue sampling for microscopic analysis can no longer rely entirely upon the eyes and fingers of the pathologist. The traditional approach to handling breast specimens should be modified accordingly, and closer cooperation with the radiologist and surgeon is necessary.

Rationale for Large-Section Technique

It may appear as a paradox that the earlier the detection of breast cancer, the larger the contiguous tissue sample needed for its comprehensive histopathological characterization. Multiple factors, such as frequent multifocality even at an early stage and the desire for less radical surgery and better individualization of therapy, as well as the need for more detailed histological description of all mammographic findings, make the larger tissue sections a rational solution. Since the large-section technique has the advantage of preserving the original morphological relationship of the lesion(s) with the surrounding tissue in one plane, including the surgical margins, the pathologist is better able to document and communicate the findings. Important morphological features, such as tumor size, multifocality, intratumoral heterogeneity and the relationship of the pathological lesion with adjacent tissue can all be evaluated and demonstrated on a single slide. This is undoubtedly the most efficient way to correlate mammographic findings with histology.

■ Prerequisites

The pathologist needs the following information for the appropriate handling of the specimen:
- Mode of detection (nonpalpable, mammographically detected vs. clinically detected, palpable)
- Type, number, size, and extent of each mammographic abnormality
- Mass lesions, solitary or multiple microcalcifications
- Architectural distortion
- Radiologist's interpretation of the findings
- Ultrasound findings
- Results of any preoperative interventional procedures, such as fine-needle aspiration, large-core needle biopsy, or open surgical biopsy
- The specimen radiograph accompanied by the radiologist's interpretation
- Orientation of the specimen according to a mutually accepted marking system

Handling of the Specimen

Fig. **8.1**-1 & 2   The surgical specimen, marked by the surgeon with sutures to ensure proper orientation, arrives at pathology together with its accompanying specimen radiograph. The longer suture marks the superficial surface of the specimen, and the shorter suture marks the surface closest to the nipple.

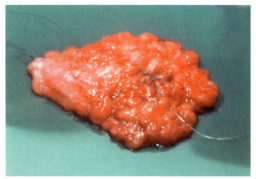

8.1-1

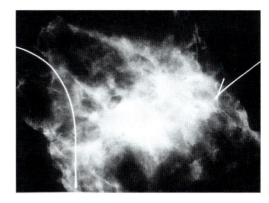

8.1-2

Fig. **8.2**   The specimen radiograph and the radiology report serve as a guide for slicing the specimen. Ideally, the specimen should be sliced when fresh, for more rapid and complete fixation of the entire tissue. Additionally, some special examination methods can only be performed on samples taken from fresh, unfixed tissue.

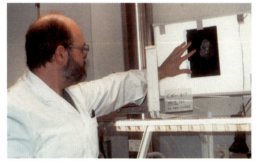

8.2

Fig. **8.3**-1 & 2   After orientation of the specimen, it is palpated and its dimensions are recorded.

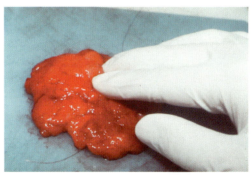

8.3-1

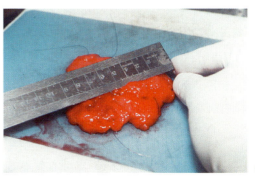

8.3-2

407

Handling of the Specimen

Fig. **8.4**-1 & 2   The surgical specimen is preferably sliced in the horizontal plane. This approach will best match the specimen radiograph, while also providing slices of largest surface area and maximum circumferential margin. If the specimen radiograph or palpation suggest the presence of more than one tumor in the specimen, an effort is made to slice in a plane that includes as many tumor foci as possible.

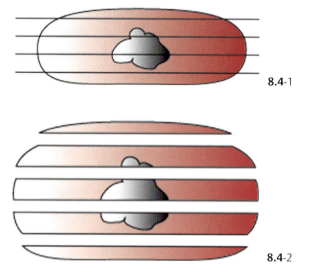

8.4-1

8.4-2

Fig. **8.5**-1   An extremely sharp, disposable knife is needed to produce slices of uniform, 3–5 mm thickness.

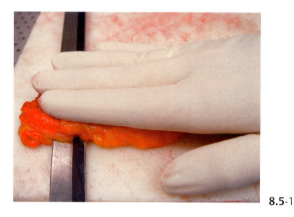

8.5-1

Fig. **8.5**-2   An even compression of the specimen can be provided by a protective, transparent plastic plate, especially when learning this technique.

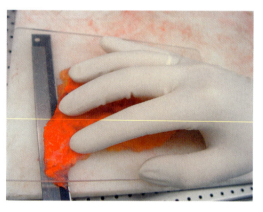

8.5-2

Fig. **8.5**-3   When slicing a mastectomy specimen, a different approach, the so-called "bread-loafing" technique should be used. The slices will then include both skin and pectoral fascia.

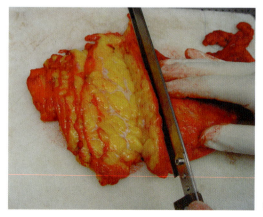

8.5-3

Fig. **8.5**-4   Serial slicing of the specimen into 3–5 mm thin slices provides an accurate, ordered display of all grossly detectable lesions within the specimen. A system for sequential numbering of the slices should be used to maintain their orientation. The slices are placed sequentially on transparent plastic films and sent for specimen radiography of the slices.

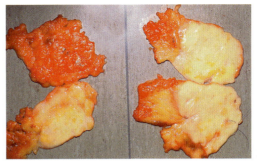

8.5-4

Fig. **8.6**-1   Specimen radiography can be done on any standard mammography unit using a low kilovoltage setting. The best results will be obtained using a specially designed specimen radiography unit. Fine-focus direct-magnification radiography at very low kilovoltage (14–17 kV using a tungsten target) will give the best results.

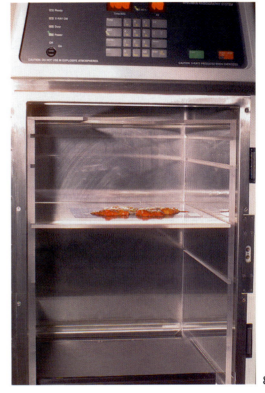

8.6-1

Fig. **8.6**-2   Radiography of these serial slices will produce images having much greater detail than radiographs of the intact specimen. These serial slice radiographs can better demonstrate additional tumor foci and can more precisely locate them for histopathological examination.

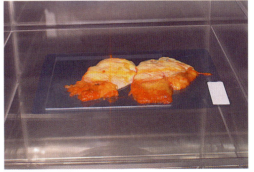

8.6-2

Fig. **8.6**-3   The radiologist marks the images containing mammographically detected abnormalities. These help the pathologist select the individual slices to be embedded in paraffin.

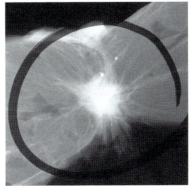

8.6-3

409

Handling of the Specimen

Inking of the entire surface of the specimen is no longer a necessity because the circumferential surgical margin can be reliably assessed both macroscopically and microscopically on the large sections.

To examine the superficial and deep surgical margins, the top and bottom slices can also be embedded for histological examination. The superficial and deep (top and bottom) slices can alternatively be sampled with small sections cut in the perpendicular plane.

The standard size large section measures 8 cm × 10 cm, which is large enough to include the entire cross section of most breast biopsy specimens. Slices from mastectomy specimens may need to be reduced in size by bisection into two adjoining slices.

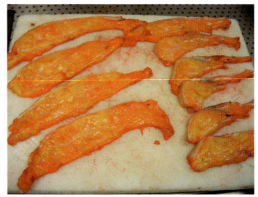

8.7-1

Fig. **8.7**-1 & 2   The cut surfaces of the slices should be carefully examined by the pathologist. As a rule, the slice with the largest tumor diameter is chosen for embedding in paraffin. In addition, slices containing other radiologically or macroscopically suspicious lesions are also selected. An average of two or three large sections is chosen from each specimen.

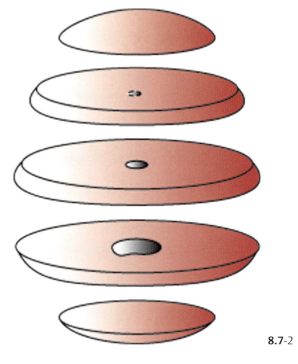

8.7-2

Fig. **8.8**   Inking can be used to mark the site of the sutures. This maintains orientation of the slices after the sutures are removed for further processing of the specimen.

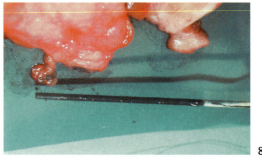

8.8

Fig. **8.9**   Fresh tissue material from macroscopically suspicious lesions can be sampled, frozen, and kept for special examinations.

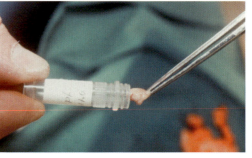

8.9

Fig. **8.10**-1 & 2 Selected slices are stretched over a cork or soft plastic board and fixed in buffered formalin. Fixation requires no more than 12 hours, which can be shortened to 30 minutes using microwave technology.

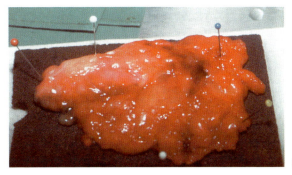

8.10-1

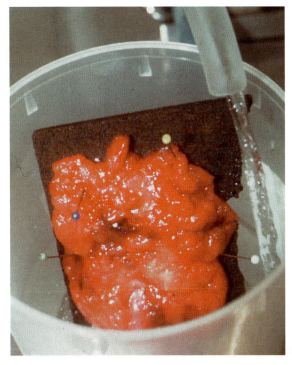

8.10-2

Fig. **8.11** Processing of the fixed tissue is essentially the same as for small tissue samples, and can be carried out in an automatic processor.

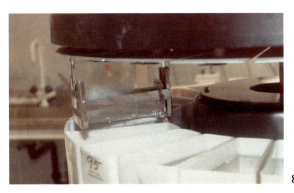

8.11

Fig. **8.12** A comparison between a large and a small paraffin block. Standard size large blocks measuring 8 cm × 10 cm may contain a tissue surface area 20 times larger than the surface area of the standard 2 cm × 2 cm sections.

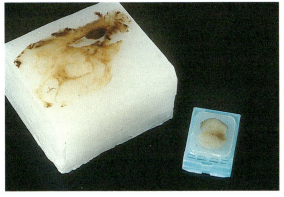

8.12

Cutting with the Macrotome

Fig. **8.13**-1 to 4   Although the macrotome is fully automated, special skill and training are needed for the technicians to produce the uniformly thin (3–4 μm) slices.

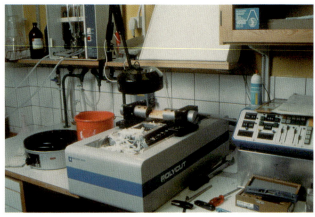

8.13-

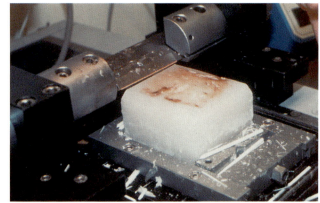

8.13-

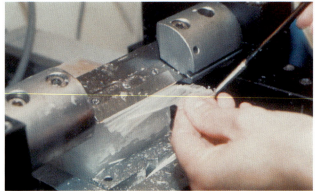

8.13-

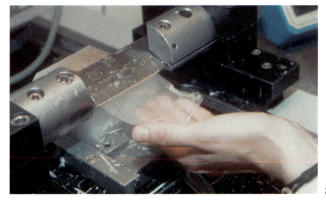

8.13-

Handling and Staining the Sections

Fig. **8.14**-1 to 3   The thin sections of paraffin-embedded tissue, initially wrinkled, are evenly smoothed out in cold and warm water baths, then caught on a glass slide.

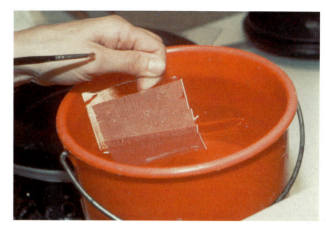

8.14-1

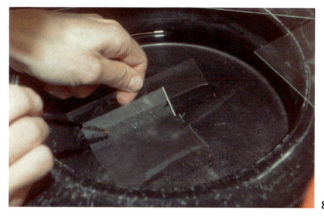

8.14-2

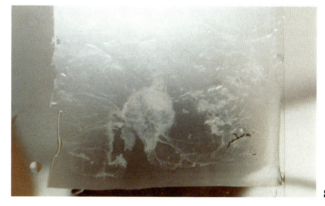

8.14-3

Fig. **8.15**   Following deparaffinization, the sections are stained in an automated stainer. After mounting, these large slides can easily be viewed on any standard microscope.

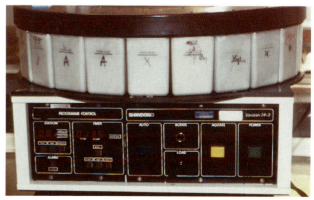

8.15

413

The Final Product: The Large-Section Slide

These slides provide the same quality of cellular detail as do smaller slides.

Fig. **8.16**-1   Large-section histology slide of a Grade 1 invasive ductal carcinoma (H&E).

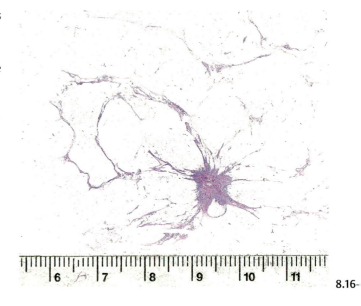

8.16-

Fig. **8.16**-2   High-power magnification of the invasive component of the tumor shown in **8.16**-1.

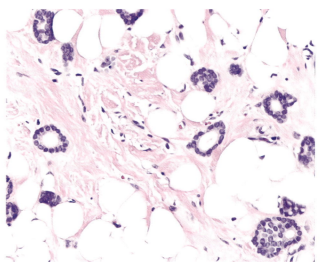

8.16-

Fig. **8.16**-3   High-power magnification of the in-situ component of the same tumor.

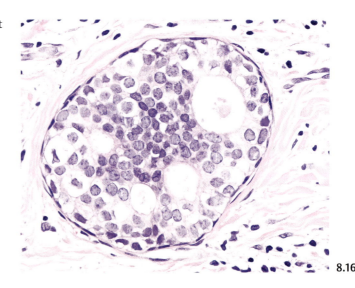

8.16-

The large-section histology technique also allows the use of special staining methods to more fully demonstrate tumor characteristics and alterations in adjacent normal tissue.

Fig. **8.17**-1 & 2 Hematoxylin–eosin stain, large-section slide and detail at medium-power magnification.

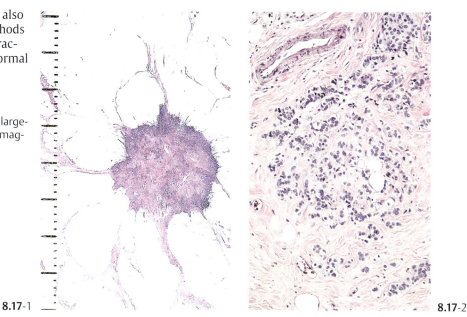

8.17-1

8.17-2

Fig. **8.17**-3 & 4 Same case, corresponding slices stained for collagen (sirius red).

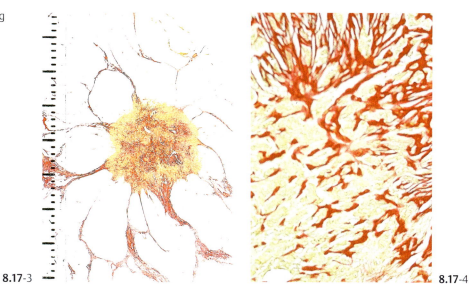

8.17-3

8.17-4

Fig. **8.17**-5 & 6 Same case, corresponding slices stained for elastic fibers (orcein stain).

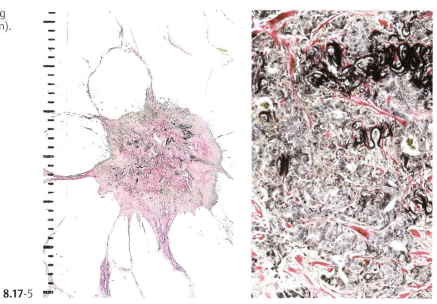

8.17-5

8.17-6

415

The Final Product: The Large-Section Slide

When viewing many small tissue pieces sampled from the operative specimen, the pathologist needs to reconstruct the operative specimen as a kind of patchwork quilt, in which the spatial relationships of the various tissue fragments may be imperfectly reconstructed. The large-section technique eliminates this unnecessary fragmentation and reconstruction of a once intact specimen.

In comparison to standard, small-block histology, the advantages of using large sections can be summarized as follows:

- Documentation of tumor size (Fig. **8.18**)
- Documentation of tumor multifocality (Fig. **8.19**)
- More accurate documentation of the extent of the disease (Fig. **8.20**)
- Documentation of intratumoral and intertumoral heterogeneity (Figs. **8.21** and **8.22**)
- More complete assessment of the surrounding tissue (Figs. **8.23** to **8.25**)
- More accurate assessment of reexcision specimens (Fig. **8.26**)

Documentation of tumor size. Taken in the plane of the largest tumor diameter, large-section slides provide a lasting documentation of the tumor size.

Documentation of tumor multifocality through inclusion of the dominant tumor mass as well as additional tumor foci in the same section is invaluable for interdisciplinary communication.

Fig. **8.18**   The full size of any tumor up to 8 cm × 10 cm, including its surroundings, is clearly demonstrated, fully documented, and available for review at any time.

Fig. **8.19**   Multiple invasive tumor foci are demonstrated, showing their relationship to and their distance from each other and from the surgical margin.

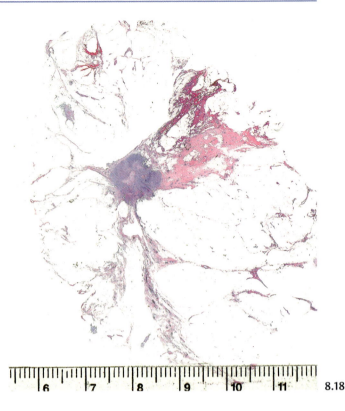

8.18

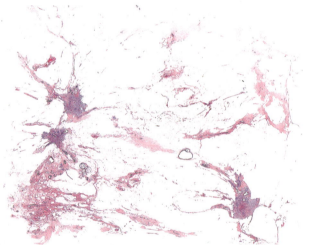

8.19

More accurate documentation of the extent of the disease. Large sections contain both the main tumor and a larger portion of the surrounding tissue, possibly containing additional foci, thus enabling more accurate assessment of the extent of the disease.

Fig. **8.20** shows an invasive breast cancer with a 90 mm × 40 mm in-situ component which required two contiguous large sections (joined at the red line) to demonstrate the full extent of the disease. More than 40 small tissue blocks would be required to cover the same area. The green marks indicate the extent of the tumor.

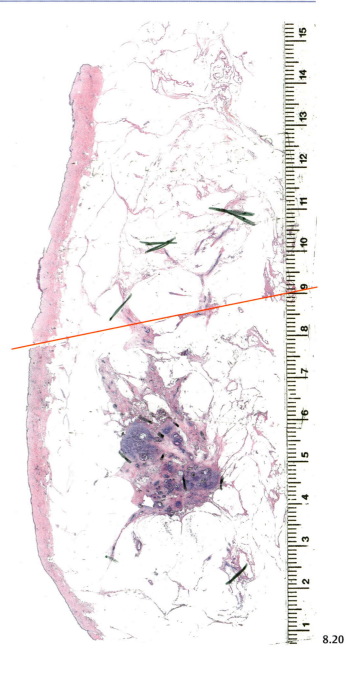

8.20

Documentation of intratumoral and intertumoral heterogeneity is more precise using large sections. Accurate demonstration of the different tumor types and their spatial relationship in multifocal tumors, as well as demonstration of the different tumor cell clones within the same tumor have important therapeutic implications.

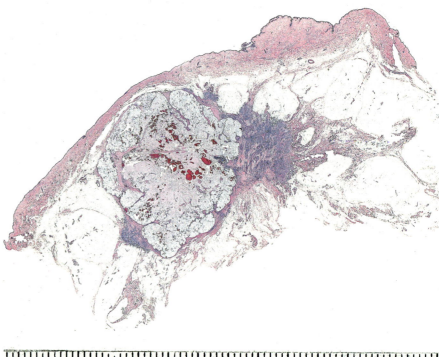

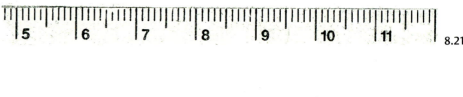

Fig. **8.21** Invasive ductal carcinoma immediately adjacent to a large mucinous carcinoma. Notice the thinning of the skin overlying the mucinous component.

8.21

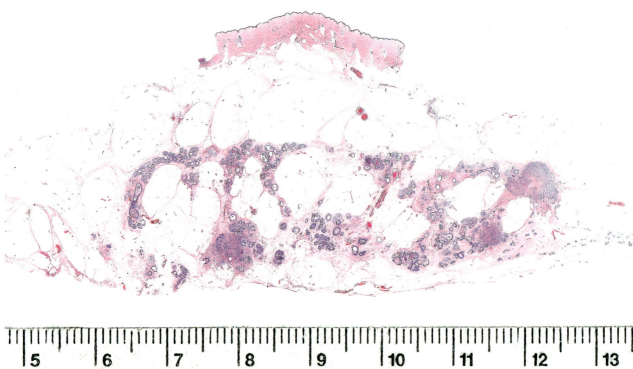

8.22

Fig. **8.22** Multiple small foci of invasive ductal carcinoma associated with extensive in-situ carcinoma spreading over an area larger than 6.0 cm in the largest dimension.

More complete assessment of the surrounding tissue. Histological evaluation of the tissue surrounding the tumor is essential to demonstrate or rule out the presence of additional tumor foci. The large-section technique, providing a larger contiguous area for review, enables the pathologist to detect changes in the surrounding tissue, such as vascular invasion, pectoral muscle or skin involvement, etc., with greater speed and higher accuracy (Figs. **8.23** to **8.25**).

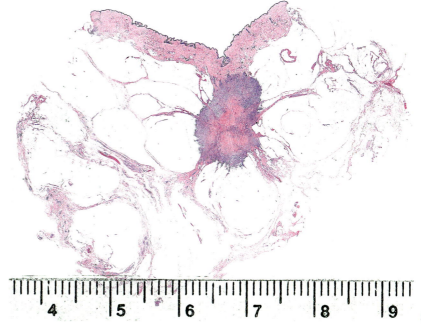

Fig. **8.23** Invasive ductal carcinoma of the breast invading the dermis and causing dimpling of the skin.

Fig. **8.24** Medullary carcinoma invading the pectoralis muscle.

Fig. **8.25** Extensive peritumoral fibrosis may give the false impression of a larger tumor diameter when only small slides are examined.

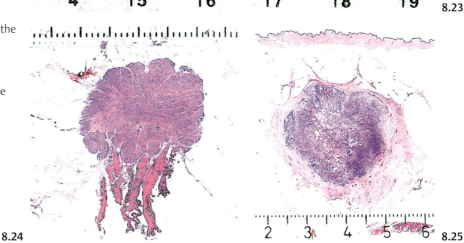

More accurate assessment of reexcision specimens. Evaluation of reexcision specimens is complicated by the healing process, which may obscure small tumor foci, making sampling unreliable and haphazard. Large-section technique provides more comprehensive sampling and improved diagnostic accuracy.

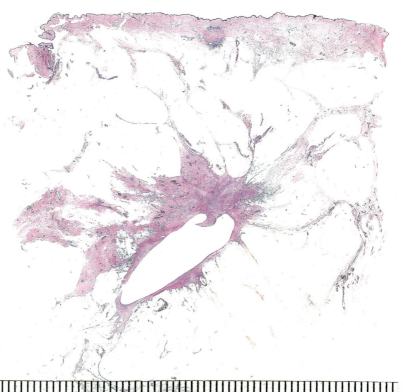

Fig. **8.26** Reexcision specimen.

Subgross, Thick-Section Histology Technique

A large, contiguous tissue sample embedded in paraffin makes an ideal source for preparing 800–1000 μm tissue slices. Following deparaffinization, clarification, and staining, the samples can be viewed with a low-power stereoscopic microscope. The major value of this technique is to bridge the gap between the low-resolution mammographic image and the high-resolution histopathology image. Viewing the breast tissue through a stereoscopic microscope provides three-dimensional visualization of normal and pathological breast structures, and is an effective teaching and communication tool for all physicians dealing with breast diseases.

■ Steps of the Technique

Fig. **8.27**-1 & 2   The paraffin block is melted overnight at 60 °C.

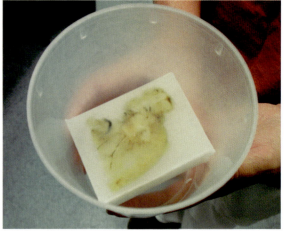

8.27-1

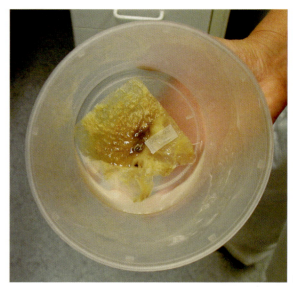

8.27-2

Fig. **8.27**-3   The tissue slice still contains some paraffin, becoming rigid at room temperature.

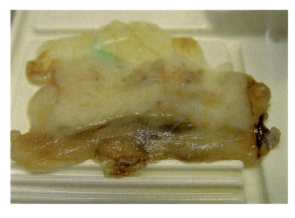

8.27-3

Fig. **8.27**-4 to 6   Using a small, sharp knife, the tissue sample is carved to a thickness of approximately 1 mm.

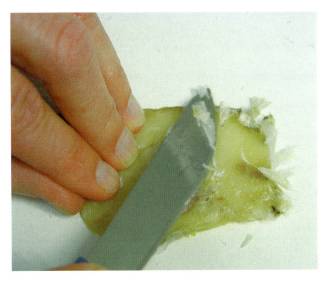

8.27-4

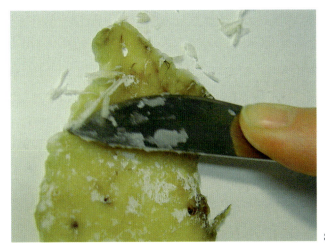

8.27-5

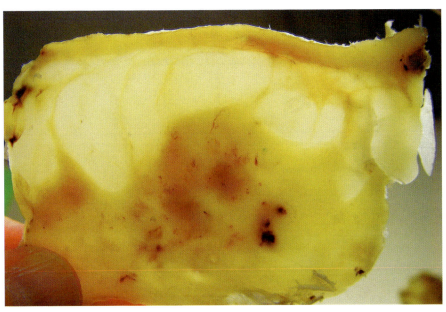

8.27-6

Fig. **8.27**-7   Deparaffinization with xylene requires several successive baths over a period of 24 hours. After rehydration in a series of alcohol baths, the slice is left overnight in a water bath.

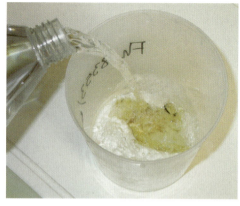

8.27-7

Fig. **8.27**-8 & 9   Staining with Harris hematoxylin. The finished sample is stored and examined immersed in methyl salicylate. If necessary, the thick-section tissue sample can be reembedded in paraffin for the production of further thin sections without damage to the cellular details.

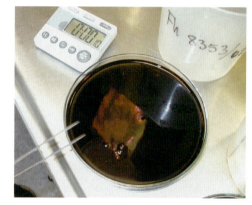

8.27-8

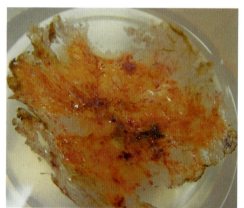

8.27-9

Fig. **8.28**   Viewing with a low-power stereoscopic microscope.

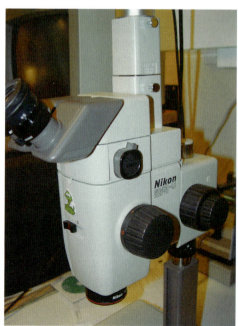

8.28

Examples of Subgross Thick-Section Histopathology Images of Breast Tissue

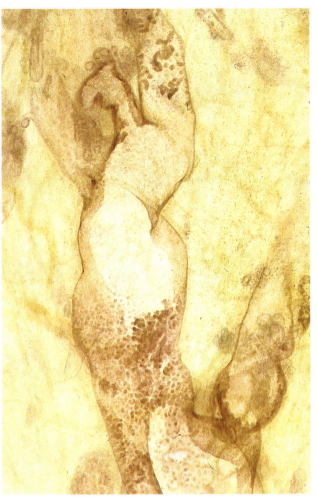

8.29

Fig. **8.29**   Distended ducts with mucin-producing micropapillary carcinoma in situ.

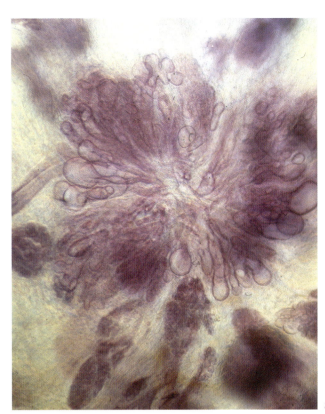

8.30

Fig. **8.30**   Radial scar.

Examples of Subgross Thick-Section Histopathology Images

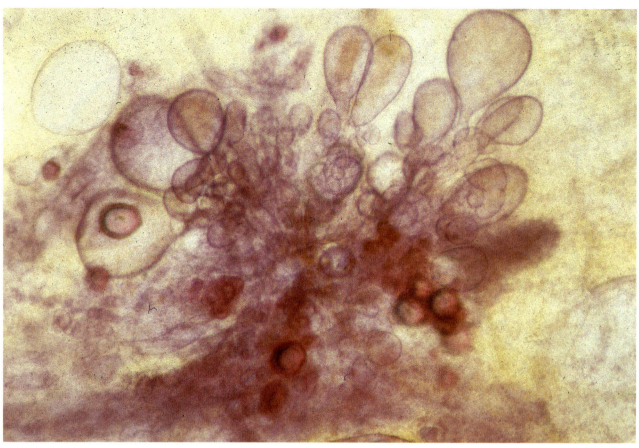

8.31-1

Fig. **8.31**-1   Microcystic dilatation of the acini.

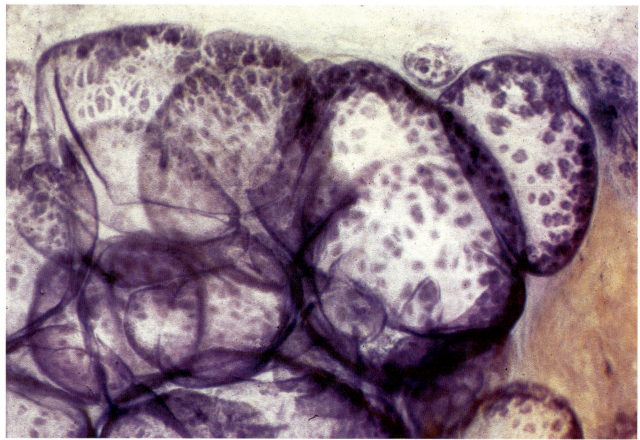

8.31-2

Fig. **8.31**-2   Typical thick-section appearance of apocrine metaplasia.

Case Demonstrations

Example 8.1

This 57-year-old asymptomatic woman was called back from screening for work-up of right retroareolar calcifications. At physical examination there was eczema of the right nipple, raising the clinical suspicion of Paget's disease.

Preoperative punch biopsy confirmed the diagnosis of Paget's disease.

Ex. **8.1**-1 & 2   Screening mammograms, details of the mediolateral oblique and craniocaudal projections.

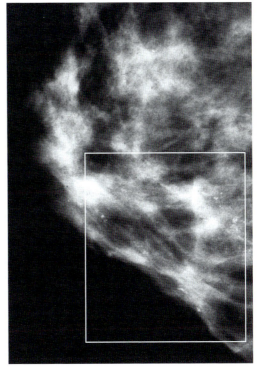

Ex. **8.1**-1

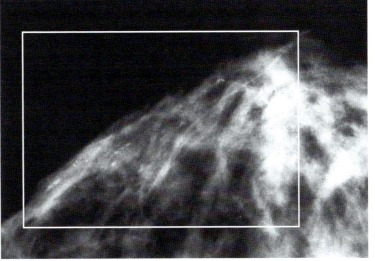

Ex. **8.1**-2

Ex. **8.1**-3   Microfocus magnification mammography shows a slightly retracted nipple and retroareolar malignant-type calcifications.

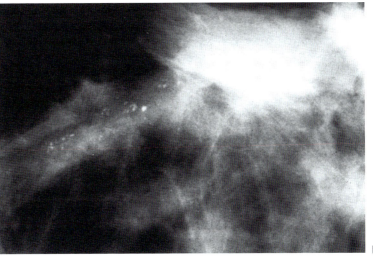

Ex. **8.1**-3

425

Ex. **8.1**-4   Specimen radiography of this large, 5 mm-thick tissue slice shows the thickened areola and dilated retroareolar ducts containing a few calcifications.

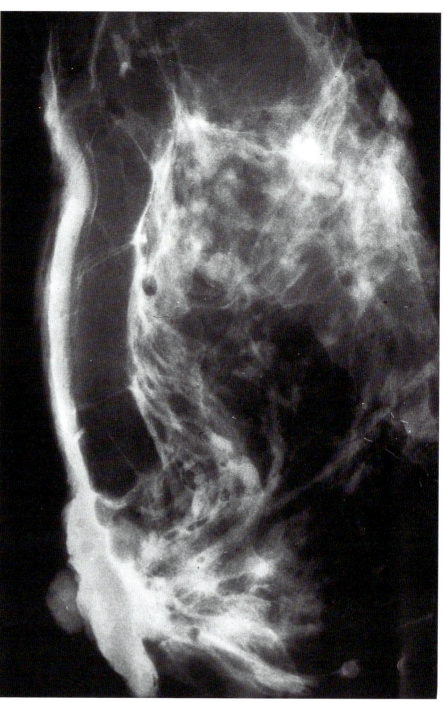

Ex. **8.1**-

Ex. **8.1**-5 & 6   Specimen radiogram and subgross, thick-section histology of the nipple and the immediate retroareolar area. Intramammillary invasive carcinoma.

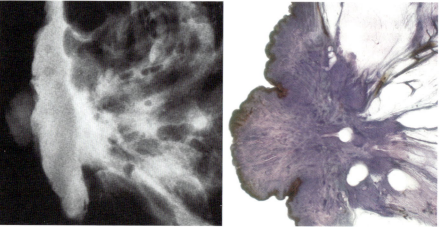

Ex. **8.1**-5

Ex. **8.1**-

Ex. **8.1**-7 Large-section histology: a 15 mm Grade 2 invasive ductal carcinoma is within and behind the nipple with associated Grade 3 DCIS and Paget's disease.

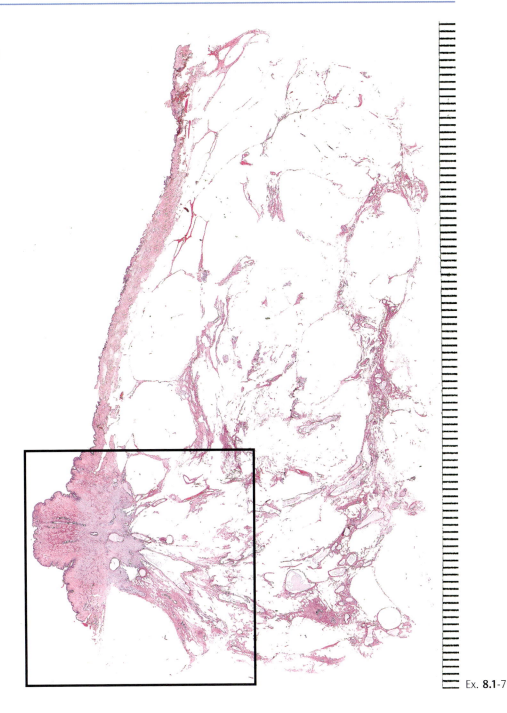

Ex. **8.1**-7

Ex. **8.1**-8 High-power microscopic magnification image histology: Grade 2 invasive ductal carcinoma.

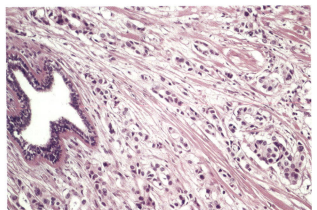

Ex. **8.1**-8

Case Demonstrations—Example 8.1

Ex. **8.1**-9 to 11 Specimen radiograph with correlative large-section histology and subgross, thick-section histology of a tissue slide adjacent to the nipple, showing a large number of retroareolar and distant DCIS foci on an area measuring 60 mm × 30 mm.

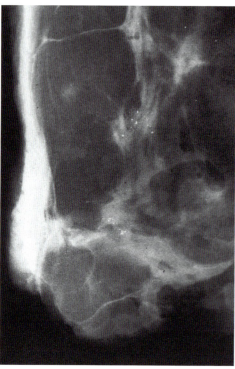

Ex. **8.1**-9

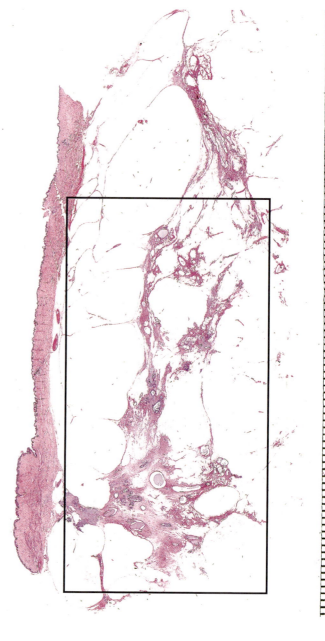

Ex. **8.1**

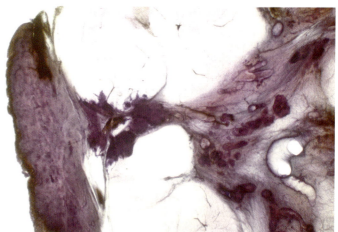

Ex. **8.1**

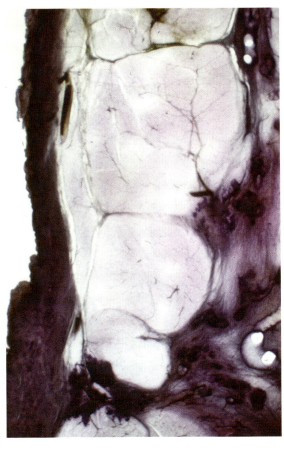

Ex. **8.1**-12

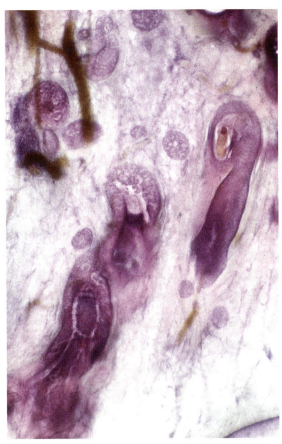

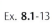

Ex. **8.1**-13

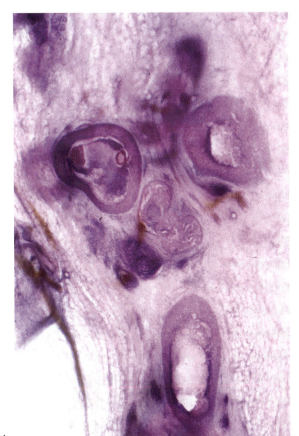

Ex. **8.1**-14

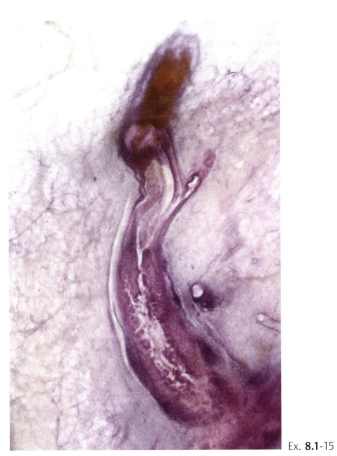

Ex. **8.1**-15

Ex. **8.1**-12 to 15   Subgross, thick-section histology demonstrating distended, tumor-filled ducts (DCIS).

Ex. **8.1**-16 & 17   Additional specimen radiograph and corresponding subgross, thick-section histology. The clusters of calcifications mark the area with Grade 3 DCIS.

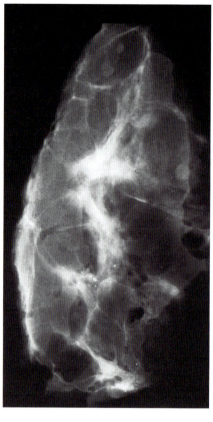

Ex. **8.1**-16

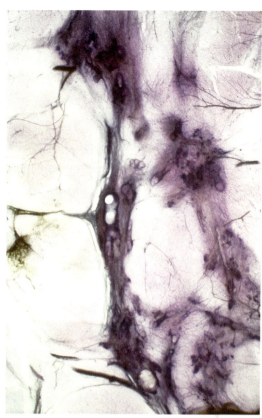

Ex. **8.1**

Ex. **8.1**-18 to 22   High-power histology images showing solid cell proliferation with necrosis and calcifications.

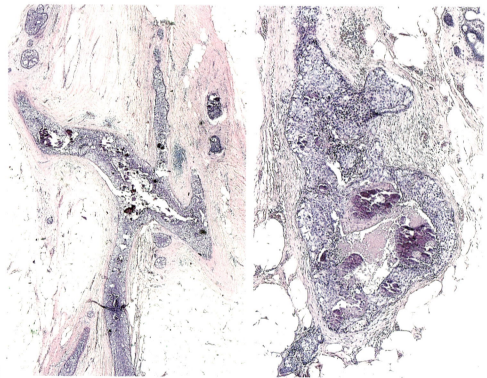

Ex. **8.1**-18

Ex. **8.1**

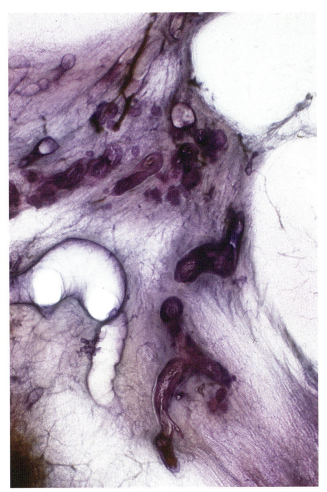

Ex. **8.1**-20

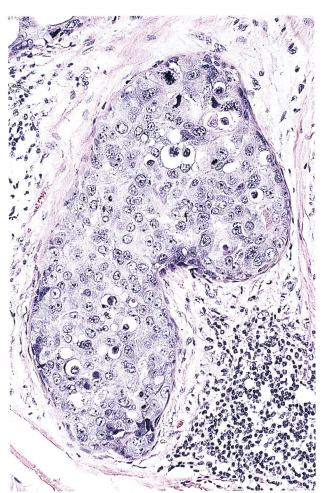

Ex. **8.1**-21

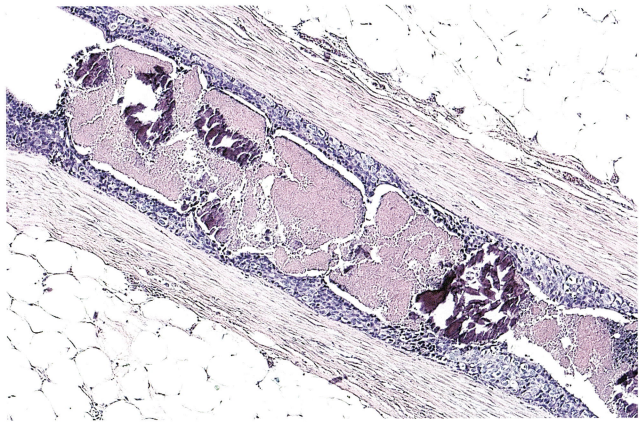

Ex. **8.1**-22

Example 8.2

An 88-year-old woman with left serous nipple discharge, but no palpable tumor.

Ex. **8.2**-1   Neither tumor mass nor calcifications are seen on the mammogram.

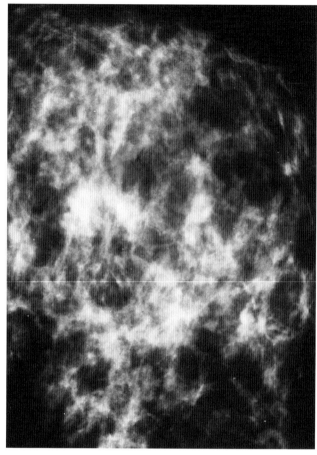

Ex. **8.2**

Ex. **8.2**-2 Galactography reveals dilated ducts branching throughout the medial half of the breast. The ducts are irregularly dilated, giving the impression of rosary beads.

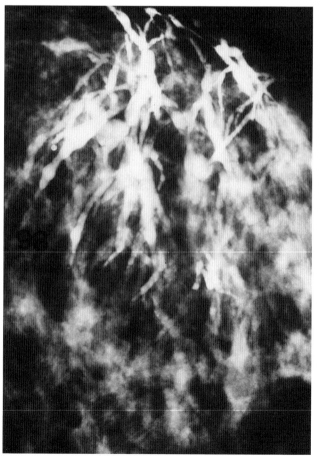

Ex. **8.2**

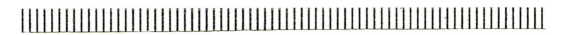

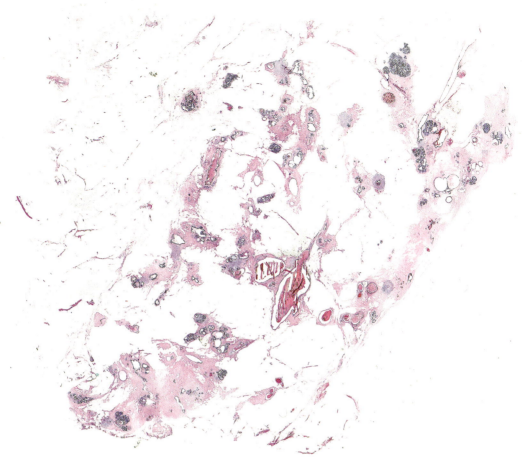

Ex. **8.2**-3

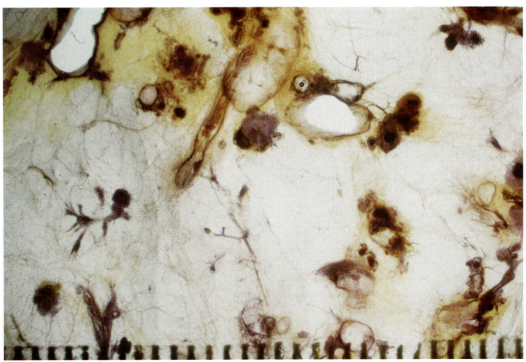

Ex. **8.2**-4

Ex. **8.2**-3   Large-section histology and subgross, thick-section histology show more than 25 tiny, 2–3 mm foci of invasive lobular carcinoma, some of which are interconnected by dilated ducts filled with micropapillary carcinoma in situ (Ex. **8.2**-4).

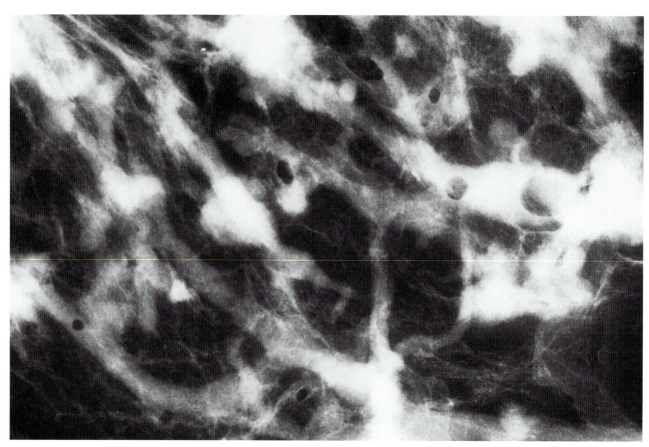

Ex. **8.2**

Ex. **8.2**-5 Radiograph of a 5 mm slice from the operative specimen. Numerous dilated ducts and several small, ill-defined tumor densities are seen.

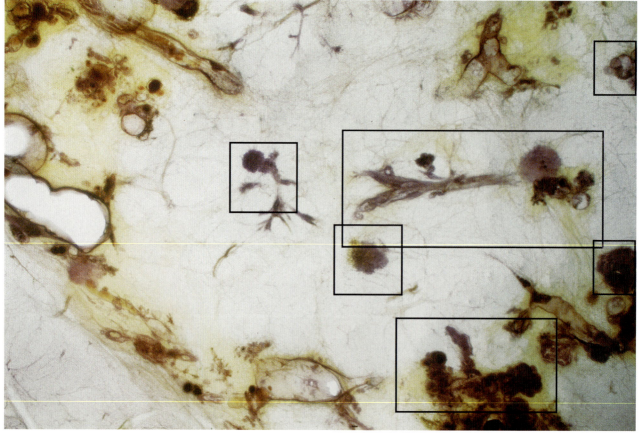

Ex. **8.2**

Ex. **8.2**-6 Subgross, thick-section histology: several tumor foci can be identified on this 1-mm-thick tissue slice.

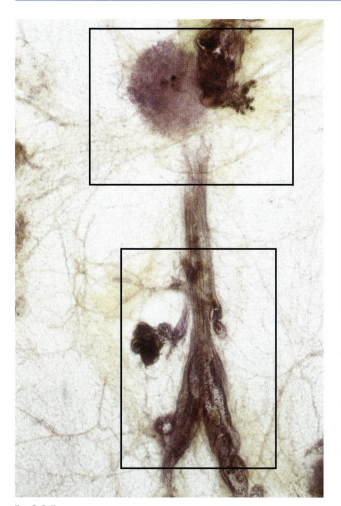

Ex. **8.2**-7

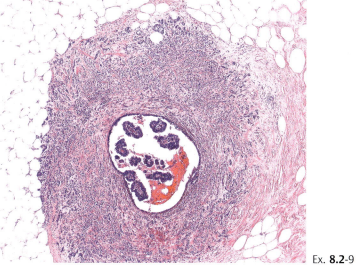

Ex. **8.2**-8

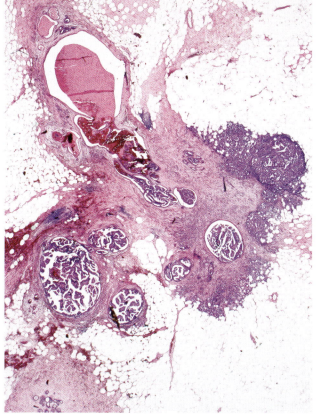

Ex. **8.2**-11

Ex. **8.2**-9

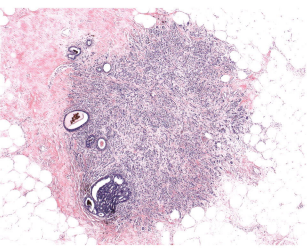

Ex. **8.2**-10

Ex. **8.2**-7 to 11   The subgross histology image is an enlargement of the area outlined by the largest rectangle in Ex. **8.2**-6. The upper rectangle in Ex. **8.2**-7 contains a small focus of invasive lobular carcinoma. The corresponding histology is seen in Ex. **8.2**-8 to **8.2**-10. The lower rectangle in Ex. **8.2**-7 contains micropapillary carcinoma in situ. The corresponding histology is shown in Ex. **8.2**-11.

435

Example 8.3

An asymptomatic 49-year-old woman called back from screening.

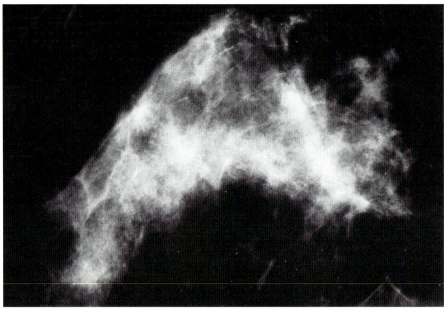

Ex. **8.**

Ex. **8.3**-1 to 3   Mammography of the left breast shows multiple stellate lesions with interconnecting bridges, some of which contain calcifications suspicious for malignancy. The corresponding specimen radiograph and large-section histology demonstrate the multiple foci of invasive carcinoma, which are interconnected by bridges containing DCIS.

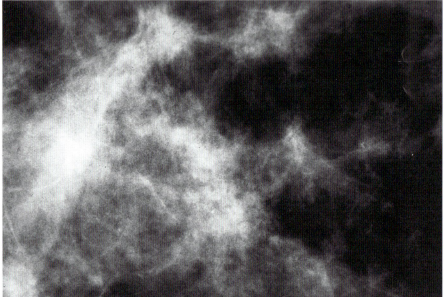

Ex. **8.3**

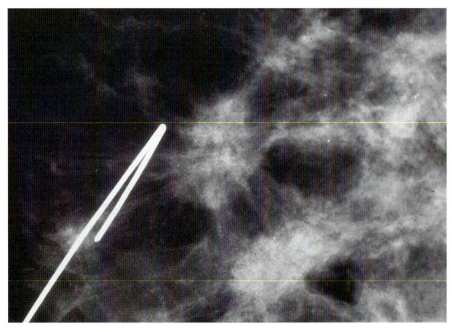

Ex. **8.3-4** to 7   High-power images of the areas marked with rectangles show that the stellate lesions are tubular carcinomas measuring up to 1 cm in diameter. The in-situ components are low-grade micropapillary DCIS.

Ex. **8.3**

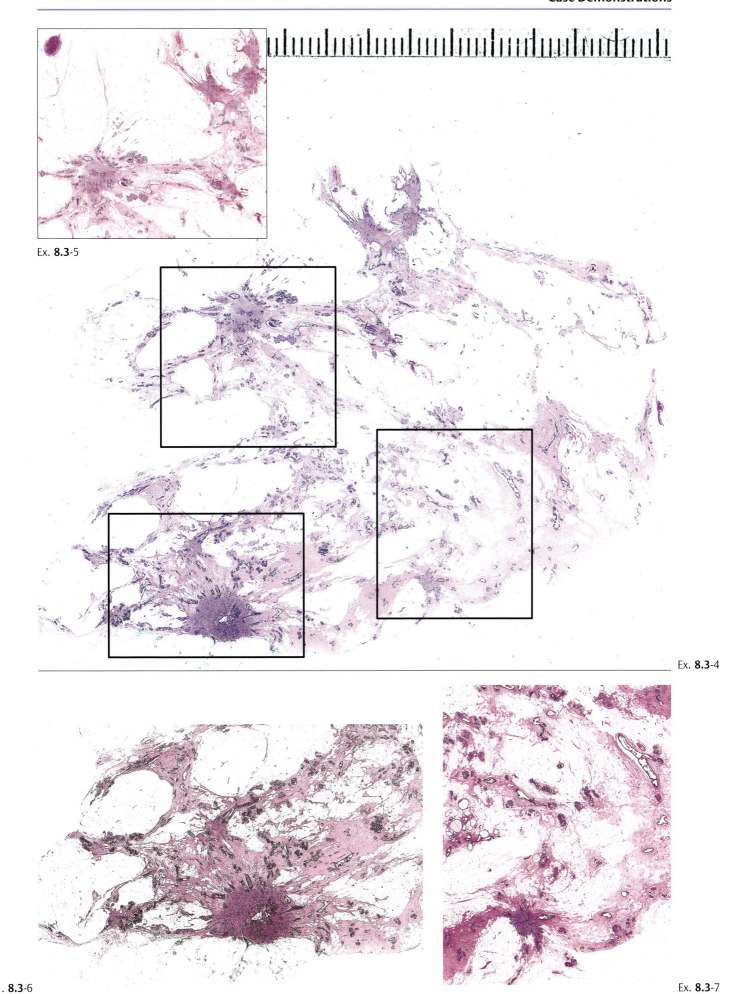

Ex. **8.3**-5

Ex. **8.3**-4

. **8.3**-6

Ex. **8.3**-7

Conclusions

The radiologist needs continuous, accurate feedback from the pathologist in order to develop her or his diagnostic skills. Without a specimen radiograph there may be no assurance that the findings described on the pathology report correspond to the preoperative mammographic findings, especially microcalcifications. Even when a radiograph of the intact surgical specimen is available, it may be difficult to correlate this image with the histological finding, especially when only small tissue samples have been taken. When the surgical specimen is serially sliced as described above, and all the slices are radiographed, the images can be directly compared with the large sections taken from the same slice that has been embedded in paraffin. A single histological large section includes the tumor(s) together with the tumor environment and the surgical margins in one plane at the same time, giving a nonfragmented image of the whole disease. Stereomicroscopic examination of specially processed thick large sections provide additional three-dimensional information about the spatial relationship of the detected lesions and the normal tissue. Both the two-dimensional and three-dimensional large sections can be directly correlated to the specimen radiographs and to the mammograms, enabling the diagnostic team to analyze, discuss, and document all the morphological findings relevant to treatment and patient care.

Chapter 9: Mammography Positioning Technique

Mediolateral Oblique Projection (MLO)
Craniocaudal Projection (CC)
Lateromedial Horizontal-Beam Projection (LM)
Cleavage View (CV)

László Tabár, Ward Parsons, Barbro Vedin, Ann Petersen

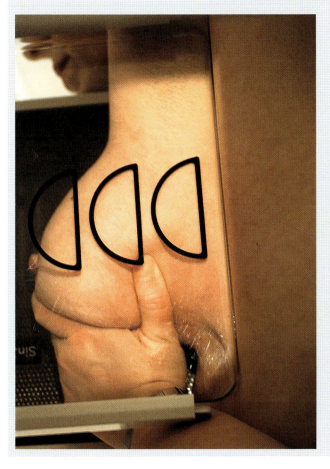
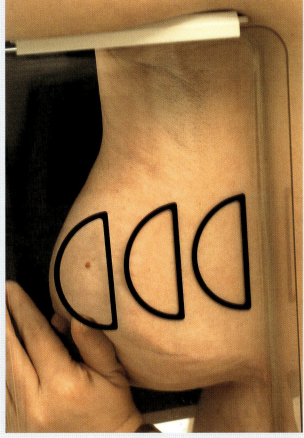

■ Table of Contents

Mediolateral Oblique Projection (MLO) 441
Aim 441
Prerequisites for Successful Positioning 442
Steps of Positioning 445
Summary of Events for Mediolateral Oblique Positioning 450
Summary of Sequence of Events for MLO Positioning of the Right Breast 454

Craniocaudal Projection (CC) 455
Aim 455
Prerequisites for Successful Positioning 456
Steps of Positioning 457
Summary of Events for Craniocaudal Positioning 460

Lateromedial Horizontal-Beam Projection (LM) 462
Aim 462
Prerequisites for Successful Positioning 463
Steps of Positioning 464
The Position Sequence with Compression Plate 465

Cleavage View (CV) 466
Aim 466

The aims of proper positioning for the MLO projection are:

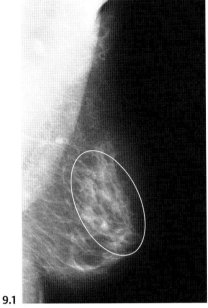

9.1

Complete visualization of breast parenchyma and the axillary nodes.

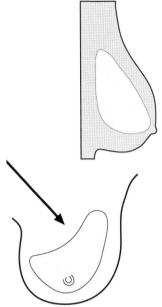

9.2

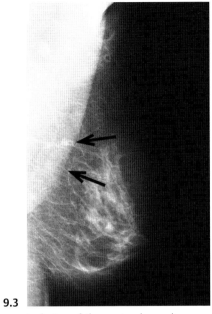

9.3

Inclusion of the pectoral muscle preferably to the level of the nipple.

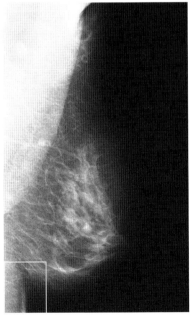

9.4

Visualization of the inframammary fold and upper abdominal subcutaneous tissue.

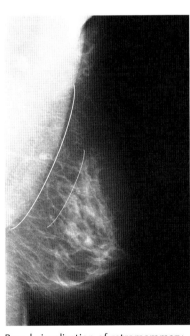

9.5

Broad visualization of retromammary fat.

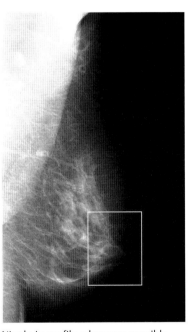

9.6

Nipple in profile whenever possible.

Mediolateral Oblique Projection (MLO)

The patient should face the mammographic unit, then turn her body away from the breast to be imaged so that her feet are approximately 45° to the chest wall edge of the cassette table.

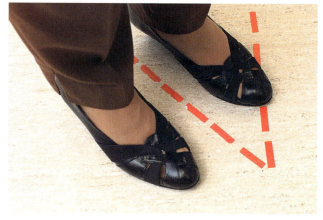

9.7

The tube angle will be unique for each patient, varying from 45° to 75°, most often about 60°.

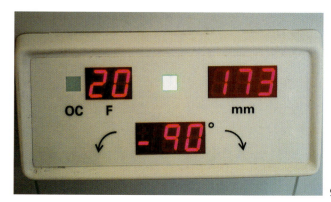

9.8

The chest wall edge of the cassette table must be parallel to the patient's pectoral muscle when the upper arm is horizontal and the shoulders are at the same level.

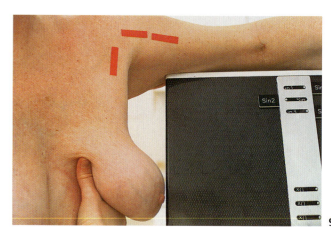

9.9

Mediolateral Oblique Projection (MLO)

The upper edge of the cassette table should be at the level of the humerus, keeping the shoulders at the same height.

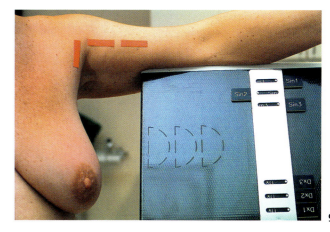

9.10

Incorrect: The shoulders are not at the same level and the cassette table is too low.

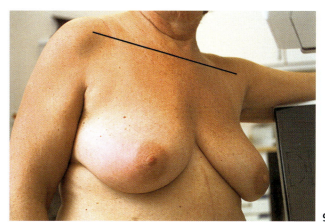

9.11

Incorrect: The shoulders are not at the same level and the cassette table is too high.

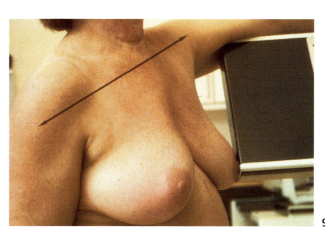

9.12

Incorrect: Although the shoulders are at the same level, the cassette table is too low.

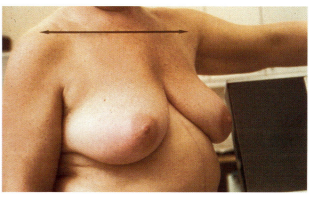

9.13

Mediolateral Oblique Projection (MLO)

The patient's hand should hold on to the lower part of the support bar. Marking it with red tape will be helpful.

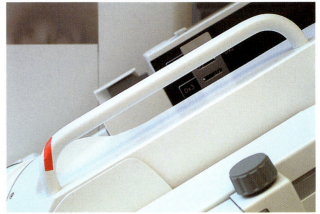

9.14

The technologist shows the patient where to place her hand.

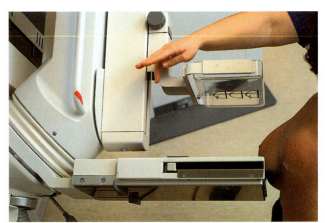

9.15

The technologist stands on the side opposite to the breast being examined. She should not allow the patient to pull herself into contact with the cassette.

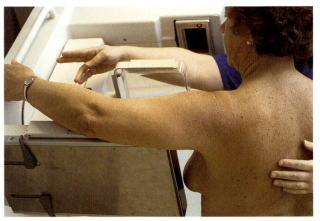

9.16

The patient's hand is now holding on to the lower part of the support bar.

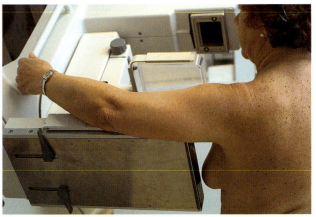

After proper preparation, the steps of positioning will follow a natural sequence, resulting in ideal images, using less effort.

9.17

Mediolateral Oblique Projection (MLO)

The technologist's flattened palm is placed vertically against the upper abdomen just below the breast.

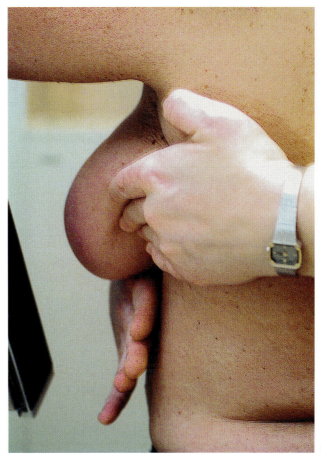

9.18

The other hand reaches around the back to assist in preparing as much soft tissue as possible for imaging.

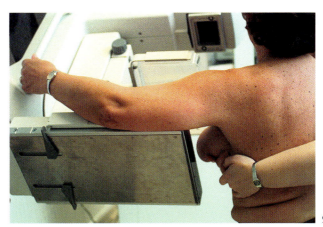

9.19

The fingers under the breast then slide upward in order to take hold of the breast from below. This maneuver
- elevates the breast;
- spreads the breast parenchyma;
- pulls the pectoral muscle away from the chest wall.

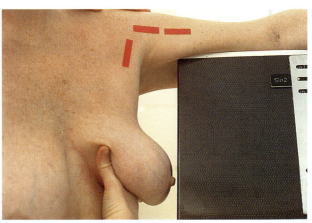

9.20

Anterior view

Posterior view

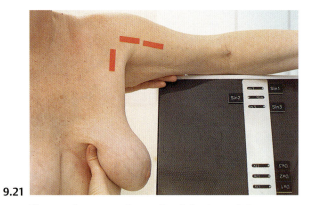

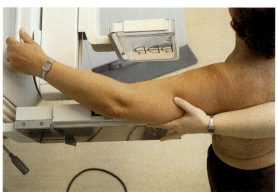

9.21   9.22

The gap between the patient's body and the cassette table is decreased by moving her directly toward the cassette table until complete contact is attained.

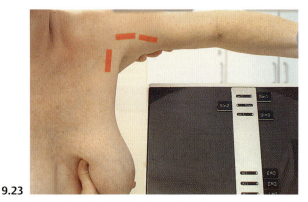

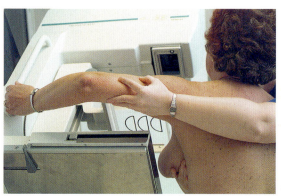

9.23   9.24

The technologist lifts the patient's upper arm and rotates it internally, then slightly rotates and flexes the patient's upper body forward, using body contact (bottom pair of pictures). This motion is designed to maximize visualization of the soft tissues of the axilla, the axillary tail, and the posterolateral chest wall attachment of the breast.

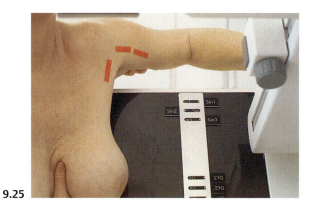

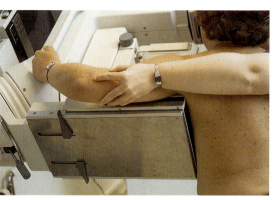

9.25   9.26

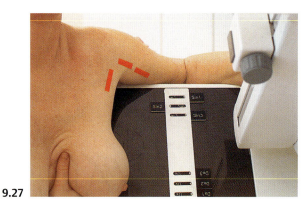

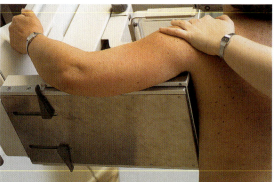

9.27   9.28

The hand on the upper arm moves to the top of the shoulder, guiding it downward and relaxing it.

Mediolateral Oblique Projection (MLO)

The fingers maintain contact with the distal clavicle to protect it from the corner of the compression plate. The technologist's other hand supports the breast over the table.

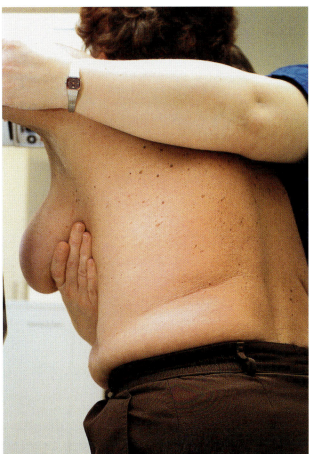

9.30

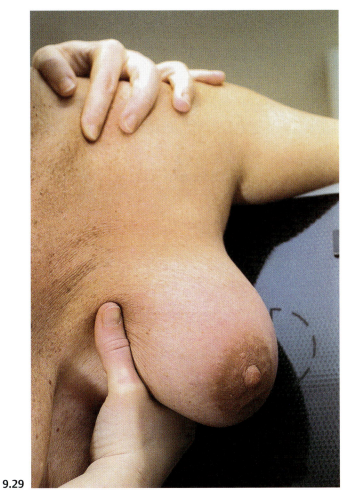

9.29

Overview of the positioning process before compression.

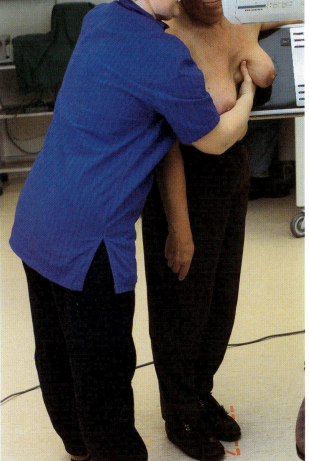

9.31

Steps of Positioning

Mediolateral Oblique Projection (MLO)

The hand supporting the breast over the cassette table lifts and pulls the breast forward and upward, using a rotational movement, spreading out the breast tissue evenly. This motion is designed to simultaneously bring the inframammary fold and a portion of the upper abdominal superficial soft tissue into the imaging field.

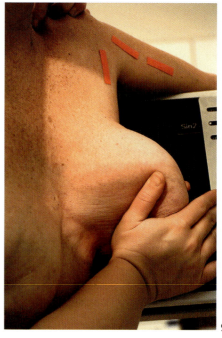

9.32

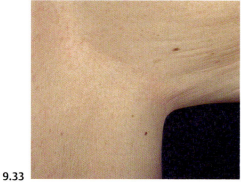

9.33

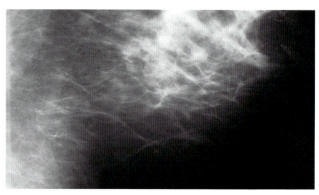

9.34

The inframammary fold and the upper portion of the abdominal subcutaneous tissue.

Finally, the patient is rotated slightly toward the mammography unit and compression is applied.

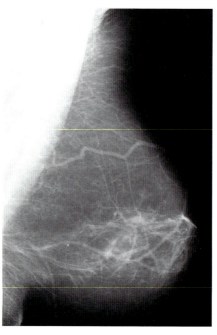

9.35

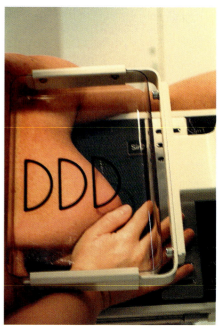

9.36

Mediolateral Oblique Projection (MLO)

A properly positioned mammogram in the MLO projection. Upper portion of the left and right mammograms in the MLO projections. A number of axillary lymph nodes are visualized overlying the pectoral muscle.

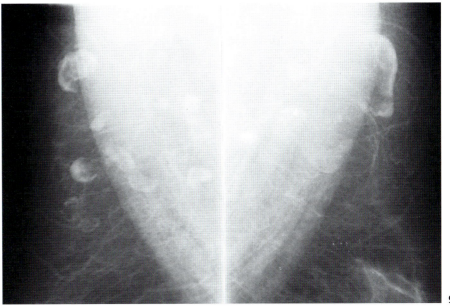

9.37

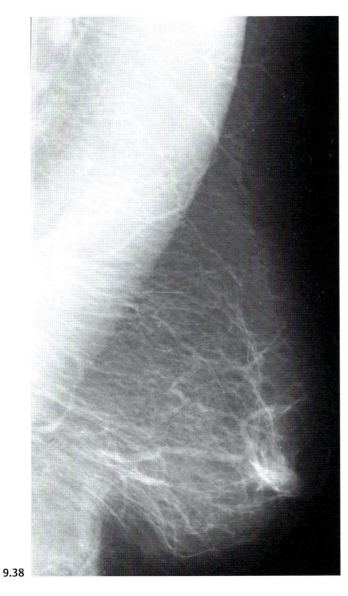

9.38

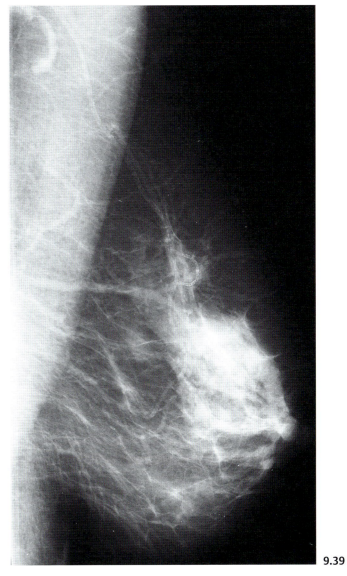

9.39

A properly positioned mammogram in the MLO projection shows the entire breast parenchyma, axillary nodes, and the pectoral muscle with a convex contour reaching to the level of the nipple, which is in profile, and the inframammary fold with the upper portion of the abdomen.

449

Mediolateral Oblique Projection (MLO)

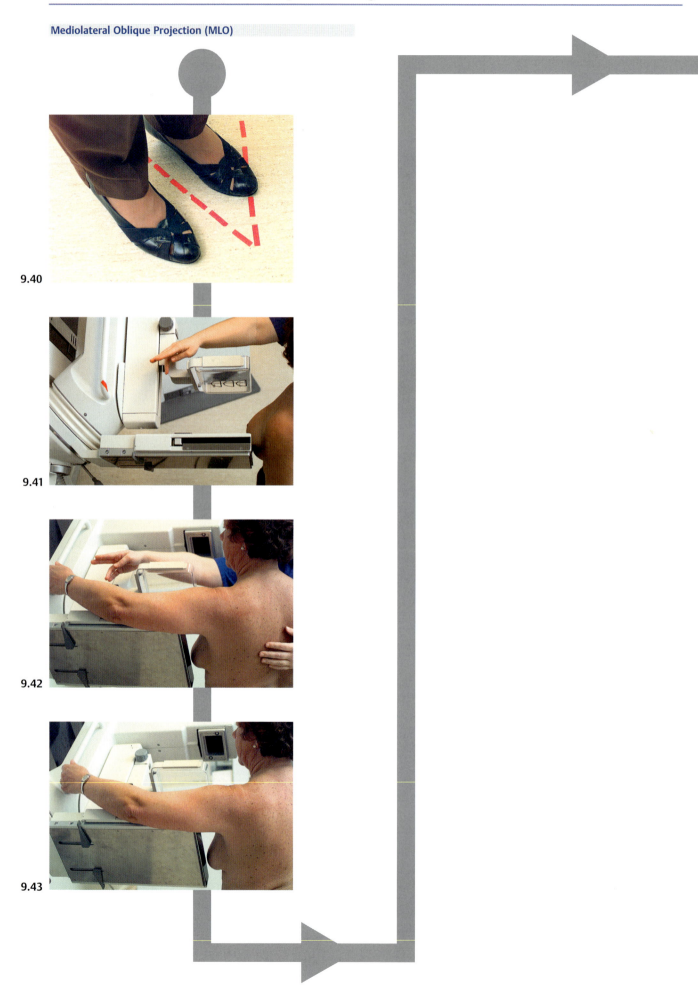

9.40

9.41

9.42

9.43

Mediolateral Oblique Projection (MLO)

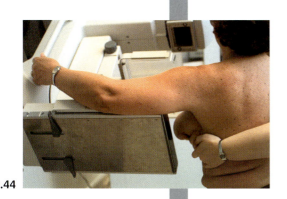

9.44

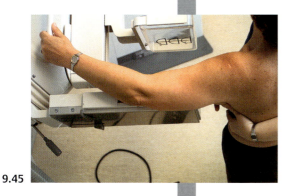

9.45

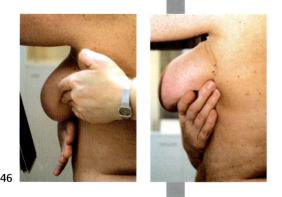

9.46

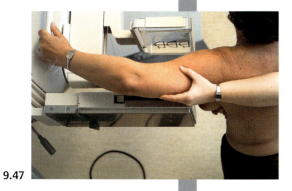

9.47

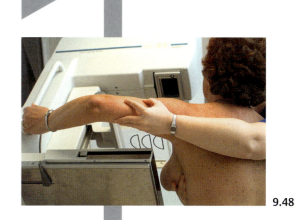

9.48

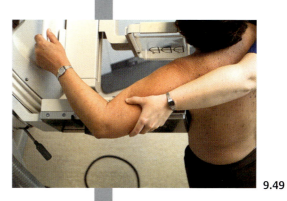

9.49

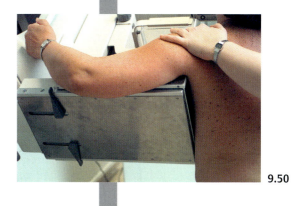

9.50

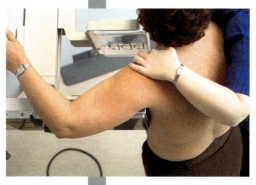

9.51

Mediolateral Oblique Projection (MLO)

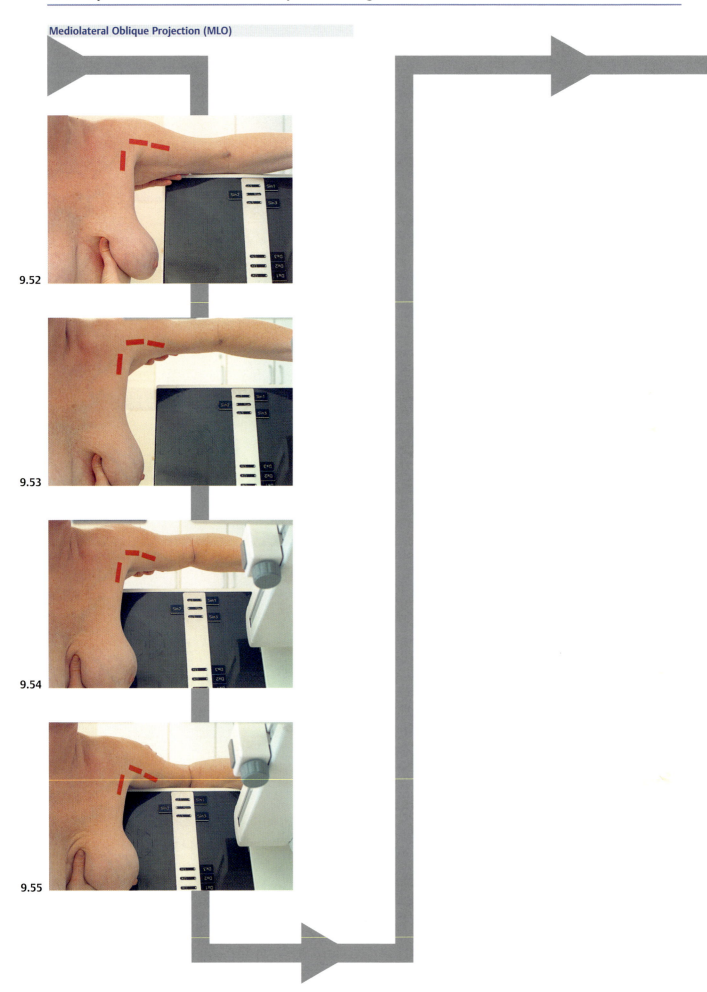

9.52

9.53

9.54

9.55

Mediolateral Oblique Projection (MLO)

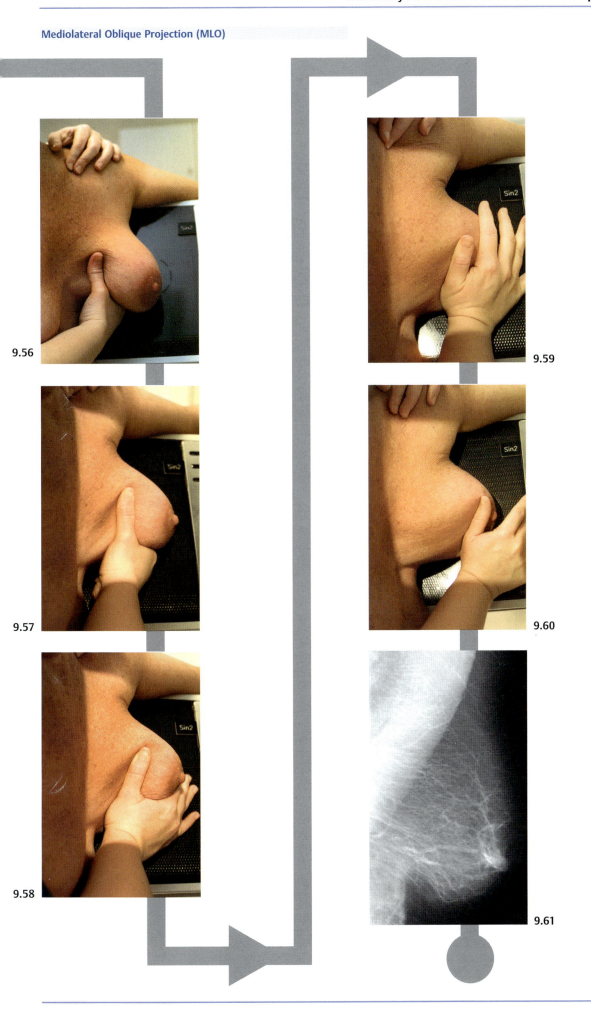

9.56

9.57

9.58

9.59

9.60

9.61

Mediolateral Oblique Projection (MLO)

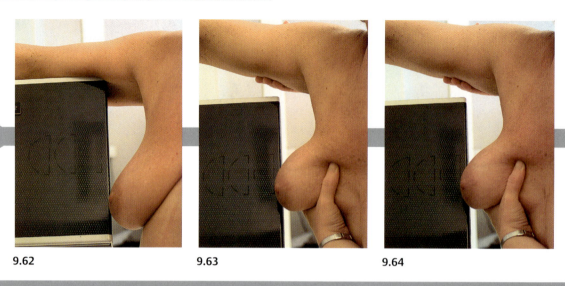

9.62

9.63

9.64

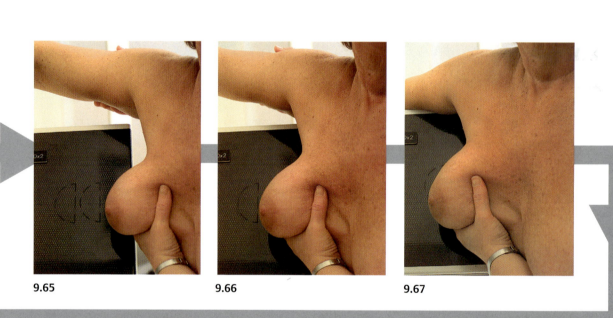

9.65

9.66

9.67

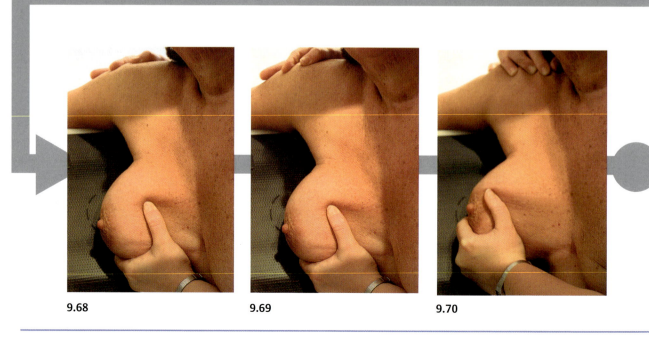

9.68

9.69

9.70

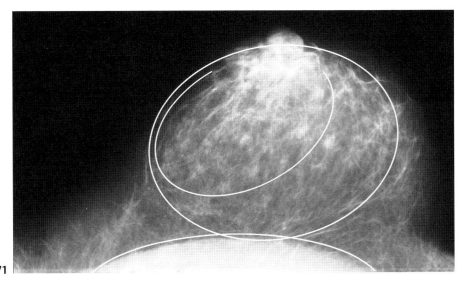

The aims of proper positioning for the CC projection are:

1 To include as much of the breast parenchyma as possible. Ideally, there should be a layer of retroglandular fat between the posterior border of the parenchyma and the pectoral muscle or the edge of the film.

2 Preferably, the posterior edge of the parenchyma and retroglandular fatty tissue as well as a portion of the pectoral muscle should be visualized.

9.71

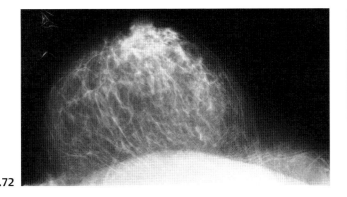

9.72

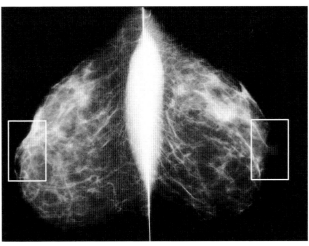

9.73

3 Include both medial and lateral portions of the breast.

4 Nipple in profile whenever possible.

Craniocaudal Projection (CC)

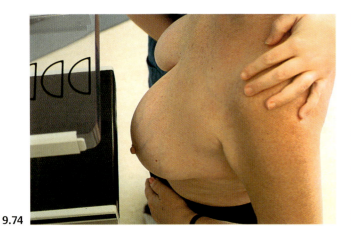

9.74

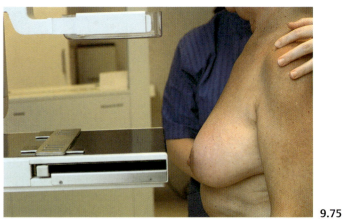

9.75

1   The cassette table is horizontal.

2   The technologist stands on the side opposite the breast being examined.

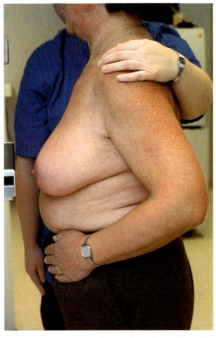

9.76

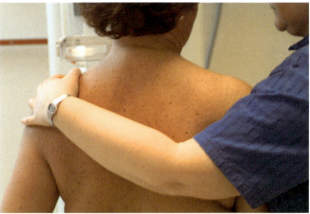

9.77

3   The patient places her hand on her abdomen below the waist on the side to be examined. This allows relaxation of the shoulder on that side.

4   The technologist places her hand on the relaxed shoulder to lower it further.
This allows inclusion of more soft tissue from the upper outer quadrant and reduces the occurrence of skin folds.

Craniocaudal Projection (CC)

1 The technologist's flattened fingers are placed vertically against the upper abdomen just below the inframammary fold.

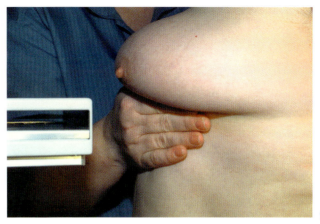

9.78

2 The fingers then slide upward, moving to the under surface of the breast, lifting it up until the little finger is just beneath the inframammary fold.
The other fingers of that hand support the breast from underneath.

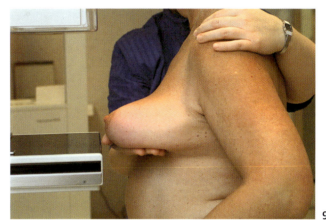

9.79

3 The edge of the cassette table should be at the height of the inframammary fold.

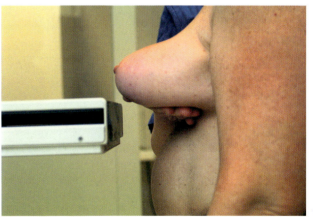

9.80

4 The breast is then lifted up and onto the cassette table. The patient is moved forward into contact with the cassette table.
At this point the technologist's little finger will touch the edge of the cassette table, *ensuring that the inframammary fold will be included in the image field.*

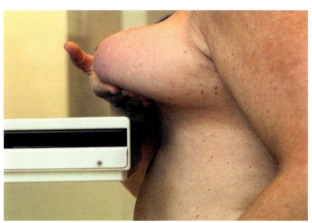

9.81

457

Craniocaudal Projection (CC)

5   The supporting hand pulls the breast forward and ensures that both the medial and lateral halves are included while the other hand moves the shoulder out of the field of view.

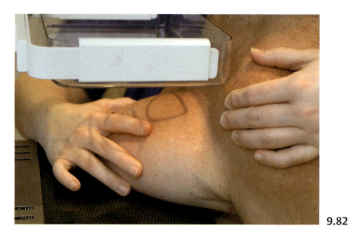

9.82

6   The technologist's hand lowers the shoulder further. This will help to eliminate the wrinkles at the lateral portion and reduces the tension of the skin over the chest wall and the upper breast.

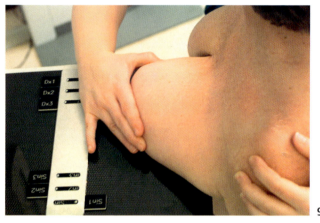

9.83

7   Before compression is applied, the technologist gently lowers the patient's shoulder while simultaneously pushing her forward. This brings in as much soft tissue under the compression plate as possible.

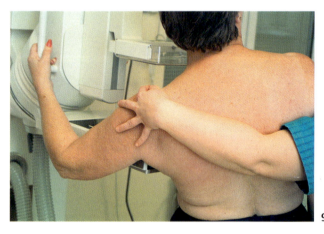

9.84

Schematic representation of the application of compression.

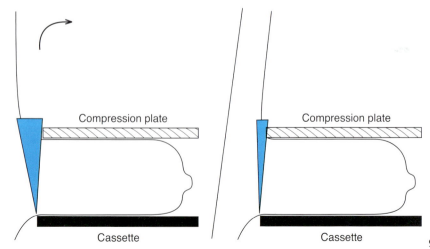

9.85

Craniocaudal Projection (CC)

8   It is ideal to maintain the cleavage portion of the opposite breast on the top of the cassette table, whenever possible.

9   The properly positioned CC mammogram (**9.86–9.88**) will include both medial and lateral portions of the breast; the nipple is in profile without deviation, and a portion of the pectoral muscle is visualized.

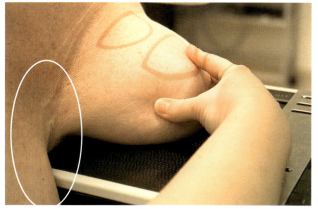

9.89

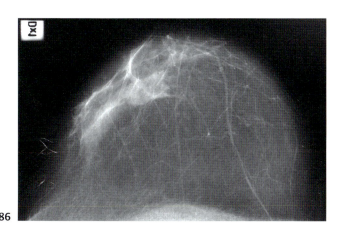

9.86

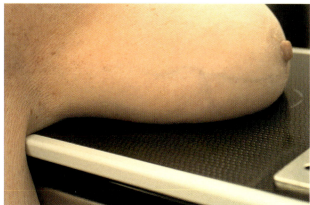

9.90

Careful attention is paid to inclusion of the medial portion of the breast.

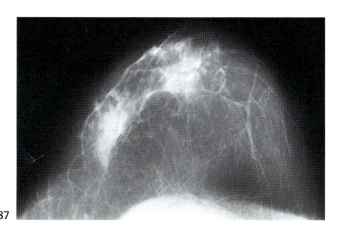

9.87

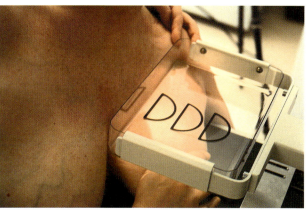

9.91

The visualization of as much as possible of the lateral portion of the breast is important because most of the breast cancers will occur here.

9.88

Craniocaudal Projection (CC)

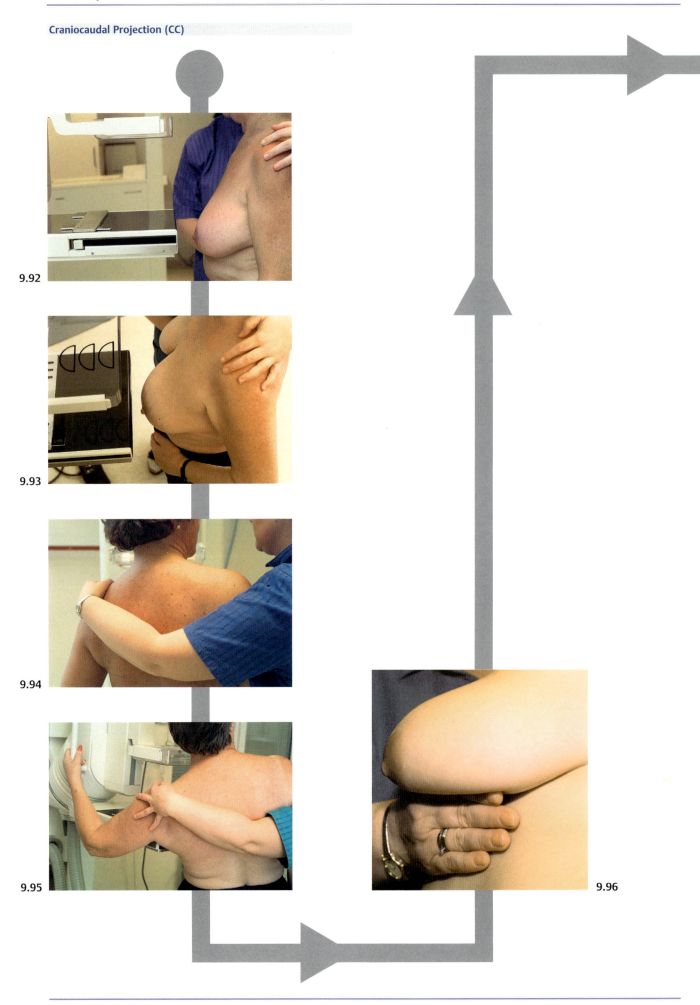

9.92

9.93

9.94

9.95

9.96

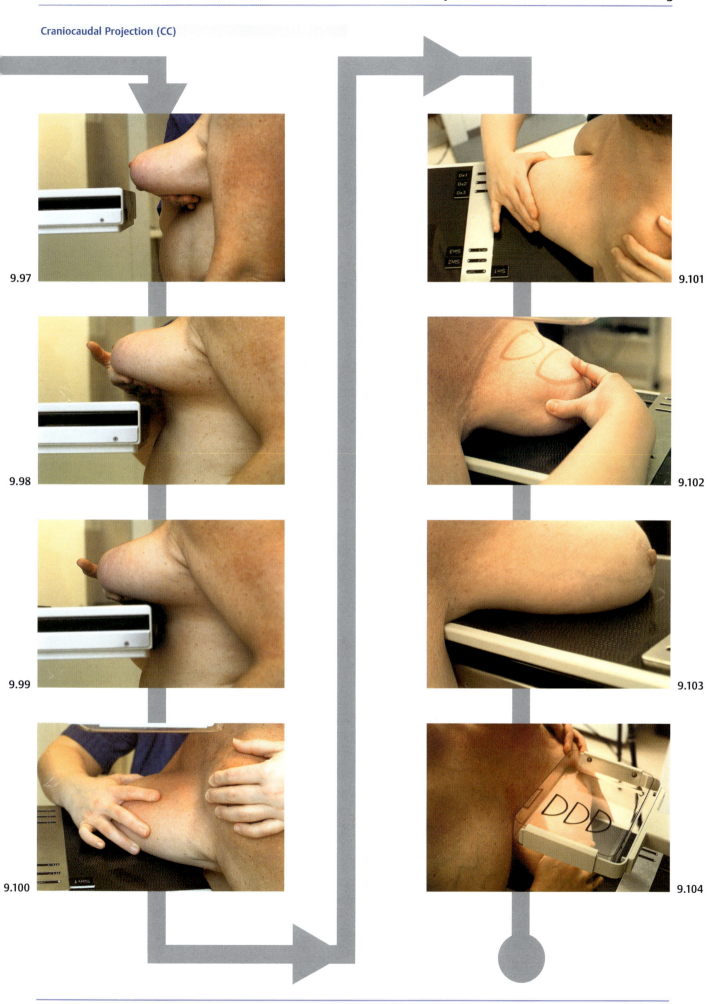

9.97

9.98

9.99

9.100

9.101

9.102

9.103

9.104

The aims of proper positioning for the LM projection are:

- To include as much of the breast parenchyma as possible.
- To give a different perspective on the parenchymal architecture of the breast.
- To enhance visualization of abnormalities localized in the medial half of the breast.
- To provide an orthogonal view of the craniocaudal projection.

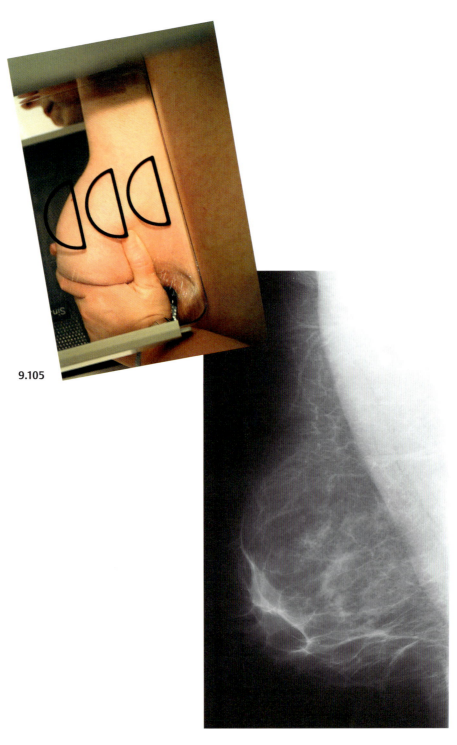

9.105

9.106

Lateromedial Horizontal-Beam Projection (LM)

1   The cassette table should be vertical. The path of the X-ray beam will then be horizontal.

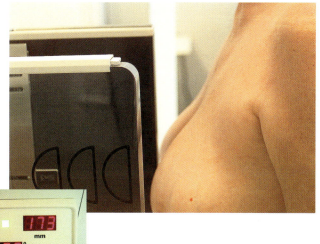

9.107

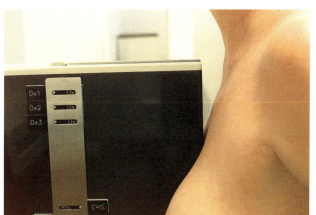

9.108

2   The patient presses her sternum against the edge of the cassette table.

9.109

3   She then leans forward until her chin is resting on the upper edge of the cassette table.

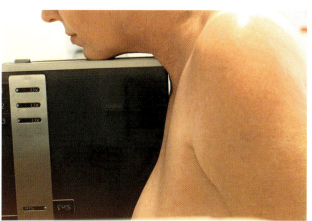

9.110

Lateromedial Horizontal-Beam Projection (LM)

1   The patient grasps the supporting edge of the cassette table, elevates her elbow, internally rotating the arm. This movement will bring the maximum amount of axillary tail tissue into the field of view.

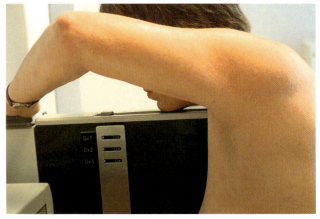

9.111

2   With her opposite hand on the patient's upper arm, the technologist rotates the patient toward the cassette table, while holding the soft tissue of the upper arm away from the compression plate.

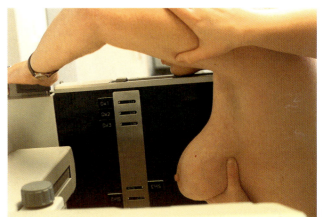

9.112

3   The hand supporting the breast from below moves forward and upward, coordinated with the application of compression. The technologist's hand maintains the proper position of the breast while this function is gradually taken over by the compression plate.

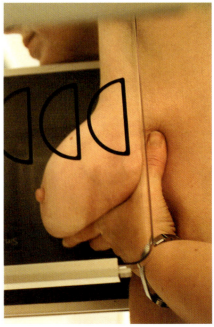

9.113

Lateromedial Horizontal-Beam Projection (LM)

4 The technologist takes hold of the breast from below, simultaneously lifting the breast and pulling it away from the chest wall.

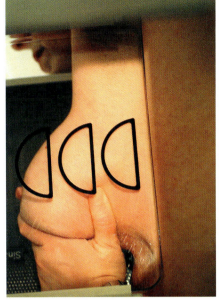

9.114

5 The technologist rotates the patient toward the cassette table. During this rotation the compression plate is used to capture and bring into the field of view as much as possible of the extreme lateral breast tissues.

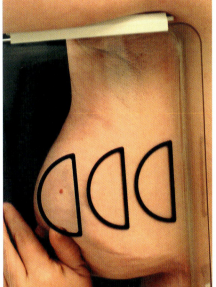

9.115

6 The lateromedial horizontal-beam projection of the left breast.

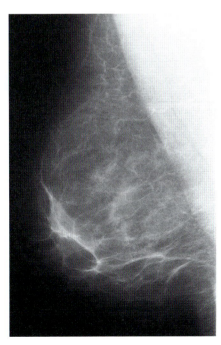

9.116

The aim of the cleavage view is to visualize the tissues and the extreme medial portions of both breasts.

The medial portions of both breasts are placed on the horizontal cassette table and compression is applied.

Note

- If the cleavage is centered, manual exposure control should be used.
- Placing the cleavage off-center may allow the use of automatic exposure.

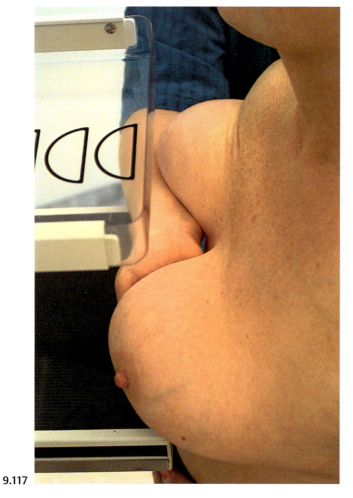

9.117

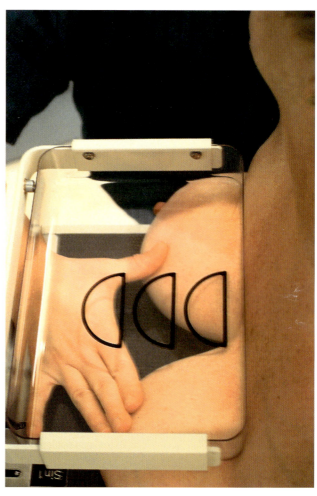

9.118

The cleavage view of a Pattern II-type breast.

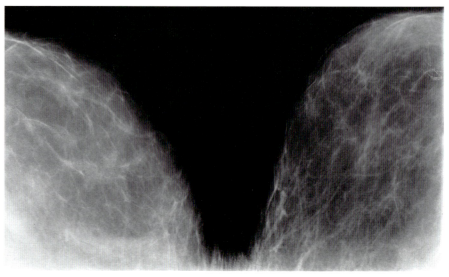

9.119

References

■ Introduction

1 Gram IT, Funkhouser E, Tabar L. The Tabar classification of mammographic parenchymal patterns. *Eur J Radiol* 1997; **24:** 131–136.

2 Ingleby H, Gershon-Cohen, J. *Comparative Anatomy, Pathology and Roentgenology of the Breast.* Philadelphia: University of Pennsylvania Press;1960.

3 Tabár L, Dean PB. Mammographic parenchymal patterns. Risk indicator for breast cancer? *JAMA* 1982; **247:** 185–189.

4 Wellings SR, Wolfe JN. Correlative studies of the histological and radiographic appearance of the breast parenchyma. *Radiology* 1978; **129:** 299–306.

5 Wolfe JN. Breast patterns as an index of risk for developing breast cancer. *Am J Roentgenol* 1976; **126:** 1130–1137.

■ Chapter 1

1 Gallagher HS. View from the giant's shoulder. The fifth annual Wendell G. Scott Lecture. *Cancer* 1977; **40:** 185–194.

2 Jensen HM. On the origin and progression of human breast cancer. *Am J Obstet Gynecol* 1986; **154:** 1280–1284.

3 Tot T, Tabár L, Dean PB. The pressing need for better histologic–mammographic correlation of the many variations in normal breast anatomy. *Virchows Arch* 2000; **437:** 338–344.

4 Vogel PM, Georgiade NG, Fetter BF, Vogel FS, McCarty KS Jr. The correlation of histologic changes in the human breast with the menstrual cycle. *Am J Pathol* 1981; **104:** 23–34.

5 Wellings SR, Jensen HM, Marcum RG. An atlas of subgross pathology of the human breast with special reference to possible precancerous lesions. *J Natl Cancer Inst* 1975; **55:** 231–273.

■ Chapter 4

1 Duffy SW, Tabár L, Smith RA, Krusemo UB, Prevost TC, Chen HH. Risk of Breast Cancer and Risks with Breast Cancer: the relationship between histological type and conventional risk factors, disease progression, and survival. *Seminars in Breast Disease* 1999; **2:** 292–300.

2 Hughes LE, Mansel RE, Webster DJ. Aberrations of normal development and involution (ANDI): a new perspective on pathogenesis and nomenclature of benign breast disorders. *Lancet* 1987; 2: 1316–1319.

3 Tabár L, Dean PB. Mammographic parenchymal patterns. Risk indicator for breast cancer? *JAMA* 1982; **247:** 185–189.

■ Chapter 5

1 Tabár L, Dean PB. Mammographic parenchymal patterns. Risk indicator for breast cancer? *JAMA* 1982; **247:** 185–189.

■ Chapter 6

1 Alexander FE, Anderson TJ, Brown HK, Forrest AP, Hepburn W, Kirkpatrick AE, et al. 14 years of follow-up from the Edinburgh randomised trial of breast-cancer screening. *Lancet* 1999; **353:** 1903–1908.

2 Aubele M, Mattis A, Zitzelsberger H, Walch A, Kremer M, Hutzler P, et al. Intratumoral heterogeneity in breast carcinoma revealed by laser-microdissection and comparative genomic hybridization. *Cancer Genet Cytogenet* 1999; **110:** 94–102.

3 Brenner AJ, Aldaz CM. The genetics of sporadic breast cancer. *Prog Clin Biol Res.* 1997; **396:** 63–82.

4 Cady B, Michaelson JS. The life-sparing potential of mammographic screening. *Cancer* 2001; **91:** 1699–1703.

5 Carlson KL, Helvie MA, Roubidoux MA, Kleer CG, Oberman HA, Wilson TE, et al. Relationship between mammographic screening intervals and size and histology of ductal carcinoma in situ. *AJR Am J Roentgenol* 1999; **172:** 313–317.

6 Chen H-H, Duffy SW, Tabár L, Day NE. Markov chain models for progression of breast cancer Part I: tumor attributes and the preclinical screen-detectable phase. *J Epidemiol Biostat* 1997; **2:** 9–23.

7 Chen HH, Thurfjell E, Duffy SW, Tabár L. Evaluation by Markov chain models of a non-randomised breast cancer screening programme in women aged under 50 years in Sweden. *J Epidemiol Community Health* 1998; **52:** 329–335.

8 Dean PB. The proven reliability of mammography screening. *The Breast* 2002; **11:** 211–214.

9 Duffy S, Tabár L, Smith RA. The mammographic screening trials: commentary on the recent work by Olsen and Gotzsche. *J Surg Oncol* 2002; **81:** 159–162; discussion 162–166.

10 Duffy SW, Tabár L, Chen H-H, et al. The impact of organized mammography service screening on breast carcinoma mortality in seven Swedish counties: a collaborative evaluation. *Cancer* 2002; **95:** 458–469.

11 Duffy SW, Tabár L, Fagerberg G, Gad A, Grontoft O, South MC, Day NE. Breast screening, prognostic factors and survival—results from the Swedish two county study. *Br J Cancer* 1991; **64:** 1133–1138.

12 Duffy SW, Tabár L, Vitak B, Day NE, Smith RA, Chen HH, Yen MF. The relative contributions of screen-detected in situ and invasive breast carcinomas in reducing mortality from the disease. *Eur J Cancer* 2003; **39:** 1755–1760.

13 European Health for All Database. WHO Regional Office for Europe, Copenhagen, Denmark.

14 Fisher B. Laboratory and clinical research in breast cancer—a personal adventure: the David A. Karnofsky Memorial Lecture. *Cancer Res* 1980; **40:** 3863–3874.

15 Fisher B., Jeong JH, Anderson S, Bryant J, Fisher ER, Wolmark N. Twenty-five-year follow-up of a randomized trial comparing radical mastectomy, total mastectomy, and total mastectomy followed by irradiation. *N Engl J Med* 2002; **347:** 567–575.

16 Gram IT, Funkhouser E, Tabár L. The Tabár classification of mammographic parenchymal patterns. *Eur J Radiol* 1997;**24:** 131–136.

17 Hakama M, Pukkala E, Heikkila M, Kallio M. Effectiveness of the public health policy for breast cancer screening in Finland: population-based cohort study. *BMJ.* 1997; **314:** 864–867.

18 Johnson A, Shekhdar J. Does breast cancer grade worsen with time? Evidence from breast screening. *Breast Cancer Res Treat* 2001; **68:** 261–271.

19 Kaufman CS, Jacobson-Kaufman L, Thorndike-Christ T, Kaufman L, Tabár L. A treatment scale for axillary management in breast cancer. *Am J Surg* 2001; **182:** 377–383.

20 Lenner P, Jonsson H. Excess mortality from breast cancer in relation to mammography screening in northern Sweden. *J Med Screen* 1997; **4:** 6–9.

21 Miller AB, To T, Baines CJ, Wall C. Canadian National Breast Screening Study–2: 13-year results of a randomized trial in women aged 50–59 years. *J Natl Cancer Inst* 2000; **92:** 1490–1499.

22 Mittra I, Baum M, Thornton H, Houghton J. Is clinical breast examination an acceptable alternative to mammographic screening? *BMJ* 2000; **321:** 1071–1073.

23 Moody-Ayers SY, Wells CK, Feinstein AR. "Benign" tumors and "early detection" in mammography-screened patients of a natural cohort with breast cancer. *Arch Intern Med* 2000; **160:** 1109–1115.

24 Nystrom L, Rutqvist LE, Wall S, Lindgren A, Lindqvist M, Ryden S, et al. Breast cancer screening with mammography: overview of Swedish randomised trials. *Lancet* 1993; **341:** 973–978.

25 Otto SJ, Fracheboud J, Looman CW, Broeders MJ, Boer R, Hendriks JH, et al. National Evaluation Team for Breast Cancer Screening. Initiation of population-based mammography screening in Dutch municipalities and effect on breast-cancer mortality: a systematic review. *Lancet* 2003; **361:** 1411–1417.

26 Richards MA, Smith P, Ramirez AJ, Fentiman IS, Rubens RD. The influence on survival of delay in the presentation and treatment of symptomatic breast cancer. *Br J Cancer* 1999; **79:** 858–864.

27 Shapiro S, Venet W, Strax P, Venet L. *Periodic Screening for Breast Cancer: The Health Insurance Plan Project and its Sequelae, 1963–1986.* Baltimore: Johns Hopkins, 1988: 59–83.

28 Sharifi-Salamatian V, de Roquancourt A, Rigaut JP. Breast carcinoma, intratumour heterogeneity and histological grading, using geostatistics. *Anal Cell Pathol* 2000; **20:** 83–91.

29 Silverstein MJ, Skinner KA, Lomis TJ. Predicting axillary nodal positivity in 2282 patients with breast carcinoma. *World J Surg* 2001; **25:** 767–772.

30 Smith RA. Breast cancer screening among women younger than age 50: a current assessment of the issues. *CA Cancer J Clin* 2000; **50:** 312–336.

31 Sundquist M, Thorstenson S, Brudin L, Wingren S, Nordenskjöld B. Incidence and prognosis in early-onset breast cancer. In: Sundquist M. *Prognostic factors in breast cancer.* Medical Dissertation No. 632, Linköping University, Sweden.

32 Tabár L, Chen HH, Fagerberg G, Duffy SW, Smith TC. Recent results from the Swedish Two-County Trial: the effects of age, histologic type, and mode of detection on the efficacy of breast cancer screening. *J Natl Cancer Inst Monogr* 1997; **22:** 43–47.

33 Tabár L, Dean PB, Kaufman CS, Duffy SW, Chen HH. A new era in the diagnosis of breast cancer. *Surg Oncol Clin N Am* 2000; **9:** 233–277.

34 Tabár L, Dean PB. The control of breast cancer through mammography screening. What is the evidence? *Radiol Clin North Am* 1987; **25:** 993–1005.

35 Tabár L, Duffy SW, Vitak B, Chen HH, Prevost TC. The natural history of breast carcinoma: what have we learned from screening? *Cancer* 1999; **86:** 449–462.

36 Tabár L, Fagerberg CJ, Gad A, Baldetorp L, Holmberg LH, Grontoft O, et al. Reduction in mortality from breast cancer after mass screening with mammography. Randomised trial from the Breast Cancer Screening Working Group of the Swedish National Board of Health and Welfare. *Lancet* 1985; **1:** 829–832.

37 Tabár L, Fagerberg G, Chen HH, Duffy SW, Gad A. Tumour development, histology and grade of breast cancers: prognosis and progression. *Int J Cancer* 1996; **66:** 413–419.

38 Tabár L, Fagerberg G, Day NE, Duffy SW, Kitchin RM. Breast cancer treatment and natural history: new insights from results of screening. *Lancet* 1992; **339:** 412–414.

39 Tabár L, Fagerberg G, Day NE, Duffy SW, Kitchin RM. Natural history of breast cancer. *Lancet* 1992; **339:** 1108.

40 Tabár L, Fagerberg G, Duffy SW, Day NE, Gad A, Grontoft O. Update of the Swedish two-county program of mammographic screening for breast cancer. *Radiol Clin North Am* 1992; **30:** 187–210.

41 Tabár L, Smith RA, Vitak B, Yen MF, Chen TH, Warwick J, et al. Mammographic screening: a key factor in the control of breast cancer. *Cancer J* 2003; **9:** 15–27.

42 Tabár L, Vitak B, Chen HH, Duffy SW, Yen MF, Chiang CF, et al. The Swedish Two-County Trial twenty years later. Updated mortality results and new insights from long-term follow-up. *Radiol Clin North Am* 2000; **38:** 625–651.

43 Tabár L, Vitak B, Chen HH, Prevost TC, Duffy SW. Update of the Swedish Two-County Trial of breast cancer screening: histologic grade-specific and age-specific results. *Swiss Surg* 1999; **5:** 199–204.

44 Tabár L, Vitak B, Chen HH, Yen M-F, Duffy SW, Smith RA. Beyond randomized controlled trials: organized mammographic screening substantially reduces breast carcinoma mortality. *Cancer* 2001; **91:** 1724–1731.

45 Tabár L, Yen MF, Vitak B, Chen HH, Smith RA, Duffy SW. Mammography service screening and mortality in breast cancer patients: 20-year follow-up before and after introduction of screening. *Lancet* 2003; **361:** 1405–1410.

46 Thurfjell EL, Lindgren JA. Breast cancer survival rates with mammographic screening: similar favorable survival rates for women younger and those older than 50 years. *Radiology* 1996; **201:** 421–426.

47 Tornberg S, Carstensen J, Hakulinen T, Lenner P, Hatschek T, Lundgren B. Evaluation of the effect on breast cancer mortality of population-based mammography screening programmes. *J Med Screen* 1994; **1:** 184–187.

48 Tubiana M, Koscielny S. Natural history of human breast cancer: recent data and clinical implications. *Breast Cancer Res Treat* 1991; **18:** 125–140.

49 Voogd AC, van Tienhoven G, Peterse HL, Crommelin MA, Rutgers EJ, van de Velde CJ, et al. Local recurrence after breast conservation therapy for early stage breast carcinoma: detection, treatment, and outcome in 266 patients. Dutch Study Group on Local Recurrence after Breast Conservation (BORST). *Cancer* 1999; **85:** 437–446.

50 Yen MF, Tabár L, Vitak B, Smith RA, Chen HH, Duffy SW. Quantifying the potential problem of overdiagnosis of ductal carcinoma in situ in breast cancer screening. *Eur J Cancer* 2003; **39:** 1746–1754.

■ Chapter 7

1 Anttinen I, Pamilo M, Soiva M, Roiha M. Double reading of mammography screening films—one radiologist or two?. *Clin Radiol* 1993; **48:** 414–421.

2 Huynh PT, Jarolimek AM, Daye S. The false-negative mammogram. *Radiographics* 1998; **18:** 1137–1154.

3 Kopans DB. Double reading. *Radiol Clin North Am* 2000; **38:** 719–724.

4 Kroman N, Wohlfahrt J, Mouridsen HT, Melbye M. Influence of tumor location on breast cancer prognosis. *Int J Cancer* 2003; **105:** 542–545.

5 Laming D, Warren R. Improving the detection of cancer in the screening of mammograms. *J Med Screen* 2000; **7:** 24–30.

6 Linver MN, Paster SB, Rosenberg RD, Key CR, Stidley CA, King WV. Improvement in mammography interpretation skills in a community radiology practice after dedicated teaching courses: 2-year medical audit of 38,633 cases. *Radiology* 1992; **184:** 39–43.

7 Liston JC, Dall BJ. Can the NHS Breast Screening Programme afford not to double read screening mammograms? *Clin Radiol* 2003; **58:** 474–477.

8 Thurfjell E, Lernevall K, Taube A. Benefit of independent double reading in a population-based mammography screening program. *Radiology* 1994; **191:** 241–244.

■ Chapter 8

1 Marcum RG, Wellings SR. Subgross pathology of the human breast: method and initial observations. *J Natl Cancer Inst* 1969; **42:** 115–121.

2 Wellings SR, Jensen HM, Marcum RG. An atlas of subgross pathology of the human breast with special reference to possible precancerous lesions. *J Natl Cancer Inst* 1975; **55:** 231–273.

3 Armstrong JS, Davies JD, Hronkova B. Backprocessing paraffin wax blocks for subgross examination. *J Clin Pathol* 1992; **45:** 1116–1117.

4 Faverly D, Holland R, Burgers L. An original stereomicroscopic analysis of the mammary glandular tree. *Virchows Arch [A]* 1992; **421:** 115–119.

5 Jackson PA, Merchant W, McCormick CJ, Cook MG. A comparison of large block macrosectioning and conventional techniques in breast pathology. *Virchows Arch* 1994; **425:** 243–248.

6 Tot T, Tabár L, Dean PB. The pressing need for better histologic-mammographic correlation of many variations in normal breast anatomy. *Virchows Arch* 2000; **437:** 338–344.

7 Foschini MP, Tot T, Eusebi V. Large section (macrosection) histologic slides. In: Silverstein MJ, ed. *Ductal Carcinoma In Situ of the Breast*. 2nd ed. Philadelphia: Lippincott, Williams and Wilkins; 2002: 148–154.

8 Tot T, Tabár L, Dean PB. *Practical Breast Pathology*. Stuttgart: Thieme; 2002: 116–123.

■ Suggested Texts for Further Reading

Barth V, Prechtel K. *Atlas of Breast Diseases*. Saint Louis: Mosby; 1991.

Bassett LW, Gold R. *Breast Cancer Detection: Mammography and Other Methods in Breast Imaging*. Orlando: Grune & Stratton; 1987.

Bassett LW, Jackson V, Fu K, Fu Y. *Diagnosis of Diseases of the Breast*. Philadelphia: W.B. Saunders; 2004.

Birdwell RL, Morris EA, Wang S-c. PocketRadiologist—Breast: Top 100 Diagnoses. Philadelphia: W.B. Saunders; 2003.

Cardenosa G. *Breast Imaging*. Philadelphia: Lippincott Williams & Wilkins; 2004.

Dronkers DJ, Hendriks, JHCL, Holland R, Rosenbusch G. *The Practice of Mammography: Pathology, Technique, Interpretation, Adjunct Modalities*. New York: Thieme Medical Publishers; 2002.

Duffy SW, Hill C, Estève J. *Quantitative Methods for the Evaluation of Cancer Screening*. New York: Oxford University Press; 2001.

Egan RL. *Mammography*. Springfield: Thomas; 1964.

Feig SA. Surveillance Strategy for Breast Cancer. *Seminars in Breast Disease*. Philadelphia: Saunders; in press.

Gallager HS. *Early Breast Cancer: Detection and Treatment*. New York: John Wiley & Sons; 1975.

Gamagami P. *Atlas of Mammography: New Early Signs in Breast Cancer*. Oxford: Blackwell Science; 1996.

Gershon-Cohen, J. *Atlas of Mammography*. Berlin: Springer; 1970.

Gold RH, Bassett LW. *Mammography, Thermography & Ultrasound In Breast Cancer Detection*. Saint Louis: Harcourt Health Sciences; 1982.

Hashimoto B, Bauermeister D. *Breast Imaging: A Correlative Atlas*. New York: Thieme Medical Publishers; 2002.

Hendriks JHCL, Holland R, Rijken, H. *MammoTrainer: Interactive Training for Breast Cancer Screening Mammography*. Berlin: Springer; 2004.

Heywang-Köbrunner SH, Dershaw DD, Schreer I. *Diagnostic Breast Imaging: Mammography, Sonography, Magnetic Resonance Imaging and Interventional Procedures*. New York: Thieme Medical Publishers; 2001.

Hoeffken W, Lanyi M. *Mammography*. Philadelphia: Saunders; 1977.

Homer MJ. *Mammographic Interpretation: A Practical Approach*. New York: McGraw-Hill; 1996.

Hughes LE, Mansel RE, Webster DJT. *Benign Disorders and Diseases of the Breast. Concepts and Clinical Management*. London: Saunders; 2000.

Ikeda, DM. *Breast Imaging: The Requisites*. Saint Louis: Mosby; 2004.

Kopans DB. *Breast imaging*. Philadelphia: Lippincott Williams & Wilkins; 1997.

Kopans DB. *Atlas of Breast Imaging*. Philadelphia: Lippincott Williams & Wilkins; 1998.

Lanyi M. *Diagnosis and Differential Diagnosis of Breast Calcifications*. Berlin: Springer; 1986.

Lanyi M. *Mammography: Diagnosis and Morphological Analysis*. New York: Springer; 2003.

Leborgne RA. *The Breast in Roentgen Diagnosis*. Montevideo: Impresora Uruguaya; 1953.

Lee L, Stickland V, Wilson R. *Fundamentals of Mammography*. Saint Louis: Harcourt Health Sciences; 2002.

Logan-Young WW, Yanes-Hoffman N. *Breast Cancer: A Practical Guide to Diagnosis*. New York: Mount Hope Publishing; 1995.

Martin JE. *Atlas Of Mammography: Histologic & Mammographic Correlations*. Philadelphia: Lippincott Williams & Wilkins; 1982.

Parker SH, Jobe WE. *Percutaneous Breast Biopsy*. Philadelphia: Lippincott Williams & Wilkins; 1993.

Pisano ED, Yaffe M, McLelland R. *Digital Mammography*. Philadelphia: Lippincott Williams & Wilkins; 2003.

Potchen J, Sierra A, Azavedo E, Svane G, Potchen EJ. *Screening Mammography: Breast Cancer Diagnosis in Asymptomatic Women*. Saint Louis: Mosby; 1992.

Rosen PP. *Rosen's Breast Pathology*. Philadelphia: Lippincott-Raven; 1997.

Rubin E, Simpson JF. *Breast Specimen Radiography*. Philadelphia: Lippincott Williams & Wilkins; 1997.

Shapiro S, Venet W, Strax P, Venet L. *Periodic Screening for Breast Cancer*. Baltimore: The Johns Hopkins University Press; 1988.

Shaw de Paredes E. *Atlas of Film-Screen Mammography*. Munich–Vienna–Baltimore: Urban & Schwarzenberg; 1989.

Silverstein MJ, Ed. *Carcinoma In Situ of the Breast*. Baltimore: Williams and Wilkins; 1997.

Stavros AT, Rapp CL, Parker SH. *Breast Ultrasound*. Philadelphia: Lippincott Williams & Wilkins; 2003.

Strax P. *Early Detection: Breast Cancer is Curable*. New York: Harper and Row; 1974.

Tucker AK, Ng YY. *Textbook of Mammography*. Philadelphia: Elsevier; 2001.

Vainio H, Bianchini F. *Breast Cancer Screening*. Lyon: IARC Press; 2002

Wolfe JN. *Mammography*. Springfield: Thomas; 1967.

Subject Index

Note:

Abbreviations

DCIS – ductal carcinoma in situ

TDLU – terminal duct lobular unit

Since the major subject of this book is 'breast cancer', entries under 'breast cancer' have been kept to a minimum and readers are advised to seek more specific entries.

A

aberrations of normal development and involution (ANDI) 125
abscess, recurring 386
accessory breast 243–245
acini 48
    atrophy 66, 144
    calcifications 85, 149
    changes during menstrual cycle 53
    cystic dilatations, calcifications in 149
    enlargement 125
    estrogen receptors 66, 67
    microcystic dilatation 424
    number during menstrual cycle 53
    subgross, thick-section histology 49
adenosis 125–126, 242
    apocrine 127
    sclerosing see sclerosing adenosis
    simple 127
adipose tissue 30, 242
    large-section histology 30–31
    mammography 30, 42–43
    Pattern I 33, 62, 63
        fibroglandular tissue outlined by 70
    Pattern II 94
    radiograph 30
    replacing fibroglandular tissue 66, 67
    subgross, thick-section histology 31, 64, 65
    surrounding retroareolar ducts (Pattern III) 120–121
advanced breast cancer, appearance 166, 171
age
    cumulative survival by 182, 183, 184
    effect on mean sojourn time 217, 218, 219
        tumor subtypes 220–227
    parenchymal patterns 160–161
        breast cancer and 163
        screening vs clinical populations 162
    tumor size and histological grade 177
apocrine metaplasia 127, 131, 281
    subgross, thick-section histology 424
architectural distortion 188–189, 358–394
    asymmetric fibroglandular tissue without 246–247
    atypical medullary carcinoma 378–385
    benefits of early detection of cancer 361
    benign breast lesions 199, 392–393
    difficulty detecting 361
    ductal carcinoma in situ 194
    fibroglandular tissue, in lobular carcinoma 134, 135
    invasive ductal carcinoma 386–391
        progression 229, 358–363, 386–391
    invasive lobular carcinoma 370–375
    lesions causing 358–394
    nonspecific asymmetric densities with 250–255
    palpable tumor with (lobular carcinoma) 370–375
    Pattern I 70, 80–81, 188
        invasive ductal carcinoma 80
        invasive malignant tumors 80, 393
        radial scars 81
    retroareolar area 359–363
    in retroglandular clear space 335
    tubular carcinoma 364–369
areolar complex
    subgross histology 6–7 see also nipple–areolar complex
asymmetric densities 240–241
    definite pathological lesions causing 256
    de-novo in "forbidden area" 329–330
    medial half of breast 318–320, 321
    in "milky way" see "milky way"
    nonspecific 307, 310
        with architectural distortion 250–255
        early malignant stellate lesions 299
        "forbidden area" 259, 262, 286–289, 307
        invasive lobular carcinoma 373–375
        surrounding mammographically malignant lesion 388
    normal fibroglandular tissue 242, 243–249
        asymmetric involution 246–247, 248
    with palpable tumor (lobular carcinoma) 370–375
    parenchymal contour change with 394–395
    retroareolar area 350
    retroglandular clear space 332–333
    systematic work-up 242
    in upper outer quadrant of breast 259
    work-up and management algorithm 258
atrophic ducts see duct(s), atrophic
axillary node positivity 263
    tumor size and grade 175

B

benign breast lesions
    architectural distortion 199, 392–393
    circular/oval-shaped lesions 201
    distracting influence on malignancy detection 342–343
    radiating structure and architectural distortion 199
benign fibroadenoma see fibroadenoma
benign hyperplasia
    powdery calcification 211
    psammoma-like bodies 281
blood vessels 17, 21, 112–113
    calcified arteries 21
    Pattern II 112–113
    subgross, thick-section histology 31
    thick-section histology 21
bone metastases 171
bracketing technique 273, 285, 304, 360, 381
breast
    accessory 243–245
    benign hyperplasia see benign hyperplasia
    regions with higher frequency of cancer 259
breast cancer
    control, paradigm shift 170
    early, nonspecific appearance 271
    extent, large-section histology 416, 417
    fibrous strands masking 20
    growth rates 216, 217
    invasiveness 178
    lesions in medial half see medial half of breast, lesions
    morphological heterogeneity see morphological heterogeneity (of breast cancer)
    mortality see mortality (breast cancer)
    palpable, downward stage shifting 178–179
    preclinical phase see preclinical breast cancer
    prevalence by parenchymal pattern 163
    previous 355–357
    as progressive disease 170, 177, 185, 216–234
    recurrence 14
    regions of breast (frequency) 259
    in retroareolar area see retroareolar area
    retroglandular clear space lesions see retroglandular clear space
    risk indicator (mammographic pattern) 32
    size see tumor size
    subtypes and frequencies 190
    as systemic disease from inception 170, 185
    upper outer quadrant see upper outer quadrant lesions
bridges, interconnecting see interconnecting bridges
building blocks 32, 40–45, 242
    homogeneous structureless densities see homogeneous structureless densities
    linear densities see linear densities
    mammographic–histological correlation 16–31
    nodular densities see nodular densities
    normal breast 32, 40–45
    in Pattern I 33
    in Pattern II 35
    in Pattern III 36
    in Pattern IV 37
    in Pattern V 38
    radiolucent areas see radiolucent areas
    in reading mammograms 239
    subgross, thick-section histology 27

C

calcification
    acini 85, 149
    apocrine metaplasia with 281
    in atypical medullary carcinoma 380
    benign, Pattern V 148–149
    casting-type 106, 194, 202, 203, 204, 205, 212
        histology 205
        invasive ductal carcinoma progression 229
        malignancy ratio 204–205
        microfocus magnification 204
        specimen radiograph 205
    crushed stone-like 194, 202, 203, 206–207
        benign 208–209, 212
        decrease with invasion of tumor 214, 215
        histology 207
        malignancy ratio 206–207
        microfocus magnification 206, 209
        multifocal invasive ductal carcinoma 267
        specimen radiograph 207
    cystic fluid, Pattern II 115
    in DCIS 383
        Grade 3 14
        high nuclear grade 106, 107
    decrease/disappearance with invasion of tumor 214, 215, 228–229
    detection vs small invasive tumor detection 179
    dilated ducts 101, 103
    distribution (frequency) 195
    diversity, upper outer quadrant 280–281
        radiographs 281
    dotted casting-type 202
    in fibroglandular tissue near DCIS 274
    indistinct amorphous see calcification, powdery
    linear branching see calcification, casting-type
    malignant 256
        missed/underdiagnosed 214–215, 228
    mammography 202–203
        frequency of types 203
    in medullary carcinoma 234
    multiple clusters 130, 145, 146, 157
        retroareolar area 360
    nonspecific, medial half of breast 319, 320
    Pattern I type breast 84–85
    Pattern IV breast 134
        sclerosing adenosis with 129–131
    Pattern V breast 145–150
    pleomorphic see calcification, crushed stone-like
    powdery 202, 203, 210–211
        benign histology 211
        malignancy ratio 210–211
        malignant histology 211
        medial half of breast 320
        upper outer quadrant 280

calcification
  retroareolar area 425–431
  sclerosing adenosis with 129–131
  "secretory disease"/"plasma cell mastitis"
    type 101
  subtypes, malignancy frequency 203
  surrounding mammographically malignant
    lesion 388
  see also microcalcifications
calcified arteries 21
call-backs 240
  for asymmetric densities 303
  convex contour 286
carcinoma in situ
  dilated duct with necrosis/calcification 99
  distending TDLU 71
  see also ductal carcinoma in situ (DCIS); lobu-
    lar carcinoma in situ (LCIS); papillary carci-
    noma in situ
castings, dotted 107
circular tumor masses 256
  benign, histology (frequencies) 201
  early diagnosis 178
  intracystic papillary carcinoma 222
  malignant, histology (frequencies) 201
  morphological heterogeneity 200–201
  stellate tumors vs (frequency) 195
classification of mammograms 32
  purpose 32
cleavage view (CV) 466
clinically referred cases 240
collagen 54
  staining for 415
colloid carcinoma 111, 191
  see also mucinous carcinoma
comet-tail 261
compound tumor
  mean sojourn time 221
  see also specific cancer subtypes
convex contours 262
  asymmetric density in "forbidden area" 286
  benign lesions 368
  circular/oval-shaped 200
  malignant lesions detection and 385
  nonspecific early stellate lesions 299
  Pattern I type 71–79
    see also Pattern I
  Pattern V type, detection 151
  terminal duct lobular units (TDLUs) 71
    pathological lesions 71–73
  tubular carcinoma 364–369
Cooper's ligament 40, 41, 56, 62
  adipose tissue outlining 31
  cysts and dilated ducts 59
  invasive lobular carcinoma of 60
  mammographic–histological comparison 57,
    58
  structure 56
  subgross, thick-section histology 59
cotton ball-like appearance 129, 130
craniocaudal projection (CC) 62, 455–461
  aims of correct positioning 455
  blood vessels in Pattern II 112
  mammographically occult lesions 86
  nodular densities 49
  normal breast 14
  patient positioning 456–459
  properly positioned mammogram 459
  radiolucent areas (Pattern I) 64
  sequence of events 460–461
cribriform carcinoma
  invasive see invasive cribriform carcinoma
  in retroglandular clear space 334–336
cribriform cell proliferation 276, 383
cyst(s) 72, 366
  air-filled 26
  Cooper's ligament 59
  fluid-filled 72
  radiograph 72
  ultrasound 24, 71, 73, 379
cystic changes, galactogram 73
cystic fluid, calcification, Pattern II 115

D

"dedifferentiation" 176, 177
"dense breasts" 32
dense structureless fibrosis 24–29
desmoplastic reaction 250, 255

discharge
  atrophic ducts, Pattern II 96
  nipple see nipple discharge
dotted castings 107
double compression method 240, 241
downward stage shifting by early detection
  178–179
duct(s) 17–19
  atrophic 95–96, 110
    galactography 95, 96
    subgross, thick-section histology 9, 96
    thick-section histology 96
  dilated 22, 28
    calcification 101, 103
    Cooper's ligament 59
    cystic changes with 73
    high nuclear grade DCIS 106–108
    Pattern V 150
    see also ductectasia
  distended fluid-filled 13, 72, 99, 100–103
    Pattern III 120
    subgross, thick-section histology 73
  fluid-filled, lactation 100, 101
  mammograms 22
  nipple/retroareolar region, subgross, thick-
    section histology 18
  normal, linear pleating 98, 99
  outlined by air (mammogram) 9
  Pattern II 95–108
  pleated, in nipple 19
  proliferating, radial scar 81
  retroareolar see retroareolar ducts
  subgross, thick-section histology 18, 19, 22–23
  subsegmental 23
  terminal see terminal ducts
  thick-section histology 17
ductal carcinoma
  advanced 198
  Grade 2, Pattern IV breast 137
  intratumor heterogeneity 193
  invasive see invasive ductal carcinoma
  spiculated invasive 114
  well-differentiated, medial half of breast 321
ductal carcinoma in situ (DCIS)
  architectural distortion 194, 358–363
    nonspecific asymmetric density with 251,
      252–253, 254–255
  atypical, architectural distortion 194
  calcification types 202
    casting-type 106, 194, 202
    crushed stone-like 194, 202
    number, appearance and extent 213
    powdery 202, 211
  central necrosis and calcification 205, 207
  comet-tail lesion 261
  cribriform cell proliferation 276, 383
  duct dilatation 99, 106–108
  early detection, mortality benefits 179
  Grade 3 383
    calcifications 14
    subgross, thick-section histology 426–431
  high nuclear grade
    casting-type calcification 106
    duct dilatation 106–108
    micropapillary architecture 107, 108
    in "milky way" 337–341
    mucin secretion 108
    solid cell proliferation 106, 147
  interconnecting bridges, medial half of breast
    322–324
  intraluminal necrosis and calcification 213
  micropapillary see micropapillary ductal car-
    cinoma in situ
  multiple foci 194
  nonspecific asymmetric density with archi-
    tectural distortion 251, 252–253, 254–255
  occult 340, 341
  "overdiagnosis" 178
  Pattern V breast and microcalcifications 146
  solid cell proliferation 202, 276
  subtypes with calcification 202–203
  upper outer quadrant 272–276
ductal remnants 133
ductal system, of lobe of breast 8
ductectasia 13, 99–108
  causes 99
  fluid causing 99, 100–103
  intraductal papillomas causing 104–105
  lactation causing 100–102
ductules 46

E

early detection of breast cancer 299
  benefits
    architectural distortion detection 361
    mortality reduction 166, 178–179
  biological factors influencing 188–235
    heterogeneity in outcome 230–231
    heterogeneity over time 228–229
    morphological heterogeneity (histological)
      190–193
    morphological heterogeneity (mammo-
      graphic) 194–215
    nature of surrounding breast tissue 188–
      189, 216
    progressive nature of cancer 216–234
  death prevention 166
  factors influencing 188–235
    biological factors see above
    human factors 188
    technical factors 188
  imaging methods 189
  indirect signs 188
    see also architectural distortion; parenchy-
      mal contour
  mechanism for effect 180–185
  outcome dependent on (medullary carci-
    noma) 232–234
  rationale and scientific evidence 165–185
  systematic viewing methods see viewing of
    mammograms (systematic method)
E-cadherin staining 357
elastic fibers, staining for 415
estrogen receptors
  acinar epithelium 66, 67
  invasive ductal carcinoma positive for 317
  invasive lobular carcinoma positive for 377
  mucinous carcinoma positive for 225
  staining 66
  tubulolobular carcinoma positive for 357
extralobular terminal duct 46

F

false–negative screening results 187
false–positive screening results 187
fat, structureless 62
fat necrosis
  crushed stone–like calcification 208
  traumatic 199
fatty replacement
  partial, lobules 66
  Pattern I 62–65
  total (Pattern II) 66
  see also adipose tissue
fibroadenolipoma 245
fibroadenoma 79
  crushed stone–like calcification 208
fibroadenomatoid change, of lobule 132
fibrocystic changes 74, 150
  crushed stone–like calcification and 209
fibroglandular tissue 30, 62, 242
  accessory 243, 244
  architectural distortion in lobular carcinoma
    134, 135
  asymmetric involution 246–247
  asymmetric without architectural distortion
    248–249
  contours 395
    normal concave 200, 242
  fatty replacement surrounding 63
  normal 242, 243–249
    asymmetric density 242, 243–249
  Pattern I 34
    outlined by adipose tissue 70
  proliferation 68
  remnants
    invasive lobular carcinoma vs 376
    pathological lesions vs 388
  replacement by adipose tissue 66, 67
fibrosis 28, 250
  architectural distortion with 250
  around invasive ductal carcinoma 241
  de-novo without trauma or inflammation 250
  dense structureless 24–29
  extensive in Pattern V 38
    invasive micropapillary carcinoma with
      157–159

focal 242, 248
interlobular 125
obscuring tumors 151–155
patchy, Pattern IV 133
Pattern 1 34
Pattern V 38, 149, 150, 153
periductal 36
peritumoral 419
postinflammatory 386, 388
retroareolar 346, 353
structureless (in Pattern V) 142
terminal duct lobular units (TDLUs) 25, 55
fibrous strands 17, 20
Pattern II 109–111
radiography and histology 20, 109
fibrous tissue 46
involuting lobule with 144
mammography difficulties 55
Pattern I 54–55
Pattern V 142
fine-needle aspiration biopsy
cautions on use 375
invasive ductal carcinoma 279
invasive lobular carcinoma 304
mammographically occult lesions 87
poorly differentiated invasive ductal carcinoma 326
retroareolar tumor 360
stellate tumors 297
tubular carcinoma 284, 297, 308
fistula 386
fluid production, nipple discharge 101
fluid retention/accumulation 53
glandular tissue 74–77
in TDLU 72
see also duct(s), distended fluid-filled
"forbidden areas" 259
asymmetric densities 259, 262, 307
de-novo asymmetric densities 329–330
see also specific regions (as given on page 259)

G

galactography 14, 17
atrophic ducts 9, 95, 96
dilated ducts 101
focal cystic change with 73
ductal carcinoma in situ (multiple foci) 194
ductectasia due to high grade DCIS 108
ductectasia due to intraductal papillomas 104
lobar anatomy 8–9
microcalcifications in Pattern II 115
micropapillary carcinoma in situ 432
normal breast 10–12, 17
Pattern I, branching ductal system 65
retroareolar ducts 121
size and extent of lobes 10–11
glandular tissue, fluid accumulation 74–77
grade of cancer see histological malignancy
grade
granular cell tumor 199
growth rates, breast cancer 216, 217
by histological type 217, 218
guidelines, screening efficacy 235
gynecomastia, asymmetric 248

H

hand-held mammography viewer 238, 239, 261,
263
Harris hematoxylin 422
hematoxylin–eosin stain 415
heterogeneity, tumor see morphological heterogeneity (of breast cancer)
histological diagnoses, at open biopsy 257
histological malignancy grade 176–177
cumulative survival by 184
Grade 1/2, low tumor size 176
Grade 3
palpable under 50 years of age 176
probability by tumor size 176–177
node status and tumor size 175
prognostic value and tumor size 180
worsening over time 228–229
histology, large-section see large-section histology
homogeneous structureless densities 16, 24–29
mammography 24

Pattern I, specimen radiograph 56
ultrasound 24
hormone replacement therapy (HRT) 32, 33, 66
asymmetric densities due to 249
transition of Pattern II to Pattern I due to 68,
69
hyperplasia, benign see benign hyperplasia

I

indirect signs, of breast cancer 188
see also architectural distortion; parenchymal
contour
inframammary fold
craniocaudal projection 457
mediolateral oblique projection (MLO) 441
palpable lump 326
in-situ carcinoma
extensive 192
see also ductal carcinoma in situ (DCIS); lobular carcinoma in situ (LCIS)
interconnected tumors
ductal carcinoma in situ 322–324
invasive ductal carcinoma in men 353
tubular carcinoma and micropapillary DCIS
436–437
interconnecting bridges
DCIS in medial half of breast 322–324
multifocal papillary carcinoma 194
tubular carcinoma and micropapillary DCIS
436–437
intertumoral heterogeneity, large-section histology 418
intracystic papillary carcinoma 192
circular/circular lesions 200, 222
with invasive ductal carcinoma 221, 222
intraductal carcinoma
high-grade 91
medial half of breast 322–324
intraductal papilloma, ductectasia due to 104–
105
intramamillary invasive carcinoma, subgross,
thick-section histology 426
intratumoral heterogeneity 176, 193
large-section histology 418
invasive carcinomas 190
aim of screening 180
cumulative survival data 180
early detection benefit 178–179, 185
noncalcified, upper outer quadrant 268–269
radial scar vs 393
size increase with time 180
see also specific invasive tumors below
invasive cribriform carcinoma
parenchymal contour changes 402–404
retroglandular clear space lesion 330–331
invasive ductal carcinoma 190
in accessory breast 245
architectural distortion (Pattern I) 80, 358–
363, 390
assessment of surrounding tissue by large-
section histology 419
asymmetric densities in "milky way" 286–
289, 310–313, 314–317, 333, 342–343
circular 194, 200
decrease in calcifications 214, 215, 228–229
evolution of small spiculated tumor 82–83
fibrosis around 241
Grade 1 414
Grade 2, subgross thick-section histology
427
Grade 3
circular 200
outcome 230
intracystic papillary carcinoma with 221, 222
intratumor heterogeneity 193
long sojourn time 217
medial half of breast 322–324
poorly differentiated 325–327
microfocus magnification mammogram 135
missed calcifications 214–215
mucinous carcinoma with 418
multifocal 15, 192, 266–267, 273, 316
parenchymal contour changes 394–395
in Pattern II breast 116–117
poorly differentiated, medial half of breast
325–327
in retroglandular clear space 332–333, 342–
343

stellate/spiculated 114, 196, 222, 311–313
tubular features, mean sojourn time 219
upper outer quadrant 310–313
early nonspecific appearance 271
lobular components 268–270, 314–317
microcalcifications 272–276
need for perception enhancement methods
290–299
nonspecific asymmetric density 286–289
well-differentiated 267
mean sojourn time 220
nonpalpable 172–173, 190, 191
ultrasound 278
upper outer quadrant 277–279
invasive lobular carcinoma
architectural distortion 370–375, 376
classic type 191, 374, 377
of Cooper's ligament 60
differential diagnosis 374, 376
mean sojourn time 226–227
parenchymal contour changes 396–397, 398–
399
Pattern IV breast 134–135, 138–139
periductal "targetoid" infiltration 377
in retroareolar area 18, 348--349, 350–351
stellate/spiculated 196
subgross, thick-section histology 433, 435
"tent-sign" 397, 398, 399
upper outer quadrant 267, 302–305
invasive micropapillary carcinoma 156–159
invasive papillary carcinoma 191
invasive tubular carcinoma 369
involution process 66–69, 388
architectural distortion in retroareolar area
359–361
asymmetric, without architectural distortion
246–247, 248
Pattern V and 142
persistent lobules 97

L

lactation, ductal distension 100–102
lactiferous ducts see duct(s)
large core needle biopsy 241
large-section histology 405–438
advantages 416
assessment of surrounding tissue 419
Grade III DCIS and Paget's disease
426–431
handling/staining of specimens 413, 415
importance 339
macrotome use 412
for multifocal tumors 317
normal breast 3
lobes 17
lobules and TDLUs 16
prerequisites 406
rationale 406
reexcision specimens, accurate assessment
419
slides and viewing 414–417
specimen handling 407–411
fixation of tissue 411
inking of surface of specimen 410
slicing technique 408–409
specimen radiography 409
lateromedial horizontal-beam projection (LM)
462–465
aims 462
correctly positioned mammogram 465
patient positioning 463–465
linear densities 16, 17–21, 46, 94, 242
adenosis in Pattern IV 126
normal breast 242, 243
Pattern II 35, 94, 95–113
Pattern IV 37
retroareolar 120
see also blood vessels; duct(s); fibrous strands
linear pleating, normal ducts in nonlactating
breast 98
lobes
anatomy 8–15
large, calcification 14
multiple papilloma 13
number in breast 8
size and extent 10
lobular carcinoma, invasive see invasive lobular
carcinoma

lobular carcinoma in situ (LCIS) 267, 305
  with invasive lobular carcinoma 377
  noncalcified 363
  occult 281
  parenchymal contour changes and 399
lobules 16, 46
  budding 52
  changes with menstrual cycle 52
  enlarged 125, 126
  estrogen receptor staining 66
  fibroadenomatoid change 132
  fluid production 101
  hormone-sensitive 49
  involuting, with fibrous replacement 144
  large-section histology 56
  mammograms 16
  partial fatty replacement 66
  persistent, in Pattern II 96, 97
  size and shapes 48, 52
lump in breast, Pattern I mammogram 78, 79
lymph node
  metastases, development, outcome change
    231
  status
    outcome 183
    preclinical breast cancer 175
  see also node-negative breast cancer

M

macrotome use 412
malignant tumors see breast cancer; specific
  tumor subtypes
mammographically occult lesions see occult lesions (mammographically)
mammographic findings, analysis 240–258
  ancillary methods and techniques 240, 241
  asymmetric densities see asymmetric densi-
    ties
  perception enhancement methods 286, 291
mammographic parenchymal patterns 32–38
  see also parenchymal contour changes; in-
    dividual patterns
mammographic techniques 238, 439–469
  cleavage view (CV) 466
  craniocaudal projection (CC) 455–461
  lateromedial horizontal-beam projection (LM)
    462–465
  mediolateral oblique projection (MLO) 440–
    454
  MLO vs CC for pathological lesions 268–269,
    332
mammography see screening, of asymptomatic
  women; specific forms of cancer
Mammospot® 240, 241
masking technique 311, 315
medial half of breast, lesions 318–327
  de-novo asymmetric density 330–331
  ductal carcinoma (stellate) 321
  interconnecting ductal carcinomas 323–324
  poorly differentiated invasive ductal carci-
    noma 325–327
  tubular carcinoma 318–320
mediolateral oblique projection (MLO) 440–454
  aims of correct positioning 441
  patient positioning 442–448
  properly positioned mammogram 449
  sequence of events for 450–454
medullary carcinoma 78, 191
  atypical 378–385
  circular 200
  invasion of pectoralis muscle 419
  mean sojourn time 223
  microfocus magnification 233, 234
  outcome dependent on early detection 232–
    234
  specimen radiography 381
men
  asymmetric gynecomastia 248
  breast cancer rarity 353
  breast cancer site 346
    retroareolar area 346, 352–354
  invasive ductal carcinoma 352–353
menstrual cycle
  breast changes 52, 53
  fluid production by lobules 101
  phases 52, 53
metachronous breast cancers 355–357
metastases

bone 171
  development, outcome change 231
  upper outer quadrant 262–263
microcalcifications 212–213, 256
  ductal carcinoma in situ (Pattern V) 146
  histology and treatment 212
  invasive micropapillary carcinoma (Pattern V)
    156–159
  Pattern II 115
  purpose of detection 202
  see also calcification
microfocus magnification mammogram 240,
  241
  architectural distortion 251
  asymmetric fibroglandular tissue 247
  linear and nodular densities 243
  normal breast 4
  tumors see specific tumors
micropapillary architecture, high nuclear grade
  DCIS 107, 108
micropapillary carcinoma, invasive 156–159
micropapillary carcinoma in situ
  mucin-producing 423
  subgross thick-section histology 432–435
micropapillary ductal carcinoma in situ 88–89,
  274, 275, 276
  duct distention 107
  medial half of breast 319–320
  in retroglandular clear space 334–336
milk ducts see duct(s)
"milk of calcium" 115
  Pattern V 149
"milky way" 259, 260, 286
  asymmetric densities 262–265, 301, 306–307,
    310, 314–317, 329–330
    high-grade DCIS 337–341
    invasive ductal carcinoma 286–289, 310–
      313, 314–317, 333, 342–343
    outlining, of benefit 264, 286, 301, 315
    retroglandular clear space and 329–330
    tubular carcinoma 344–345
  nonspecific appearance of early breast cancer
    271
morphological heterogeneity (of breast cancer)
  190–215
  histological 190–193
    intratumor 193
  large-section histology 418
  mammographic 194–215
  over time 228–229
mortality (breast cancer)
  DCIS, early detection benefits 179
  in men 353
  reduction
    downward stage shifting by early detection
      178–179
    screening of asymptomatic breast cancer
      168–169, 178, 186–187
  in UK vs Denmark 185
  before vs after screening introduction 186
  see also survival
mucin 225
  secretion, high nuclear grade DCIS 108
mucinous carcinoma
  circular 200
  ill-defined, fibrous strands 111
  intratumor heterogeneity 193
  invasive ductal carcinoma with 418
    in male 354
  lobulated 194
  mean sojourn time 224–225
  ultrasound 225
  unifocal 171
mucin-producing micropapillary carcinoma in
  situ 423
multifocality of tumors 66, 272, 276, 355–356
  documentation by large-section slides 416
  invasive ductal carcinoma 15, 192, 266–267,
    273, 316, 324
  papillary carcinoma, interconnecting bridges
    194
  screening rule to keep searching 276, 282,
    284, 317
  see also specific histological subtypes
myoepithelial layer 369

N

nipple
  craniocaudal projection 455
  ducts 18
  pleated ducts 19
  retraction 425
  subgross, thick-section histology 6–7, 18, 19
nipple–areolar complex
  invasive lobular carcinoma 350–351
  mammogram 6
  subgross histology 6–7
nipple discharge
  bloody 104
  micropapillary carcinoma in situ 432–435
  normal fluid production 101
  Pattern III 121
  serous 105, 108
node-negative breast cancer
  detection difficulties 181
  outcome 166
node-positive breast cancer, outcome 166
node status, cumulative survival by 183
nodular densities 16, 46–52, 242
  adenosis in Pattern IV 126
  normal breast 242, 243
  Pattern IV 37, 124, 125
normal breast
  asymmetric densities 240, 242–249
  building blocks see building blocks
  changes with menstrual cycle 52, 53
  lobar anatomy 8–15
  mammogram 3, 4
  microarchitecture 50
  normal diversity 16
  skin and areolar complex 6–7
  subgross anatomy 3–15
  subgross, thick-section histology 3, 4, 6–7

O

occult lesions (mammographically)
  architectural distortion due to 250
  Pattern I 86–91
  Pattern V 151, 152–153
open biopsy
  histological diagnoses 257
  radial scar 393
orcein stain 415
outcome of breast cancer
  heterogeneity 230–231
  of medullary carcinoma 232–234
  see also mortality (breast cancer); survival
oval shaped tumors 256
  benign, histology (frequencies) 201
  malignant, histology (frequencies) 201
  morphological heterogeneity 200–201
  see also circular tumor masses
"overdiagnosis" of breast cancer 178

P

Paget's disease 425
papillary carcinoma
  intracystic see intracystic papillary carcinoma
  invasive 191
  multifocal, interconnecting bridges 194
papillary carcinoma in situ
  biopsy 87
  large-section histology 88
  with necrosis but without microcalcification
    87
papilloma
  crushed stone–like calcification 208
  intraductal 104–105
  multiple 13
    intraductal, ductectasia due to 104–105
    nonspecific asymmetric density with archi-
      tectural distortion 253
parenchymal contour changes 394–404
  concave, fibrosis 242
  convex see convex contours
  as indirect sign 188
  invasive cribriform carcinoma 402–404
  invasive ductal carcinoma 394–395
  invasive lobular carcinoma 396–397, 398–399
  Pattern I 56–61
    see also Pattern I

Pattern V 151–155
perception of lesions with viewer 283
tubular carcinoma 400–401
pathological lesions
characteristics 358–404
see also architectural distortion; parenchymal contour changes
indirect signs 188
nonspecific appearance (small) 262
types 256
in upper outer quadrant 259
pattern(s)
breast cancer prevalence by 163
distribution by age 160–161
screening vs clinical referred populations 162
relative frequency of types 160–161
Pattern I 32, 33–34, 40–91
architectural distortion see architectural distortion
building blocks 40
proportions 33
calcifications 84–85
characteristics 40–42
concave contours 62
mammographically occult carcinoma 86–91
convex contours 70
fibroadenoma 79
invasive ductal carcinoma 83
medullary carcinoma 78
diagnostic threshold problems 188
dynamic nature 66
fatty replacement 62–65
fibroglandular tissue outline by adipose tissue 70
fibrosis with 34
fibrous tissue 54–55
involution 358
nodular densities 46–53
normal 40–69
parenchymal contour 56–61
importance of subtle changes 82–83
scalloped border 56
pathological lesions 70–91
regression to Pattern II/III 66
relative frequency of types 160
spiculated tumor evolution 82–83
subgross thick-section histology 34
transformation of Pattern II to 68, 249
Pattern II 32, 35, 93–117
atrophic ducts 95–96
building block proportions 35
frequency of types with age 160
linear densities 94, 95–113
blood vessels 112–113
duct dilatation 95–108
fibrous strands 109–111
microcalcifications 115
pathological lesions 114–117, 277
persistent lobules 96, 97
radiolucent adipose tissue 94
transformation of Pattern I to 66
transformation to Pattern I by HRT 68, 249
Pattern III 36, 119–121
frequency of types with age 160
Pattern IV 37, 123–139
adenosis 125–127
age-related constancy 124, 161
breast cancer prevalence 124
diagnostic threshold problems 188
fibroadenomatoid change of lobule 132
frequency of type with age 161
occurrence 124
patchy fibrosis 133
pathological lesions 134–137
sclerosing adenosis 128–131
Pattern V 141–163
age-related constancy 143
calcifications 145–150
benign 148–149
malignant 146–147
diagnostic threshold problems 188
frequency of type with age 161, 162
invasive micropapillary carcinoma 156–159
involuting lobule with fibrous replacement 144
noncalcified lesions, perception 151–159
"tent-sign" 151, 152
pectoralis major muscle
male breast cancer infiltration 346

mediolateral oblique projection 441
medullary carcinoma invading 419
upper outer quadrant lesion screening 259, 260
perception enhancement methods 286, 291
periductal connective tissue, proliferation 120
perimenopausal women, proliferation of fibroglandular tissue 68
peritumoral fibrosis 419
"plasma cell mastitis" 101
postmenopausal women
mammographic patterns 160
sojourn times 216, 217
preclinical breast cancer 174–177
duration and tumor size at detection 216
early detection see early detection of breast cancer
impact of screening see screening
nonpalpable 167, 172–173
outcome 167
progression prevention 168–169, 170–171, 187
pregnancy, involution process 66
premenopausal women
Pattern I 33
sojourn times 216, 218
premenstrual phase 52, 53
preoperative localization techniques 339
prognostic factors, histological, cumulative survival 180, 181
psammoma-like bodies 85, 128, 129
benign hyperplastic breast changes 281
powdery calcification relationship 210

R

radial scar 363, 392–393
histology 4–5, 199
invasive carcinoma vs 393
mammogram 4, 199
proliferating ducts causing 81
subgross, thick-section histology 423
radiologists
requirements 438
tasks 269
radiolucent areas 30–31, 40, 62–65, 242
oval-shaped 65
ovoid 64
Pattern I 62–65
Pattern II 94
see also adipose tissue
radiopaque densities 40, 46–53, 62
convex contours (Pattern I) 71–79
see also fibrous tissue; linear densities; nodular densities
randomized control trials, mammographic screening and mortality reduction 186
reexcision specimens, large-section histology 419
retroareolar area, lesions 346–357
architectural distortion 359–363
breast cancer in men 346, 352–353
calcification 425–431
invasive ductal carcinoma 353
mucinous component 354
invasive lobular carcinoma 18, 348–349, 350–351
malignant change 18
tubulolobular carcinoma 355–357
tumors 346, 347
detection methods 348
retroareolar ducts 18, 19
dilated 19
distended fluid-filled 120
Pattern III 36, 120–121
pleated 17
surrounded by adipose tissue 120–121
retroareolar fibrosis 346, 353
retroglandular clear space 135
architectural distortion 250
fibroglandular tissue protrusion 282
lesions 328–345
asymmetric density 332–333
cribriform and micropapillary DCIS 334–336
high-grade DCIS 336–341
invasive cribriform carcinoma 328–331
invasive ductal carcinoma 332–333
retromammary fat 441
roman arches 274

S

sclerosing adenosis 128–131
with calcification 129–131
powdery calcification 211
without calcification 128
sclerosing duct proliferation 81
screening, of asymptomatic women (by mammography)
analysis of findings see mammographic findings, analysis
beneficial effects, mechanisms 180–185
benefits for younger women 177
call-backs 240
cumulative survival by prognostic factors 180, 181
double reading of mammograms 235
functions/aims 180, 185, 238
impact, mechanism 174–177
histological malignancy grade 175, 176–177
node status 175
tumor size 174, 175, 176
impact on mortality 186–187
mortality reduction 168–169, 178
importance 185
scientific foundation 165–185
invasive ductal carcinoma 172–173
invasive micropapillary carcinoma 156–159
morphological heterogeneity see morphological heterogeneity (of breast cancer)
optimization, guidelines for efficacy 235
optimization of factors 185
pathological lesion in Pattern II breast 116–117
pathological lesion in Pattern IV breast 134–137
philosophy 237
preclinical phase, mortality reduction 168–169, 178, 186–187
prerequisites 237
service programs 186
viewing of mammograms see viewing of mammograms (systematic method)
sebaceous glands, subgross thick-section histology 6
service screening programs 186
sirius red stain 415
skin
nipple region, radiograph 7
normal breast 6
retraction 166, 198
sojourn time 168, 216
age influence on 217, 218, 219
tumor subtypes 220–227
duration by histological type 216, 218
compound tumor 221
invasive ductal carcinoma 217
invasive ductal carcinoma (well-differentiated) 220
invasive ductal carcinoma with tubular features 219
invasive lobular carcinoma 226–227
medullary carcinoma 223
mucinous carcinoma 224–225
tubular cancer 219
postmenopausal women 216, 217
premenopausal women 216
specimen radiography 409
spiculated lesions/tumors 256
advanced ductal carcinoma 198
central tumor mass with spicules 194
circular tumor masses vs (frequency) 195
distribution (frequency) 195
ductal carcinoma (Grade II) 136, 137
early diagnosis 178
evolution 82–83
intratumoral heterogeneity 193
invasive ductal carcinoma 114, 311–313, 322–324, 387
in retroglandular clear space 332–333
malignancy frequency 368
mammographic appearance 196
medial half of breast 322–324
morphological heterogeneity 196–197
multiple 266
Pattern V breast 154
retroareolar, in men 346
retroareolar area 350–351
tubular carcinoma 309, 367

spiculated lesions/tumors
    in upper outer quadrant 265, 293, 294, 303, 309
    see also stellate lesions/tumors
spot compression 240, 241, 265, 387
staining of specimens 413, 415
stellate lesions/tumors 307
    benign, histology 199
    cytology not recommended 294
    de novo after invasive ductal carcinoma 296
    early nonspecific density 299
    invasive ductal carcinoma 222, 292, 306–309
    malignancy ratio and histology 196, 197
    mammographic appearance 196
    in medial half of breast 318–320
    micropapillary DCIS 436–437
    near parenchymal contour 397
    Pattern V 151
    in retroglandular clear space 335
    size 307
    in upper outer quadrant
        invasive ductal carcinoma 306–309
        tubular carcinoma 282–284
    yield from breast cancer screening 259
subgross, thick-section histology 420–424
    Grade III DCIS with Paget's disease 426–431
    image examples 423–424
    micropapillary carcinoma in situ 432–435
    technique 420–422
    tubular carcinoma and micropapillary DCIS 436–437
    see also specific tumor subtypes
subsegmental duct, subgross thick-section histology 8, 48, 51
surgical scars 393
survival
    after screening introduction 186
    by age 182, 183
    by breast cancer size 182
    by histological malignancy grade 184
    by histological prognostic factors 180, 181
    of invasive carcinomas 180
    of medullary carcinoma 232
    by node status 183
    solitary tumor (tubular carcinoma) over 10 mm 345
    see also mortality (breast cancer); Two-County (W-E) Swedish Trial
sweat duct, subgross thick-section histology 7
sweat gland, subgross thick-section histology 7
Swedish Two-County trial *see* Two-County (W-E) Swedish Trial

"tent-sign" 151, 152, 188, 397
    invasive lobular carcinoma 397, 398, 399
    tubular carcinoma 367

terminal duct lobular units (TDLUs) 46
    appearance/structure 46
    atrophic 23, 28
    behind nipple 18
    carcinoma in situ distending 71
    convex contour 71
    cystically dilated 25, 72, 73
        subgross, thick-section histology 51, 71, 73
    fibrosis around 42
    fibrosis obscuring 55
    fluid accumulation 72
    galactogram 44, 49
    histology 44
    hyperplastic 127
    increased fluid production 99, 100–103
    involution 66, 97, 144
    lactating 100
    mammogram 16, 22, 44, 50
        fibrous tissue causing difficulties 55
    "milk of calcium" in 25, 115
    nodular densities 16, 242
    normal 242
    pathological lesions, convex contours 71–73
    subgross, thick-section histology 8, 22–23, 46, 47, 48
    thick-section histology 49
terminal ducts 46, 48
    extralobular 46
    subgross thick-section histology 48, 49
"thickening" (of tissue)
    architectural distortion and 370–375
    palpable 280–285
    tubular carcinoma, upper outer quadrant lesions 280–285
tubular carcinoma
    architectural distortion 364–369
    asymmetric densities in "milky way" 344–345
    invasive 369
    mean sojourn time 219
    in medial half of breast 318–320
    parenchymal contour changes 400–401
    powdery calcification 211, 284
    in retroglandular clear space 344–345
    stellate/spiculated 196
    subgross, thick-section histology 436–437
    in upper outer quadrant 282–285, 297–299, 306–309
tubulolobular carcinoma 117
    retroareolar area 355–357
tumor size
    cumulative survival by 182
    documentation by large-section slides 416
    histological grade and prognosis 180
    impact of screening 174–175, 176
    radiologist's goal for detection 185
    small, early detection benefits 181
    solitary tumor and survival 345
Two-County (W-E) Swedish Trial 167, 168–169,

185
    cumulative survival after screening introduction 186
    survival by node status and age 183
    survival by tumor size and age 182

ultrasound 241
    benign fibroadenoma 79
    cysts 71, 73, 379
    homogeneous structureless densities 24
    invasive ductal carcinoma 293, 315, 387
        well-differentiated 278
    invasive lobular carcinoma 398
    invasive micropapillary carcinoma (Pattern V) 157
    mucinous carcinoma 225
    multifocal invasive ductal carcinoma 15
    retroareolar ducts 121
    retroareolar tumor 360
    tubular carcinoma 284, 297, 401
    tubulolobular carcinoma 356
upper outer quadrant lesions 259, 260–317
    ductal carcinoma in situ 260–261
    invasive ductal carcinoma
        with lobular components 268–270
        moderately differentiated 286–289
        well-differentiated 264–267, 277–279, 290–299, 310–313
    invasive lobular carcinoma 302–305
    metastatic tumor 262–263
    micropapillary DCIS 272–276
    multifocality 264–267, 272–276
    nonspecific asymmetric density 286–289, 303
    subtle asymmetric densities 271
    "thickening" due to tubular carcinoma 280–285
    tubular carcinoma 297–299, 306–309
    see also "milky way"

vessels *see* blood vessels
viewing large-section slides 416
viewing of mammograms (systematic method) 237–404
    conditions for 238
    perception of subtle abnormalities 238
    philosophy and prerequisites 238
    side-by-side, step-by-step 239, 395